Aging Wisely...

Wisdom of Our Elders

Irving I. Silverman   Ellen Beth Siegel

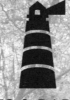

JONES & BARTLETT
LEARNING

World Headquarters
Jones & Bartlett Learning
5 Wall Street
Burlington, MA 01803
978-443-5000
info@jblearning.com
www.jblearning.com

Jones & Bartlett Learning books and products are available through most bookstores and online booksellers. To contact Jones & Bartlett Learning directly, call 800-832-0034, fax 978-443-8000, or visit our website, www.jblearning.com.

Production Credits

VP, Executive Publisher: David D. Cella
Publisher: Cathy L. Esperti
Editorial Assistant: Carter McAlister
Director of Production: Jenny L. Corriveau
Associate Marketing Manager: Alianna Ortu
VP, Manufacturing and Inventory Control: Therese Connell
Composition: S4Carlisle Publishing Services
Project Management: S4Carlisle Publishing Services
Cover Design: Michael O'Donnell
Director of Rights & Media: Joanna Gallant
Rights & Media Specialist: Wes DeShano
Media Development Editor: Troy Liston
Cover Image (Title Page, Part Opener, Chapter Opener): © James Whitesmith/Moment/Getty
Printing and Binding: Edwards Brothers Malloy
Cover Printing: Edwards Brothers Malloy

Library of Congress Cataloging-in-Publication Data
Names: Silverman, Irving, 1920- editor. | Siegel, Ellen Beth, editor.
Title: Aging wisely... wisdom of our elders/edited by Irving I. Silverman, Ellen Beth Siegel.
Description: First edition. | Burlington, Massachusetts : Jones & Bartlett Learning, [2018] | Includes bibliographical references.
Identifiers: LCCN 2017012933 | ISBN 9781284141733 (paperback : alk. paper)
Subjects: | MESH: Aged--psychology | Aging--psychology | Life | United States | Personal Narratives
Classification: LCC QP86 | NLM WT 145 | DDC 612.6/7--dc23
LC record available at https://lccn.loc.gov/2017012933

6048

Printed in the United States of America
21 20 19 18 17   10 9 8 7 6 5 4 3 2

Dedication

To my loving wives, Henrietta and Nancy,
who spiritually motivated me
to continue living and aging after they left me;
to my children, Suzy, Ellen, Bill, and Peggy;
to my grandchildren, Jolie, Deb, David, Erica, Daniel,
and Johana; and to my new great-grandchild, Catie,
all of whom inspire me to keep on aging.

—IIS

To my husband (and helpmate), Don;
my beloved children, Jolie, Deb, and David;
my mother, Henrietta, who died way too soon;
and my father, Irving, still alive and kicking at 97;
to my dear "sisters born from different mothers,"
Sherri and Sharon;
and to all the contributors
who made this book possible.

—EBS

Contents

Foreword

Stephen Colwell, MBA
Executive Director, NewBridge on the Charles
Dedham, MA

As the Executive Director of a truly creative and erudite senior living community, I have had the pleasure of meeting authors, inventors, and even individuals who have scientific formulas named after themselves. When one of these amazing residents, Irving Silverman, told me about his intention to create a book about aging and longevity, I was enthusiastic about its prospects. Irving decided to include stories and thoughts on a variety of subjects, drawing in part from the lives of our residents and staff at NewBridge on the Charles. The breadth and depth of these experiences give us all a chance to look into the world of thousands of years of individual histories. This is a book of insights, as told by our living legacies.

While many books on aging and longevity have been published recently, no book expresses the voices of seniors the way this book does. The opinions of our seniors have been shaped by the Depression, World War II, McCarthyism, the Cold War, the emotional upheavals of the civil rights movement, the moon landing, etc., etc. These seniors are living historians. Yet the chapters that they have written are not about significant geopolitical events or life-altering moments in time. The stories contained herein are about the *views* that were shaped by this history.

Irving originally titled this book *How to Live to 120.* He was inspired to write this when he saw a *National Geographic* cover story (May 2013) that showed a cherubic child with a headline suggesting that "this baby will live to be 120." Living to 120 for today's seniors may be a bit unrealistic, so Irving decided the book would be called *Aging Wisely . . . Wisdom of Our Elders,* and hopes to have it function as a guide for students of the aging process—and for all of us as we get older.

I see this as a collection of insights from the wise and experienced. I think back to my own history and recognize how often I've said to myself, "If only I knew then what I know now." This is a collection of "know-nows" for those of us open enough to learn young. After all, if we live by the wise words contained herein, we may see the other side of 120.

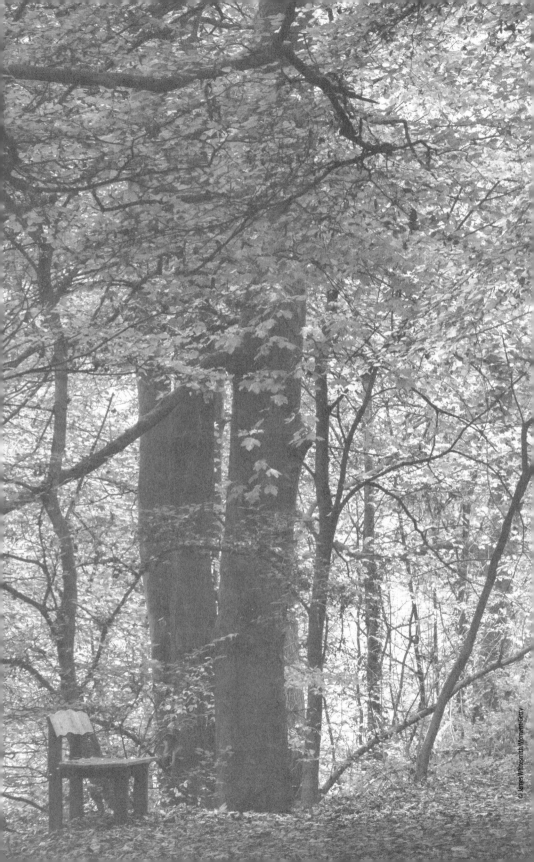

About the Authors

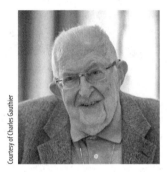

Courtesy of Charles Gauthier

Irving I. Silverman was born in 1920, the son of immigrant parents, and has been visually handicapped from birth. He attended a special sight conservation class in elementary school, and then went on to high school and the City College of New York's Baruch School of Business, where he majored in advertising and publishing.

Following his graduation from college, Irving began a 45-year career at the National Knitwear Association (NKA), a trade association in the knitting industry. But his proudest achievements came in his community service. After the death of his first wife, Henrietta, at the age of 35, he established and led the Long Island chapter of Parents Without Partners; and it was through that organization that he met Nancy, his second wife. At age 56, he became President of the New York Region of United Synagogue, the governing body of the Conservative Jewish movement, and in 1980, he led an effort to allow Jews to emigrate from the Soviet Union.

After retiring from NKA, Irving created the Kosher Food and Jewish Life Expo, which "brought kosher out of the closet." He also indulged his collector instincts by establishing collections of antique printers' wood type, lighthouse replicas, and giraffe figurines.

Along with Nancy, Irving vacationed in Maine for almost five decades. Nancy had a lighthouse built on their property, and following her death in 2002, Irving designated the lighthouse as a wedding chapel, officiating at 35 wedding ceremonies there.

Irving's previous book, *A Trilogy . . . Three Hearts . . . One Soul,* contains his autobiography and tributes to each of his wives. He now lives at NewBridge on the Charles in Dedham, Massachusetts, and is 97 years old.

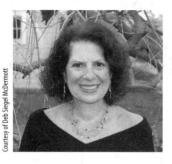

Courtesy of Deb Siegel McDermott

Ellen Beth Siegel, JD, PsyD, is a clinical psychologist and a former lawyer. She is a graduate of the University of Pennsylvania, Harvard Law School, and William James College (formerly the Massachusetts School of Professional Psychology) and currently serves as a Teaching Associate in Psychology at Harvard Medical School. For many years on staff at Cambridge Health Alliance in Cambridge, Massachusetts, she now maintains a private practice with offices in Cambridge and Newton, Massachusetts. She is on the Advisory Board of the Endowment for the Advancement of Psychotherapy at Massachusetts General Hospital and the Alumni Advisory Board of William James College.

Ellen is also a poet. Her poems have been published in *Bellowing Ark, The Christian Science Monitor, Concrete Wolf, Poetpourri,* and *The Warwick Anthology.* A nominee for a coveted Pushcart Prize, she is a co-editor of *Do Not Give Me Things Unbroken* (2002), a poetry anthology, and co-author of *Unlocking the Poem* (2009), a collection of poetry "assignments" illustrated by selected poems, both her own and from 101 other poets. Ellen's chapbooks *Remembering Endymion* and *The Sweet Moth Kisses Never Traded* have been finalists in various chapbook contests and are looking for a publisher; she is also hoping for enough time to put together a full-length volume of her poems.

Ellen lives in Waban, Massachusetts, with her husband, Don, and has three grown children who delight her every single day. She is also Irving Silverman's daughter.

Acknowledgments

This book would never have seen the light of day without the support and encouragement of many people. I especially want to thank the management team at NewBridge on the Charles, Lou Woolf and Steve Colwell; all the elders, caregivers, academics, and other professionals who have collaborated in this project by contributing chapters on their experiences and views of aging; the students and faculty of William James College, who contributed chapters as an extension of their new specialization in geropsychology; and my dear friends Nancy Lelewer Sonnabend and Muriel Trask Davisson-Fahey, who led me to several of the contributors to the book. My daughter, Ellen Beth Siegel, devotedly and professionally assisted me in creating this book, and well deserves being listed as co-author. Cathy Esperti, my very capable editor at Jones & Bartlett Learning, interpreted my continuing publishing requests and made this book possible, along with her dedicated team, Carter Cathleen McAlister, Manjusha Chandrasekaran, Juna Abrams, Alianna Ortu, and Wesley DeShano. I am also grateful to my computer helpers, Arthur Wood and Mariah MacKenzie. Most of all, I want to thank *you,* the readers, who hopefully will find this book a useful guide to aging.

—IIS

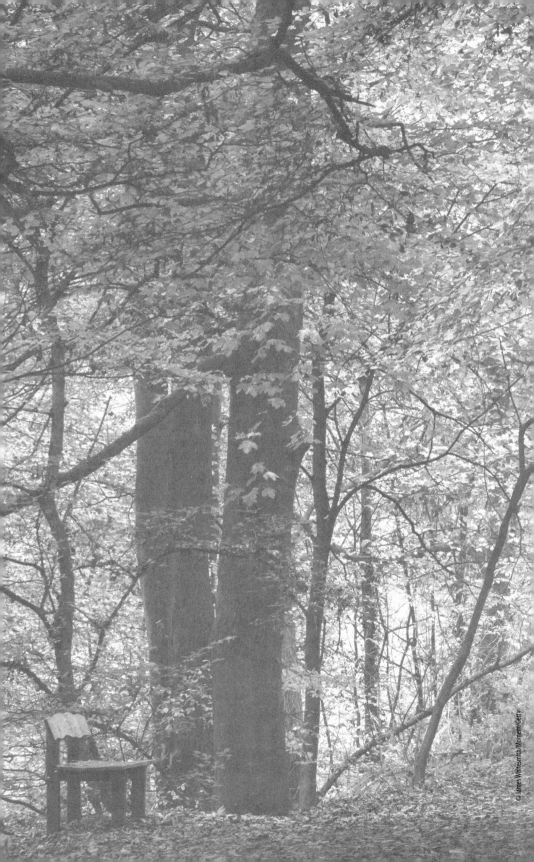

Introduction

If we are lucky—if we have good genes—if we take good care of ourselves—all of us have a good chance for a long life.

This is a book about aging. As people live longer, aging takes on increased relevance to society, and society has more reason to seek out the voices—and the wisdom—of elders who are not sitting around waiting for "the end," but rather are living full, vibrant lives. Like Tony Bennett, the singer and entertainer, who—at age 90—published a memoir entitled *Just Getting Started,* today's seniors are showing that people who are older can also be "just getting started . . .," and they can offer a lot worth listening to for students planning to work with seniors, for other seniors, and for those of us who aspire to reaching our own senior years.

My father, Irving Silverman, the principal author of this book, is not an academic or an expert in gerontology, but at 97, he *is* an expert in the art of aging. He was 95 when he conceived the idea of assembling a book filled with his own thoughts about aging and the thoughts of other elders. His goal was to provide insight into what it is like to live a long life in today's world. He first solicited contributions from other seniors living in NewBridge on the Charles, the retirement community that he moved to at age 90. There was an enthusiastic response, and several staff members asked to participate as well. He next approached William James College, a graduate college of psychology with a newly created specialization in geropsychology. The faculty and students there were pleased to contribute chapters, leading to additional contributions from colleges, universities, and hospitals.

By the time he was done, he had contributions from 73 collaborators, dispersed all across the United States. And these collaborators are a diverse lot. Many are elders, aged from 68 to 103. They are lawyers, doctors, and nurses; entrepreneurs and Wall Street executives; educators and researchers; social workers and psychologists; chemists and physicists; stay-at-home moms; CEOs; novelists and poets; and rabbis, ministers, and priests.

The chapters in this volume are diverse too. Opening with the life stories of some inspiring elders, we move to the biology of aging, emotional responses to aging, and issues around the changes that aging might cause. From there, we turn to chapters that look at using both our internal strengths and the resources of the world around us to age better. Other chapters look at interpersonal relationships; overcoming obstacles; issues in such fields as work and retirement, housing, driving, and money; the many meanings of success; and finding fulfillment in our later years. We next explore what can be derived from religion, prayer, and spirituality, and then some of the soberer topics connected to aging: end-of-life issues; coping with loss; and how we hope to be remembered. Finally, we conclude with some special words of wisdom.

The book grew beyond my father's initial expectations, and he enlisted my help to organize its contents and prepare it for publication. Sharing in this enterprise is a gift that I'm grateful to give him . . . and getting this book out and into the hands of others thinking about aging is something I too have become passionate about.

Please read the multitude of voices collected here. It's a chance to see how rich and fulfilling our older years can be; a chance to benefit from the collected wisdom of this group of experts in aging; and for those of you who are students of the aging process, it's a chance to hear directly from the seniors that you want to help.

—EBS

Learning Through the Creation of This Book

Mariah MacKenzie
Senior, Needham High School
Needham, MA

Even the process of creating this book involved sharing with a younger generation and passing on a wealth of experience. In this story, a high school student who volunteered to help make the book a reality reflects on what she learned and how she grew from the process, as well as on the contribution that she sees this book making to younger generations.

What she has written gives useful insights into what young people can learn from older generations, and how "youngs" and "olds" can help each other.

One of our greatest tools in life is experience, a chance to learn. That is what this process has been for me. Being a part of the creation of this collaborative work has been a privilege, allowing me to learn, piece by piece, the way that Mr. Silverman and his peers see the process of aging, something incredibly foreign to me. There is a vast difference between growing up and growing older. As someone who has only been part of this world for a fraction of the time that a majority of these other contributors have, I cannot provide much insight on that process. But working to bring their knowledge to life in the form of a book has been fascinating, and I am honored to be a part of it. There is so much to learn from listening to and reading through the stories and knowledge of each of these people; I invite you to see for yourself how unique each of their perspectives is.

I remember when Mr. Silverman first told me that he wanted to undertake this work. I had only known him for a few weeks, and I didn't know what to expect. I had read his previously published work: *Three Hearts, One Soul,* and thus I knew that he was a gifted writer, but the idea of helping to create a completely new book baffled me. It was not that I didn't think it could be done; if there's one thing about Mr. Silverman that I have come to know, it is the astounding extent of his determination. However, I still didn't know how the creation of this book could happen. It seemed off in the distance, and I never imagined we would get this far so soon.

My role has changed with each part of this project. Early on, I helped reach out through email to residents of NewBridge on the Charles, the community where Mr. Silverman lives. I also took part in the physical writing of Mr. Silverman's contributions. As a seasoned user of technology due to my generation, I can type and work a computer with ease, and Mr. Silverman often dictated his chapters to me. I had been able to type from his dictations before, but this experience was different. These stories and recollections were more extensive, more in depth—his opportunity to share what has been most important to him as he has gone through his life.

One by one, other people showed interest, and contributors accumulated. It was a chance for them to speak, to share their stories, their unique input on what it means to age and remain true to yourself. It was an opportunity to express opinions on how you can still grow, mentally and emotionally, as an older person, and it was a richness of stories of why aging shouldn't stop you from enjoying and taking in all there is to life.

Once submissions started coming in, my role again shifted. We needed to sort through and format them, as well as perform a quick edit. This provided me with a chance to get a glimpse of some of the things that these contributors have accomplished, experienced, and thought about in their lifetimes. In addition to elders, contributors come from the academic world, adding yet another perspective on aging. These are people who work with elders and are professionally educated on health, and therefore are knowledgeable on how aging works.

An extensive amount of thought and effort has gone into the creation of this book, particularly on the part of Mr. Silverman. It has grown out of his desire to continue to add his input and ideas to the world and to express himself yet again in a published work. It has grown into so much more than what it started as, due to the efforts of everyone who has helped along the way.

I would like to add a message to younger readers—maybe not as young as me, but young enough that they haven't experienced the aging process in the same way as the elders represented here. First, people who are not yet of older age can still gain important knowledge from this book. The growing and aging process is part of our entire lives.

Many of the lessons outlined in this book are not solely applicable to older generations. We could all benefit from learning to accept help when we need it, to accept people and their differences, and to experience life while we still can. Older people in our society can teach us so very much. They have seen and been through so much more than we can imagine. One day that will be us, but for now, we need to listen to them, let them give advice, appreciate their perspective, and value their contributions to society. Anyone older than you has more years of experience, and often a more thorough knowledge about our world. We cannot let their voices go unheard.

PART **I**

Life Stories

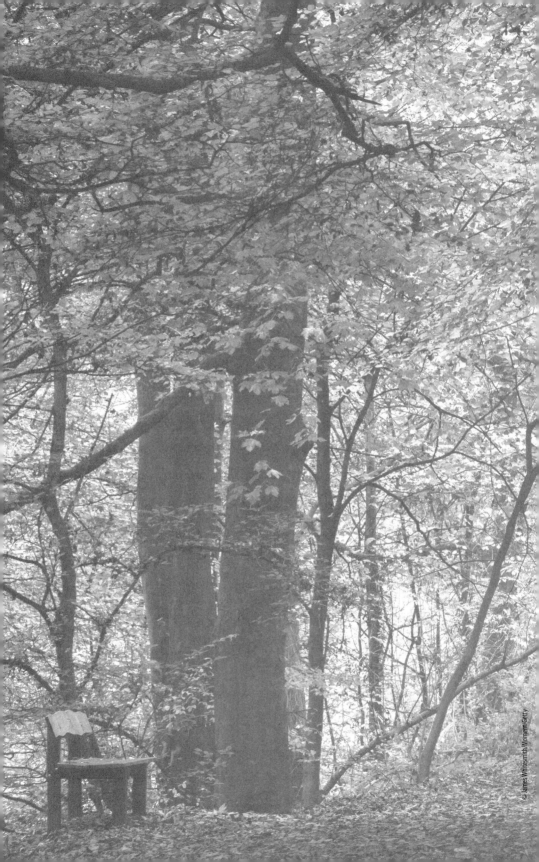

CHAPTER 1

Sharing Our Stories: Emotional Comfort for Survivors

Melissa M. Kelley, PhD
Associate Professor of Pastoral Care and Counseling
Boston College School of Theology and Ministry
Chestnut Hill, MA

For many elders considering (or perhaps actively confronting) their own dying, a great concern may be how their loved ones will fare after their death. This concern might lead to concrete advance planning, such as making financial arrangements for survivors or distributing cherished possessions to those for whom they will be meaningful. What may seem harder to plan for are the survivors' emotional responses. Is there anything that elders can do to support their survivors' emotional well-being after their deaths? Of course, this is a hugely complex question, given the enormous range in factors such as people's temperaments, ways of grieving, cultural or religious backgrounds, histories of loss, and particular ways of relating to their elders.

Given this tremendous variation, I must be modest in what I suggest here. I think that for some survivors, a source of additional sadness or struggle in their grief when a loved elder dies may be the question of whether the elder was largely at peace with his or her life. A specific way to frame this question is whether the elder understood his or her life as meaningful in significant ways. I have sometimes had this concern when some of my loved elders have died, and not knowing how they would respond to this question has indeed added sadness to my experience of grief. Flowing from this concern, I would like to propose one concrete idea, addressed directly to elders: you might attend to your survivors' emotional well-being following your death by attending *before* death, in an intentional, focused way, to the story—or narrative—of your life and the meanings that emerge from this story.

3

In the contemporary world of grief research and theory, work that considers our lives in terms of narrative or story has become an important focus (see, for example, Neimeyer, Harris, Winokuer, & Thornton, 2011; Neimeyer, 2001). Here, I will say a bit about what this focus encompasses. All humans are people of stories. That is, we often think and communicate about our lives in the form of stories, or narratives. For instance, when beginning a new relationship, we often share parts of our personal stories with one another, such as interesting aspects of our childhood and significant moments in our work lives or in our journeys as parents or grandparents. Although we certainly communicate with others in ways besides stories, it seems that across time and across cultures, humans instinctually tend to think and communicate about their lives in the form of stories (Polkinghorne, 1988). The stories that we form and share about our lives contain story elements like those that we might have learned in elementary school. That is, our stories have plots (sequences of events from beginning to end), characters (major and minor characters, protagonists and antagonists), and themes (the essential or unifying message or heart of the story), among other elements. All these elements come together to form the stories or narratives that we know and share about our lives.

Why does this matter? Of critical importance is the connection between story and meaning. The stories that we know and tell about our lives are an essential way that we understand and express what is most important to us; we might think of this as the meaning or meanings of our lives.

Meaning is a complex term. Elsewhere, I have offered the following definition of *meaning:*

> [M]eaning is the deep sense we make of things, the way we understand the world, how we articulate the overarching purpose or goal of our lives, the significance we seek in living, the core values by which we order our lives. Meaning also includes theological dimensions such as how we understand God's activity in the world, God's feelings about and responses to us, and God's role in suffering. Meaning, including theological meaning, helps to create order, sense, and purpose out of experiences and events that could otherwise seem random, nonsensical, disordered, or chaotic.
>
> (Kelley, 2010, p. 75)

Story and meaning are inextricably linked. Our life stories reflect and shape how we understand the meaning of our lives (Mishler, 1986;

Polkinghorne, 1988). If we want insight into how we make meaning of our lives, it is important to consider how we tell our life stories.

As we age and/or contemplate our own dying, we may find ourselves naturally looking back over our lives and carefully reviewing parts of our life stories. For those interested in reflecting in intentional ways on their life stories, a structured process to guide this reflection may be helpful. There are many print and online resources available for this sort of process, often using the terminology of *life review*. In doing life review, we might consider specific questions that invite us to reflect on elements of our life stories in careful ways. For instance, what would we highlight as a peak experience, or high point, in our life stories, and what might we consider a nadir experience, or low point (McAdams, 1993)? Some of these moments may have been what Robert Neimeyer, a researcher and psychologist who works extensively in grief, has described as "narrative disruptions" (Neimeyer, 2000, p. 207) because they disrupt the narratives or stories that we were living or hoped to live. What impact did these events have on our stories, and what do they suggest about who we used to be or are now (McAdams, 1993)? These are examples of ways to reflect both on our stories and the meanings that emerge from these stories.

It seems clear that those who engage in a structured life review sometimes experience great benefits, such as increased self-esteem, a sense of mastery, and an enhanced sense of well-being (see, for example, Lamers, Bohlmeijer, Korte, & Westerhof, 2015; Westerhof & Bohlmeijer, 2014). This process can help us to see—perhaps for the first time—how our life stories "come together" and make overarching sense. Events that once might have seemed random or disconnected might, with the benefit of hindsight and active reflection, emerge as aspects of a connected whole. Even those experiences of narrative disruption, which once may have seemed senseless or unwelcome intruders in our stories, can upon reflection stand out as important, perhaps even cherished, dimensions of our overall narratives.

For instance, some people come to feel that the times of greatest challenge in their lives have led to the most important personal growth. For those with a faith perspective, this process may allow one to see where God has been present throughout one's life, even if one did not notice or feel this presence at certain moments. And given the inextricable link of story and meaning, we may find that our reflection on the arc of our life narrative also enables us to see more clearly or to name anew the central meanings of our lives. Perhaps this sounds a bit like Monday morning quarterbacking, whereby one "rewrites" one's story to make it more satisfying or to ensure that its elements fit neatly together. This is not what I intend to suggest. This process can be quite challenging, and there is no clear blueprint for how it will unfold.[1] Yet it offers the possibility of coming to understand our lives in fuller, richer, and more meaningful ways, and this could be one of the greatest gifts that we ever enjoy.

Life review also may constitute a great gift for one's survivors in multiple ways. I will directly address elders as I highlight four of these ways. First, and perhaps at the most fundamental level, survivors often cherish the opportunity to learn more of their elders' stories. Sometimes children, grandchildren, or friends know your story only from the time they entered it. Often they are eager to learn more about the earlier plot material of your life and feel greatly enriched by this material. Second, your survivors' stories, of course, are linked in important ways to your own. As your survivors come to know you in deeper, fuller ways through your reflection on your life story, they come to know their own stories in deeper, fuller ways as well. This potentially enlarged self-understanding could be a great source of emotional strength and comfort after your death. Third, parts of your reflection—perhaps especially your ways of making meaning of loss, challenge, and narrative disruption—may become an invaluable part of the legacy that you leave to your survivors and a source of strength, hope, and comfort for them as they face their own inevitable struggles in life. They will have your example on which to reflect and from which to draw, again and again. Your example may come to mean different things to them at different moments in their lives.

All these points lead to the fourth, which is that your intentional reflection on your story may help your loved ones to feel a sort of ongoing connection—or continuing bond (Klass, Silverman, & Nickman, 1996)—with you after your death. Through sharing your story and your ways of making meaning in life, you may enrich and strengthen the connection that your survivors feel with you. As certain stories that we read or hear move us profoundly and then live on in a deep place within us, so your survivors may continue to feel a vibrant and deeply felt connection to you through your reflections on your life story. In all these ways, and perhaps more, your wisdom, perspective, and ways of making meaning of your life may provide rich and ongoing emotional sustenance and comfort for your loved ones, in their grief and beyond.

---

[1] An important caution is in order. Those with a very difficult or traumatic life history may do well to discuss with a trusted professional (such as a counselor, physician, or religious leader) the question of whether life review would be a helpful process. If they do embark on a life review, they might do well to seek professional assistance in this process.

Reflections for Readers

1. Elders who share their life stories with family and friends may bring greater peace of mind to the loved ones who survive them, as this author suggests, because it will give the survivors greater understanding of the meanings of their elders' lives. What will sharing their stories contribute to the elders?

2. What are the risks and benefits of a structured life review? What do we stand to learn about the meanings of our lives through such reviews, and how might we use that knowledge? If we do undertake a life review process, how might we apply what we learn in ways that will help and support our loved ones?

3. People who believe in God often frame their understanding of their lives' meaning in terms of theological considerations of God's role in the world that we inhabit—questions, for instance, about whether God is responsible for everything that happens. For people without belief in such a deity, what alternative structures might help them find meaning in the universe or consolation in randomness?

4. This author writes, "Some people come to feel that the times of greatest challenge in their lives have led to the most important personal growth." Can you locate such experiences in your own life? What about them caused you to grow, and how did they create or foster that growth?

5. Why would a continuing bond with a deceased loved one enrich the lives of survivors, and how would it do so? Might it also enrich the end phase of life of the deceased? In what ways?

6. How might reading or otherwise sharing the life stories of people we don't know—such as the stories contained in this volume—add to our store of meaning-making for our own lives?

References

Kelley, M. M. (2010). *Grief: Contemporary theory and the practice of ministry.* Minneapolis, MN: Fortress Press.

Klass, D., Silverman, P., & Nickman, S. (1996). *Continuing bonds: New understandings of grief.* New York, NY: Taylor & Francis.

Lamers, S. M. A., Bohlmeijer, E. T., Korte, J., & Westerhof, G. J. (2015). The efficacy of life-review as online-guided self-help for adults: A randomized trial. *Journals of Gerontology: Series B: Psychological Sciences and Social Sciences, 70*(1), 24–34.

McAdams, D. P. (1993). *The stories we live by: Personal myths and the making of the self.* New York, NY: William Morrow and Company, Inc.

Mishler, E. G. (1986). *Research interviewing: context and narrative.* Cambridge, MA: Harvard University Press.

Neimeyer, R. A. (2000). Narrative disruptions in the construction of the self. In R. A. Neimeyer & J. D. Raskin (Eds.), *Constructions of disorder: Meaning-making frameworks for psychotherapy* (pp. 207–242). Washington, DC: American Psychological Association.

Neimeyer, R. A. (2001). *Meaning reconstruction and the experience of loss.* Washington, DC: American Psychological Association.

Neimeyer, R. A., Harris, D. L., Winokuer, H. R., & Thornton, G. F. (2011). *Grief and bereavement in contemporary society: Bridging research and practice.* New York, NY: Routledge.

Polkinghorne, D. E. (1988). *Narrative knowing and the human sciences.* Albany, NY: State University of New York Press.

Westerhof, G. J., & Bohlmeijer E. T. (2014). Celebrating fifty years of research and applications in reminiscence and life review: State of the art and new directions. *Journal of Aging Studies, 29,* 107–114.

CHAPTER 2

Burn and Rave[1]

Ben Slomoff, MA
Business Executive, Mediator, and Arbitrator (retired)
Walnut Creek, CA
Age 103

I was born on November 16, 1913, in Pittsburgh, Pennsylvania, the son of immigrants who had escaped from Lithuania, then a part of Russia. Facing Russia's pogroms, its ethnic and religious persecution, and the Russian army's draft, they fled to the United States in 1900. My parents met and were married in the United States. Our home had a European flavor.

My early youth, growing up in New Kensington in western Pennsylvania, was wasted in a futile quest for fulfillment. I strived for a sense of belonging. I played all the high school sports on the first team, yet I did not fit in culturally with the majority group, who were from a different faith and background. Their parents were hard-working, hard-drinking immigrants who mined coal, made steel, or worked in the aluminum factory that dominated the town. Unlike those others, we did not have a Christmas tree or Easter bunny; rather, we lit candles for Hanukkah, celebrated Purim, observed Shabbat every Friday night, and occasionally had a kosher chicken dinner without white gravy. Ham, pork, and shellfish were considered forbidden.

We were the odd family in a mostly Welsh and Slavic Christian community. We also were mired in the great economic Depression of the 1930s: mills, mines, and factories, the economic engine of the region, were all shutting down. My parents lost everything that they had acquired from years of hard work and savings. All around us, working men were being laid off, staying unemployed for long stretches. Banks closed and the entire town was foreclosed on. Fortunately, my father was

---

[1]Dylan Thomas—"Old age should burn and rave at close of day."

able to rent a house and keep the family together. My mother did sewing and sold coffee house to house to survive.

Public school and education in general were offered at the lowest possible level of quality, with low expectations for students. Most teachers were poorly trained political appointees. They had very little interest in teaching, and students responded in kind; neither cared—a waste in so many ways. Education beyond high school was economically difficult. With money from a series of low-paying jobs, I enrolled briefly in the University of Pittsburgh. I then applied for officer training, was accepted, and was commissioned as a second lieutenant, intending to serve one year of active duty in 1940–1941. The assignment was to build (along with the Corps of Engineers) an air base in Dothan, Alabama, to train British pilots. My year was up in December 1941, but Pearl Harbor was attacked on December 7 of that year, and I was transferred to the newly established Air Force and remained on active duty for six more years. I later did 10 additional years in the Reserves, retiring as a staff officer with the rank of lieutenant colonel.

Before the war, I had been hired as a trainee by the Brown Shoe Company in St. Louis, Missouri. The training involved all aspects of the shoe industry: manufacturing, sales, promotion and advertising, factory operations, buying leather and materials, finance, credit—all intended to prepare me for management. After the war, I bought the Milford Shoe Company, a small New England manufacturing company, and developed it into a large domestic and international company. In 1968, I sold my company to my largest customer and did consulting for a few years.

At the age of 75, I retired and enrolled in the University of Massachusetts to complete my education, which had been interrupted by the Great Depression. I had been taking special courses at the Harvard Extension School in poetry, playwriting, and literary criticism, as well as studying Shakespeare for a year with Professor Marjorie Garber. At UMass Boston, I was given credit for these courses and earned a BA in Public and Community Service in 1993, at the age of 80, followed by a Master's in Conflict Resolution, Human Security, and Global Studies in 1997, at the age of 84. At that point, my life truly began anew. I immediately applied for arbitration and mediation training with the Financial Regulatory Authority (FINRA). After much training and rigid testing, I was accepted as an Arbitrator and Mediator for NASDAQ and the New York Stock Exchange.

After I received my Master's degree from UMass Boston, my wife and I founded a Symposium in Conflict Resolution at the University of

Massachusetts, which brought in such brilliant leaders as Senator George J. Mitchell, Morton Deutsch, Herbert Kelman, and Ambassador Dennis Ross to lecture to graduate students on the world's major political and religious conflicts. I have continued supporting the symposium with great success for the last sixteen years.

When I lived in Connecticut prior to Boston, I conducted a Mortimer Adler Great Books class at the Federal Correctional Institution at Danbury for many years. Not only was it gratifying, but it gave me great insight into and knowledge of classic literature and philosophical exposure. In 1999, I worked as a mediator on the planning of the air rights of the extension of the Mass Turnpike as part of the "Big Dig" in Boston. As a reward for this effort, Mayor Thomas Menino declared a "Ben Slomoff Day" in Boston and stated that no matter where I lived, I would always be an honorary Bostonian.

In 2000, I moved to the Bay Area in California and offered my services to the Contra Costa Superior Court Small Claims Division as a pro bono mediator. For the next nine years, I performed several hundred mediations and was nominated as Mediator of the Year in 2010, at the age of 97. At the age of 102, I published my second book of poetry, *Never Enough.* (My first book, *Stalwart Bends,* was published in 2012 when I was 99.) I also wrote and produced a play in Boston titled *Don't Catch the Rabbit.*

I am very proud of my family. Sylvia and I were married for 69 years until her death in 2007. My son, Mark, is a physician at the Emergency Department at John Muir Hospital in Walnut Creek, California. My daughter, Judith, is a psychotherapist in London. I am active in writing clubs and a poetry group called the Ina Coolbrith Circle, founded in September 28, 1919. I also belong to a luncheon club and the Diablo Club, in which world affairs and public policy are discussed. We are now working on Stephen Hawking's cosmology book, *A Brief History of Time.* I have won many poetry prizes, including a first prize of $300 in a citywide contest.

In spite of many surgeries over the years, including a heart valve replacement in 1999, I am in generally good health and live independently. I do not use a walker or cane, and I attend a fitness center regularly to focus on balance exercises. I have a longtime companion, Rheta Daggs, who keeps me very socially active. I am also working on my third book of poetry and contributing my best to improve our very conflicted society. On November 16, 2016, I turned 103. I still drive, day or night— but carefully.

One of my poems, about the process of aging, appears here:

Ode to Aging

What a struggle to stay the same

When fleeting time's to blame.

Inside I'm filled with hope and fear

To stave off failure, keep life dear,

Keep up appearances year by year.

A child's disappointment adds stress,

Old fading love hurts—no less.

Acceptance, dependence conflict my days,

Bloating my calendar in foolish ways.

Wanting what I may never get,

Hiding frustrations—goals not met.

Then . . . the pleasure at last as things go well,

Good news to make my old heart swell

Aging: you have a good story to tell.

Reflections for Readers

1. In what ways is this author's experience of aging similar to and different from other older adults you've interacted with?
2. What does this narrative suggest about the importance of life-long learning and community service?
3. The poem "Ode to Aging" presents both the difficulties and the rewards of growing older. What do you see as the primary difficulties and rewards of aging?

CHAPTER 3

Serendipity

Nancy Lelewer Sonnabend
Associate in Neurology, Harvard Medical School
(retired), and nonfiction author
Boston, MA
Age 82

I have lived my life by allowing doors to open and being willing to enter wherever they led. This essay describes just a few of those openings and how they took me in unexpected directions.

I dedicated most of my married years to my husband and four children, several of whom have learning disabilities—a couple have attention deficit hyperactivity disorder (ADHD) and one is on the autism spectrum. In order to help my children, I developed manipulative materials and brought two of the programs to market. Because of the materials that I developed and patented, a book that I wrote on learning disabilities, and my service on many boards dealing with dyslexia and other learning disabilities, I was invited to lecture at many conferences and universities.

By the time I was in my late forties, I was divorced, and one of my children was married, one was living in California, and two were in college. I found myself alone and at loose ends for the first time in my life. So when life hit a low ebb, I entered a six-week program for women who wanted to switch jobs or go into the workforce for the first time. The program wasn't particularly productive, but a potluck dinner party that I had for Sarah Lawrence alumnae led to a number of fascinating adventures.

The day of the potluck, I had a bad cold and a fever. I wished that I had not offered to have the dinner at my apartment. At 10 p.m., I was ushering my last guest, Deborah Hermann, to the door. "I understand you know a lot about dyslexia," she said. "Can you tell me about it?"

I felt so awful that I just wanted her to leave, so I said, "Sure, perhaps we can have lunch sometime and talk."

"Well, it's really my husband who is interested."

"Fine, have him call me." I gave her my numbers and shooed her out the door.

A week later, I received a phone call from a gentleman who identified himself as Dr. Howard Hermann. I had no idea who he was until he said, "My wife met you at the Sarah Lawrence gathering last week. I'd like to meet you and talk about dyslexia. Could I pick you up next Tuesday at 9 p.m. and take you to MIT?"

I tried to talk Dr. Hermann into meeting earlier, and at my apartment, but he insisted on our going to the Massachusetts Institute of Technology (MIT), so I finally agreed.

Tuesday evening, Dr. Hermann picked me up at 9 p.m. When we reached the Center for Space Research, he fumbled in his pocket and eventually said, "I didn't bring the right key. Don't worry, there is a lock on a nearby building that I can open with my knife and we can get in that way."

We moved on to another building. With a little finagling, he got the door open, and we proceeded to go up and down stairs and through long, dark corridors until we came to the basement of the Center for Space Research. Throughout the walk, I was thinking, "This is not smart. You are with a man you know nothing about, he has a knife, you're in dark halls, and no one knows where you are." Once we arrived, Howard put on the lights, pointed to a large object in the center of the floor, and said, "This is one of the first flight simulators ever made. Would you like to try it?"

I replied, "I don't understand. What's that got to do with dyslexia?"

"Nothing."

"So, what do you want to know about dyslexia? I'm dyslexic and have raised dyslexic children. Do you want to test me?"

"No, I know all about you and your work with dyslexic children. I'd like you to work with me on a project studying eye movements in dyslexics. I don't know about dyslexia, and you could help me. I think I could teach you to be a researcher. There's no money for salaries now, but you would learn a lot. After we run the pilot project, we may be able to get NIH funding."

"Can I just waltz into MIT and do research? I have a liberal arts degree from Sarah Lawrence College and that's it."

"You'd need to turn in your CV and have an interview with Larry Young, head of the lab."

"What's a CV?"

"Curriculum vitae."

"What's that?"

"It tells what you've done."

"Oh. I have a 1-page résumé."

"Great. Make it 25 pages and you have a CV."

The research sounded interesting, and the program that I was in seemed to be leading me nowhere. I decided to finish the remaining weeks of the program and, at the same time, work on a CV. I called a friend who was a professor at Boston University and asked for help. She came over, and in no time, I had a respectable CV. What I hadn't realized was that my patents, copyrights, trademark, and the places where I had lectured could, and should, be listed on my CV. They had not been part of my résumé.

In 1983, after an interview with Larry Young, I became a research affiliate in MIT's Man/Vehicle Lab, Department of Aeronautics and Astronautics. I shared an office with Dr. Hermann (who, by that time, was Howard to me) and, much to my wonder, the astronaut Byron Lichtenberg.

The day that I started as a research affiliate, Howard took me into the room where the research was to be done. One of the technicians asked me, "Do you know how to calibrate the bifurcation paradigm?"

"Not yet," I said.

When we got back to the office, I promptly told Howard that I hadn't understood a word the technician had said. Howard laughed and explained that one of the issues that the research was designed to examine was whether dyslexics, like normal readers, have a biological preference to look in one particular direction when lights are shown so far on the periphery that both lights cannot be seen without moving the eyes from one light to the other. This reaction happens so quickly that people are not conscious of it. To examine the issue, Howard said, a subject's head would be secured, and the movements of both eyes were recorded as the subject, seated in a dark room, watched a perimeter screen.

For the pilot experiment, several dyslexics and a control group of normal readers were chosen. A center light would appear on the screen, followed by the projection of either a single light appearing randomly on the left or the right side of the screen or the projection of two lights, one on the left side of the screen and one on the right of the screen. All the lights had the same luminance, and when two lights came on, they were always an equal distance from the center light. Over time, our research found that dyslexics make a more random choice of where they first look when lights are bifurcated (a light on the left and one on the right simultaneously) than do normal readers.

Howard taught me how to be a researcher. In turn, I taught him about dyslexia. Together, we made a great team. He was not good about keeping things organized, but that is my forte. One of my jobs was to file all the papers before Howard lost them. In return, Howard, who reads rapidly, would put papers in three piles for me: papers I didn't need to read, papers for which I needed only to read the summary, and papers I needed to read completely. When we were writing up our research, I would frequently ask him how to spell a word. He'd tell me and go right on reading. It was heaven. My spelling is so poor, I couldn't always find the word that I wanted in the dictionary. (This was before spell check.) In September 1986, three years after I began work at MIT, the first article with my name on it appeared in *Cortex*. A second article followed later that year.

Although I shared a desk with Byron Lichtenberg, he was rarely present. When I began work, I was told to put his pictures of outer space and the things he had in the drawers in the building's storage area. I did so, and a month later a young, handsome man appeared at my desk. "Is this your desk?"

I jumped up and said, "You must be Byron Lichtenberg. If you need the desk, I'll move someplace else."

"No, I don't need the desk. I'm just wondering what happened to all my pictures and the stuff that was in the drawers."

"It's all in storage. Do you want me to get it?"

"No. What are you researching?"

When I told him, he laughed. "It's appropriate that we share a desk. You're studying inner space, and I'm studying outer space." And with that, we became friends.

Byron was the first true scientist to become an astronaut. All those before him were astronauts who then learned something about science. During my first year at MIT, Byron was launched into outer space on Space Lab One. Larry Young was the chief investigator on the experiments that Byron carried out during his mission, so all communications were downlinked into our lab. I remember sitting for hours listening to Byron and the others as they carried out their duties while circling the Earth every hour and a half. In 1992, after all three of us had left MIT, Byron went up again. This time, he invited me to the launch. It was one of the most dramatic events that I've ever experienced. Knowing Byron was on board, listening to the countdown, hearing "You're green to go,

Godspeed," and feeling the ground shake under me like an earthquake reduced me to tears.

Howard and Brian weren't the only interesting people I met at MIT.

One day while I was working in the lab, a large man shuffled into my office. He was grossly overweight, his clothes were disheveled, and his beard was unkempt and showed the remnants of his last meal. He poked me in the arm and said, "You Nancy?"

"Yes," I said reluctantly.

"I've been looking for you. I'm having a conference next month at my monastery, Villa Musso, on the Italian Riviera and will be bringing together top scientists from all over the world to discuss dyslexia and learning differences. I'd like you to come."

"Thank you, but I can't get away next month," I replied politely, while thinking, "This guy is a street person and a crazy one at that. How do I get him out of my office?"

He turned to leave and then turned back to say, "Now that I've seen you, you will help me start my wheelchair company in the U.S."

"No, I don't do wheelchairs," I said firmly.

"Sure you do. You'll see."

He ambled out, and I forgot about him. Two nights later, at 3 a.m., my phone rang. I picked it up and heard a foreign language.

"Who is this?"

"Per Udden."

"Who? Speak English."

"Remember, I was in your office a couple of days ago. I want you to come to my conference and start my wheelchair company in the U.S."

"It's 3 in the morning. Please don't call me again." I hung up.

The phone rang again immediately. "You're rude. Don't hang up on me."

"Look, I don't know you, and its 3 in the morning."

"It's not 3 a.m. here."

"If you call me again in the middle of the night, I'll call the police. Now, I'm hanging up."

Over the next several days, as I asked around the lab if anyone knew a man named Per Udden, Per continued to call me, but during the daytime. From fellow workers, I learned that Per was a Swedish doctor who, along with Axel Wennerblom, an engineer, discovered the sticky material that holds sanitary pads to women's underpants. The two men sold the license for their invention to Stille-Werner, a company in Sweden that sells sanitary pads throughout Europe. Per used some of the money that he received to buy Villa Musso, his Italian monastery, and some to start an electric wheelchair company, Permobil A.B., in Sweden. At some point during various conversations about Per, I learned that he was dyslexic, which, of course, intrigued me.

I did not go to the conference that Per first invited me to, but I have gone to many since then, in various parts of the world. And I helped him establish Permobil of America, Inc. in the United States (now renamed Permobil USA). I spent a month in Sweden learning how Permobil wheelchairs were made and serviced, and then I became a founding director of Permobil of America. In fact, the company's first U.S. office was in my apartment. So good were the Permobil chairs that shortly after they began appearing here, U.S. and foreign companies started to copy their features. Today, Permobil is the leading provider of power wheelchairs with mobility products for complex injuries and disease in the world.

It was through my work with Permobil that I met Princess Marianne Bernadotte. During the month that I spent in Sweden learning about Permobil A.B., I was introduced to her. Later, she, Per, and I spent a few days in Wilmington, Delaware, to promote Permobil at the Dupont Institute. I still remember the day that I introduced Marianne to the New York City bus system. We came out of Tiffany's that day, only to discover that it was pouring and there were no taxis available.

"Have you ever ridden a public bus?" I asked.

"No."

"Well, you're going to now," I said as I handed her quarters and pushed her in front of me. The bus that we got on was already quite full. We found ourselves standing in the aisle, squashed between bodies in front and behind us. The driver was one of those who like to accelerate and then jam on the brakes, throwing everyone backward and forward with each jerk.

"How do you like riding this bus?" I asked.

"I like my chauffeur-driven limo better."

She got even. One evening, we were walking down the street on the Upper East Side when Marianne noticed people going to an art opening party.

"Come on, let's go," she said.

"We can't just walk in there."

"Sure, we can," she said as she pulled me into the party. We drank champagne, ate hors d'oeuvres, and looked at the pictures. No one even noticed us. As we left, we thanked the man at the door.

When I became a founding director of Permobil of America, Per sent me to Edward L. Bernays for advice on marketing Permobil in this country. Dr. Bernays, whom I came to call Edward, was gracious with his time, helpful, and fascinating. There was an entire wall of pictures of him with every President, Head of State, and Chief Executive Officer (CEO) of a major corporation that I could imagine. I learned from others that he was the nephew of Sigmund Freud, one of the first to attempt to manipulate public opinion using the psychology of the subconscious, and many considered him to be the originator of modern public relations. He was named one of the 100 most influential Americans of the twentieth century by *Life* magazine. I remember noticing a new painting of him over the fireplace one afternoon and saying, "Edward, that's a wonderful new portrait of you. I like it. Did you just decide to have it painted?"

"No," he said. "It's for the National Gallery in DC, but there is some rule that they can't hang it until ten years after I die, so I told them they'd have to wait; and in the meantime, I wanted to enjoy it."

Per was a collector of people. It was because of Per that I was able to work in Frank Duffy's Brain Electrical Activity Mapping (BEAM) laboratory at Harvard Medical School as an associate in neurology, and because of Per that I could assist in other projects, including Heidelise Als's kangaroo box studies.

One of Per's scientific projects was the Ober 2 eye tracker. Jan Ober, from Poland, had developed a new eye tracker with Per. When the eye movement project at MIT did not receive funding from the National Institutes of Health (NIH), Per paved the way for Jan and me to use the Ober 2 eye tracker with some of the dyslexic youngsters and their matched controls on which Frank was running BEAM studies. I was grandfathered into the lab as an associate in neurology, and Jan and I ran eye movement studies on Frank's dyslexic subjects for six weeks. Later, Per sent me to Poland to spend a week in Jan's lab in Poznan.

The Ober project led to me assisting on a number of projects, including some by Heidelise. My job for her kangaroo-in-a-box studies was to keep the mother and child in the center of each video lens as I taped their movements. I also administered the Wechsler Intelligence Scale for Children—Revised (WISC-R) to eight-year-olds who were part of Heidelise's longitudinal population of preemies and spent many months in a room working the computers and keeping one child per day happy and involved as a technician recorded the child's brain waves.

As far as I know, Per was the first person to bring together neurologists, geneticists, and specialists in temporal processing, as well as other medical specialists, to discuss reading, learning differences, and dyslexia. Per and Professor Ragnar Granit founded the Rodin Remediation

Academy in 1984 to promote multidisciplinary research on dyslexia and other learning disabilities. Rodin Remediation Academy conferences are by invitation only and usually include about 100 people. Participants present their research findings and then have the opportunity to discuss their work with colleagues from different disciplines, as well as different countries.

In 1994, a Rodin conference held on the island of Malta introduced me to Montserrat Estil-les. As I studied the program for the conference, I noticed that one of the women attending the conference, Montserrat Estil-les, was from Spain. Later, after the first day's papers had been given, I spotted Montserrat Estil-les on an excursion boat that we had all boarded. From what I could observe, she didn't seem to speak much English. As the conference was held in English, I asked her in Spanish, "Do you understand what is being said at the conference?"

Thrilled to find someone who spoke her language, she replied in Spanish, "No, I don't understand. I have a clinic for dyslexics in Barcelona and I'm here to learn. Can you come to my room tonight and explain everything that has been said today in Spanish?" That was the beginning of our friendship. That night, and every night until the end of the conference, I translated all that I could remember of the day's events into Spanish for her, and then we would discuss the events and papers in detail. To this day, we keep in close contact. We have visited each other's homes on several occasions and communicate by phone and e-mail frequently.

All this opened the door to a new career and new friends. I went from wife and mother—always mother—to a research affiliate at MIT, where I shared a desk with a brilliant doctor and an astronaut, to a founding director of Permobil of America with friends around the world, to an associate in neurology who attended world-renowned conferences on dyslexia and learning differences. This was an amazing beginning, offering new worlds to conquer.

As the years passed, my hearing deteriorated, so I resigned from all the boards on which I was serving and eventually left Harvard Medical School. But again, new doors opened. I wrote another book, this one about my family, and am now in touch with many family members I never knew I had. I once went to a benefit for homeless women and sat next to a woman who was on the Asperger board, and she said that she wanted me to talk to the executive director of what today is the Asperger/Autism Network (AANE). The following week, the executive director came to my home and spent two hours with me, and the next thing I knew, I was on a committee to reorganize their board. Today, I serve on the Executive Advisors' board of AANE.

I also received a call asking if I would consider serving on the national board of the Hearing Loss Association of America (HLAA), which is headquartered in Bethesda, Maryland. I've been on that board for seven years, and I'm its oldest member.

Back in 2000, I called a friend but got her husband, who was rushing out, instead. I asked where he was going. He said, "I'm going to class at Harvard Institute of Learning in Retirement. You should join. The classes are great." So I applied to HILR, was interviewed by two people for over an hour, and have been attending classes there ever since.

All you have to do is put yourself out there, and good things happen.

Reflections for Readers

1. What are the challenges to letting life carry you serendipitously? What are the benefits?
2. What does one gain or lose by sticking to a life plan?
3. Are there personality traits that make one more open to unanticipated opportunities?

CHAPTER 4

Exercising One's Mind; Counting One's Blessings

Helene Oppenheimer
Director, Tax Library, BDO Seidman, 1983–1993 (retired)
Dedham, MA
Age 82

I remember from the time I was a little girl of three or four years of age, thinking about my life and what it meant to have elderly grandparents with whom we spent so much time. Every weekend, my parents, my brother, and I would take a streetcar across the city to spend the day at my mother's parents' house. I remember thinking about their lives—my mind was moving constantly between their world and mine. How did they manage to keep their love alive when they had been apart for five years early in their marriage?

My grandfather would tell me that using your mind, thinking about your life, was something to be done every day, throughout the day. I would ask my mother about this and how she managed to "get through her day" because I remember being worried about everyday living—daydreams (sometimes scary) would take up a part of my waking hours.

My mother told me I was "too young to worry about things." That is when I thought to myself that I had to involve myself and my mind in things that mattered to me. I began asking for books—which at that age were coloring books—and progressed to easy picture books, in order to make up stories that were pleasing to me. My life began to be filled with reading books, going to concerts and art museums with my parents, going to the public library, and then taking lessons in tap, ballet, and toe dancing.

All this took place while I was in elementary school, where I was chubby and awkward. There was little I could do about my appearance, but I discovered that my mind could roam into imaginative narratives that took me out of myself. I could make up stories. I could do puzzles. I easily memorized words, and I learned to use a dictionary. When I would question my dad (my mother was too busy to deal with all my questions), he would give me an answer that led to more questions, and that made me eager for more information, so more questions would follow.

My dad then must have thought I should have some way to look up answers myself, because he bought a set of *The Book of Knowledge,* with yearly updates. The wonderful hours spent searching for answers to all my questions made dull days fly by quickly. Another activity for my mind that I enjoyed was working on picture puzzles. They were a challenge, as I progressed from simpler to more complicated ones, but I lost interest when I found them too easy to do.

As I grew up through elementary school, I never lost my wonder at life. The more I learned, the more I wanted to learn, and I spent hours at the Enoch Public Library whenever a parent could take me there. I was not allowed alone downtown until I was about nine years old. I did walk to elementary school sometimes with neighborhood friends, who left me behind as I dawdled, watching for any little creature that might scurry from behind a bush or burrow into the dry hills along the path we walked.

And school itself was a wonder: so much to learn. I loved the one teacher for each grade until sixth grade, where we rotated to a separate teacher for each subject, and where this became even more exciting because each teacher had a different style, and I found it a challenge to remember what was required by each one. I loved the details of geography, learning about the rivers, lakes, and mountains. We learned about Maryland history and the city of Baltimore.

Those days flew by in a blur of learning and activity. And after school, walking home, looking forward to my milk and cookies, rushing so I could go out and play in the neighborhood—Step Ball and Territory were my favorite games. There was a gang of us in the neighborhood always out playing until dinner and bedtime. I was usually tired enough not to complain when my mother said it was time for bed, for bedtime became my thinking time: to review the day's activity, just as waking early allowed me to listen to the sounds outside and think about the day ahead. My mind was always working, whether noticing the freshness of the air, breathing in the smell of a spring shower, looking at the clouds, or wondering at rainbows and sunsets (I was never up early enough to see a sunrise). I loved being outside. So "Up and out" became an early motto.

And then came summer camp. At a very young age, I was sent off to camp—another life, away from the stringent rules of home and school; a relaxed way of being and a learning experience all its own: living in close quarters with 2 counselors and 10 girls in a bunk. My mind took off: sounds, sights, and smells were different. I loved the morning bugle call, for it meant the start of another exciting day ahead; then the flag raising and those wonderful breakfasts. Hiking, swimming, archery, color wars, "backwards day," cookouts and sleep-outs, never-ending activity throughout the day with a pause after lunch for nap time. I resented nap time, but I still found ways to use that time to savor the activity just finished and the one ahead.

Then, after a full afternoon of other activities—sometimes a hike into "town" to mail our weekly letter home, or sometimes a nature walk, rather than a spirited hike—we had dinner and an evening sing-along before flag-lowering. Then, the calm of hearing "Taps" at sunset, the cool of the evening air, another day ending, and another night of rethinking the wonderful day and looking forward to the bugle call for a new day to begin.

It was at camp that I listened to the rustling leaves and the songs of birds and the clicking of insects, where I learned to make a campfire and watched with wonder as marshmallows melted into a gauze of liquid sugar . . . I learned that food dropped on the ground was still okay to eat. Then there were the sudden summer showers, bursts of rain leaving puddles for me to float downed leaves and twigs in, feeling the hard raindrops that felt like crushed ice bursting on my skin, and then marveling at the disappearance of moisture and learning about evaporation. The summers ended all too quickly.

I was disappointed when I knew the summer was ending, but I also rejoiced when my parents came with my favorite uncle to bring me home, to begin preparations for school and the Jewish High Holy Days. There again, something new had been introduced when my parents decided that I should attend Hebrew School to learn Jewish history and to learn to read Hebrew to follow the services. This was not my favorite thing to do, but it has not hurt me—it only took me away from my love of playing outdoors.

Junior high passed in a maze of new learning and socializing, but it was when I entered high school and began science classes that I realized that too much social activity would interfere with my love of learning, with my mind growing and playing catch-up with the world. I decided that to anchor my day, I needed to participate in the sports program at my high school, which was only a 15-minute walk from home.

Little did I know that my mind would be as involved as my body! Learning a sport is more than engaging in physical activities. I had to question the reasons behind how to shoot a basket from varying angles; I had to know how to direct a ball in tennis and ping-pong and bowling. Volleyball took its own understanding of working with a team. I learned all those techniques and helped my teammates as well, so that we could become a cohesive and winning force. I loved my high school, and I did not look forward to leaving and heading in a new direction, but I knew I did not want to stay home and work.

Applying to college in those days was easy. I applied to only three schools and chose Simmons College because it was a small women's school in a city. High school graduation came, and suddenly I was embarking on a new adventure. What stress I experienced on the overnight train to Boston!

BOSTON! Where I would fall in love with a school and a city that would stretch my mind, where I would make lifelong friends, where I would be prepared for a life filled with more learning than I ever could have imagined in one lifetime. My academic education at Simmons College was matched and enhanced by the offerings of the city's culture: the Museum of Fine Arts, the Boston Symphony, the Metropolitan Opera that came to perform locally each year, and my most beloved Isabella Stewart Gardner Museum. I had to soak everything in quickly and fully because I knew that at the end of four years, I would have to return to Baltimore, find employment, and once again live at home. My parents expected that.

In a short time, I had a job in the media department of the largest advertising agency in Baltimore, and became engaged to the man I thought I would spend the rest of my life with . . . but my mind knew me better than I did, and after much agonizing, I broke the engagement when I understood that a conventional Baltimore Jewish marriage was not for me. One blessing that I had not thought about was my parents' support. They told me it was my life to live; they would not advise me, but would support any decision I made.

After my broken engagement, I had a lively social life. I dated interesting men, and I decided to attend Shakespeare classes in night school at Johns Hopkins. This led to attending plays at the Stratford Shakespeare Festival in Connecticut and going to theater in New York City. I relished all this adventure.

And then I met the love of my life, Martin, and moved with him to Washington, D.C., where he worked as a tax attorney. Another blessing, another family to love, as Martin and I were close with both sides of our families, and we spent many weekends together with one family or the other because it was easy to travel between the two cities. Married life was exciting, and Washington was a happening place to be.

New joy came with the arrival of our first-born son, Alan. And having our families nearby was more than a blessing because I knew I was not ready to be a mom, so both families pitched in to help. Having a baby was an exciting learning experience for both Martin and me until the novelty wore off, and I decided that being with a baby all day was not my idea of fun.

I decided to get a volunteer job, found a competent babysitter two afternoons a week, and went off happily to the Corcoran Gallery of American Art. We did not know then that a move to New York was in our future. We enjoyed our nearby family and new friends with their young babies. We were blessed with a sometimes too challenging baby and had lots of fun together.

Martin decided after seven years working in government to practice in New York City with a large law firm. So off we went happily to another life. We encountered a new challenge when our twins were born, and we realized that we could not raise three children in New York City. We moved to a suburban town in New Jersey where we could walk to town, own a dog, have good public schools, join a synagogue, and have an easy commute for Martin.

We settled in, but I did not sit still for long. I joined our temple's board as the first woman Vice President, became active in the local chapter of the National Council of Jewish Women, and served on the Lay Committee of Education, which conducted studies on education and advised the local Board of Education. I volunteered at the Child Care Center and at a newly formed organization to help the elderly in the area. I did finally return to work when the children went off to college, and I found an entirely different way of life for a number of years.

Now after many years of an active life, here we are at NewBridge on the Charles, still active. I am still stretching my inquiring mind and still counting my blessings.

Reflections for Readers

1. Exercising one's mind is related to learning new things. This author mentioned several ways that she found to exercise her mind as a child, including creating stories, reading, doing puzzles, and asking questions. What would you add to her list? Are any of these activities limited to young people, or can they be applied to seniors too? Do seniors have a different set of ways to exercise their minds?

2. For this author, childhood and youth were times filled with wonder. How does experiencing such a sense of wonder translate into "counting one's blessings"?

3. This author referred to some events as "not my idea of fun," but she found ways to take something positive from the experience or transform the experience into something personally fulfilling, no matter what it was. Can you think of times in your own life when you have used one of these means to convert a negative experience into a positive one?

5

Elwood and His Golden Nature

Laurie Schreiber
Freelance writer/editor
Bass Harbor, ME

At one time, Elwood Banfill was awarded the *Boston Post* Cane for being the oldest citizen in his community. It wasn't a gift he particularly wanted.

"It puts me in mind of Clarence Harding," he told a group of town officials and family members who met at his house to make the ceremony an occasion. "He was to be the recipient of the cane, and he said to my wife, 'Oh, I don't want that. Everybody who gets that cane dies.'"

Elwood was 99 at the time. He had a smile that lit the room. "As the old saying goes, you might as well laugh as cry," he said. He turned to an admirer and brandished the gold-headed ebony cane. "You remember King Midas and his gold? This is like his scepter."

The story goes that the *Boston Post* Cane was a marketing invention of Edwin Grozier, the *Boston Post*'s publisher, who in 1909 sent fancy canes to 700 New England towns, with the request that they be presented with the newspaper's compliments to the oldest citizen. Upon that person's death, the cane would be transferred to the next oldest citizen.

Elwood wasn't really put out by the gift. He had a sunny nature and a loving family. His beloved wife, Elvira, had died several years earlier, during the seventieth year of their marriage. Elwood recalled when they met, in the early 1930s. He had just been called home after his freshman year at the University of Alabama to assist the family as the Great Depression deepened. "We began to double date," he said. "That's the spark that started the fire. She had so many good qualities,

I'm telling you. She was very talented in many ways." Hung on the walls around the house were some of Elvira's watercolors, oils, and charcoal drawings. She was also an excellent cook, and she learned how to make beautiful clothes from her mother, who was an excellent seamstress in an era when women's clothes were handmade. "We had an extremely happy life," Elwood said.

Elwood also recalled his productive career. As a young man, he worked for a company in Ashland, Massachusetts, called Warren Tel-echron, whose founder invented a self-starting, synchronous motor designed to provide accurate timekeeping. "There had been electric clocks for a long time," he said, "but if the power failed, the clock just sat there; it didn't start. So this old gentleman, Henry Warren, found out how to make a simple change in the little motor that ran the electric clocks so that they became self-starting. As a consequence, these clocks were in great demand. And General Electric never overlooks a good deal, so they immediately bought the whole business."

Elwood's first job was in the clock-testing department. When he began taking night courses on electricity, his supervisor saw that he wanted to get ahead, so he was shifted to the department that tested timed motors—the sort that could be used, for example, to allow a bank vault door to be opened in the morning. "If the bank vault opened at the wrong time, big trouble," he said.

Soon enough, Elwood became a supervisor. Then the Japanese bombed Pearl Harbor. He decided to sign up for the U.S. Air Force as a civilian employee. "I was motivated because I was young enough, I was in my 30s, I had no children, and I knew that it wasn't going to be long before Uncle Sam grabbed me," he said. Given his expertise in the testing of timed instruments, he was immediately accepted, and shortly afterward, he was shipped off to Bridgeport, Connecticut, where he worked for a manufacturer of aviation instruments for wartime flying. "Bridgeport was a beehive of activity for the war," he said.

He spent 17 years in the Air Force, subsequently spent several years with a Reynolds Metals Company subsidiary, and retired in 1973. He always felt fortunate to have been a witness to an important part of the twentieth century.

The couple enjoyed their time in Connecticut. Their home was in a pleasant enough location. Unfortunately, construction of the Connecticut Turnpike changed all that. There were no pollution controls on cars at the time. So although the turnpike was several miles from their home, the prevailing westerly wind wafted fumes to their doorstep. "We'd sit out on the patio and we'd say, 'Well, this isn't so good,'" he recalled.

They decided to move. First, they thought about North Carolina. "It was beautiful country and everything," he said. "It was nice, but my wife said, 'There's no seashore.' So I said, 'I know what you're thinking about.'"

What she was thinking about was Mount Desert Island, in midcoast Maine. In 1941, the summer before Pearl Harbor, the couple had vacationed in Canada and returned through Maine. They camped in Acadia National Park. "We went to Seawall. Oh, my wife was crazy about the place. She did some sketches, and we finally ran out of time. I had to get back to work. So we said, 'Oh, we're coming back here next vacation.' But it was wartime—no travel."

Then the couple started a family and stayed in Connecticut. But they never forgot Maine. In 1972, Elwood bought a looseleaf spiral notebook. He cut out real estate ads from the newspapers and pasted them in the notebook. When they got the chance, they drove back to Maine to check out the various places. They landed at Mount Desert Island and found a house that they loved, but they were told that it had just been sold. That evening, they returned to their inn and prepared for the drive back to Connecticut the next morning. They woke to an ice storm. "I said, 'Oh man, we've got to drive back in this mess,'" he recalled. "We got packed up, went out to the office, the guy out there says, 'Good morning,' and I say, 'I don't know how good it is.' And he says to me, 'Mister, any day that you can get out of bed, stand on your own two feet, and take a deep breath is a good morning.' And I say, 'You are so right. I will consider it as a good morning.' That always stayed with me."

The couple returned the following spring to continue their house hunt, and lo, the first house was still available. Mission accomplished. They moved in 1974, the day before the Fourth of July, loading as much as they could in their Plymouth. Their son-in-law towed up a U-Haul. At first, they only had an old wooden crate to sit on. But eventually they put everything in order.

"We spent a lot of happy hours here," he said. "We walked a lot. We walked just about every trail on this side of the island and probably went to the Wonderland trail about every day, and to Ship Harbor and Western Mountain. On Western Mountain, the National Park Service maintains a little book; our signatures are in there."

Just the other morning, he said, he was thinking about something that his mother taught him. "I don't understand why she concentrated on this, but she taught me that life is filled with disappointments and that you must learn how to deal with disappointments and not let them get you down," he said. "That one thing is outstanding in my recollection.

I guess it's a good thing to be able to handle disappointments because I guess they're bound to come."

At 99, energetic and cheerful, this was a man who seemed to go beyond such excellent but sober counsel. Before the gold cane presentation, Elwood was at his kitchen table, peeling an apple. The door to his home was framed by towering lilac bushes, with the scent drifting into the front room. He had a pot of coffee going and a load of laundry in the washing machine. Around the neighborhood, he was known for his baking. Friends loved his biscuits, pies, and strawberry shortcake.

He sat down with a visitor and showed off a photo album of the renovation of his daughter Nancy's historic home in New Jersey. Then he pulled out a large-format Ansel Adams calendar—one of many from over the years, which were stacked beside his easy chair—to find the date of the most recent visit from his daughter and her family, who traveled to Maine every couple of months. Each day's square was filled with Elwood's tidy script; this was where he kept a log of his activities—haircut, church, cleaning lady. There were details as well, such as what time he got home from church and how many people attended the service.

Elwood was 103 when he died. Up until then, he was pretty close to fit as a fiddle, still driving himself around and shopping for his own groceries, although he sometimes asked a friend to go along. "I don't go, say, to Ellsworth without somebody with me," he said, a few years before he died. "Poor eyesight. You have to kind of play it by ear, how you feel. You don't want to be taking chances."

He did plenty of walking by virtue of doing chores around the house—so many chores that he was thinking of buying a pedometer just to see how many miles he racked up. The newspaper and TV news kept him up on current events. "I tell people I'm still turning the crank," he said. "The old catch phrase—use it or lose it. And that applies to your brains and your muscles and everything."

Reflections for Readers

1. What are the benefits of maintaining a positive mindset?
2. How can someone develop positivism?
3. What techniques might someone use to handle disappointments?

CHAPTER **6**

Reflections at Age 95

Adrienne G. Richard
Writer, poet, and Lecturer
Weston, MA
Age 95

Poetry is how I express myself, how I look in on my life—past, present, and future. I was born in 1921, north of Chicago. I remember Schlosser's Market, Wilson's Bakery, Zick's Department Store, Mr. Ilg the florist, the woods around our house, the Horace Mann School, dog paddling in Lake Michigan, Skokie Junior High, New Trier High School, the farmland, the great prairie to the west. I was learning, observing, finding my way as a writer, starting in journalism, through war and the loss of friends.

Birds of the Spirit

Birds may have been just birds once,

but the change came so early on,

no record exists, only deepest memory.

Little birds at first perhaps:

tree swallows in migrating flocks

that wheel against September

light, disappear and reappear.

Herdsmen knew they must start again
on the great journey, go down to
warmer meadows, need and desire
and fear converging.

Big birds came into their own, perhaps,
as dreams grew: think of the eagle,
its size, its courage, its daring, seated on
a million flag poles, gilded on
the church lectern, the Gospel side.

Think of the raven atop its totem pole, staring
out to sea, maker-destroyer-protector-judge.

Think of the stork, the red-tailed hawk,
the white pelican migrating alone,
the albatross following the square rigged ship,
its life sacred to every life on board.

Think of the great blue heron, its enviable
serenity, its flight overhead sometimes
with companions, sometimes alone, breath
rasping in the long throat, its silent tiptoe through
pond water at dusk, substance merging with the night.

Think of your bird that accompanies you
on the journey from birth to death.

We know they are not just birds.

I graduated from the University of Chicago in 1943. There, I met my husband, Jim, who rode east from Miles City, Montana on a cattle train to go to college. We were together 49 years until his death in 1992; we were separated for only two years, during World War II. I was a wife, a mother of three sons, and a writer—publishing four novels (*Pistol, The Accomplice, Wings*, and *Into the Road*), and a medical book, *Epilepsy: A New Approach.*

Trailing Arbutus

Leaving the flower show one late winter day my friend

said, "Look what I got at the wild flower booth!"

I peered into her brown bag, at a green plant, and said,

"What is it?" She said, "Trailing Arbutus! I had one. But it died!"

I saw one, once, hiking in early June, in New Hampshire's

White Mountains. We were almost at the summit

of some so-called peak when across the trail at my feet

lay a green vine, tiny white blooms shining among dark leaves.

"Is that Trailing Arbutus?" I cried out to my companion, but

he didn't know—he was scanning peaks. In my childhood,

my mother had told me about them—in her childhood,

she loved to come upon them in the woods—in Ohio perhaps, or

in the Georgia mountains near Tallulah Falls—I don't know
    where—

but I can see it lying in front of the toes of her Buster Brown boots.

I thought, I must call her, in Tucson, and tell her, "I have seen
a Trailing

Arbutus in bloom." But I didn't. I wrote her a long letter.

I found my letter, unopened, on her desk—she had died a few
days earlier.

I did not know the great gulf of death until I saw it.

In 1992, when Jim died, I was 70, and I faced the redesign of my life.
I wanted to get back to some creative work, but I feared the long days
of writing novels, closed off in my library for a year or more. I needed
projects that took me out into the world, engaged me with people; and
the brevity of a poem appealed to me. Unlike a novel, it didn't take two
years to write one.

The Crematory

I stand behind the velvet rope

alone and not alone

in the back room

where the ovens are

Men in green work clothes

bring in his body

in a cardboard box

like long-stemmed roses

They place it on the conveyor

that moves it slowly

through steel doors

into the fire

Outside the August sun

is a copper disk

stuck

in a pewter sky

The road

hot as fire leads away

to some new place

I do not know

I get lost

on my

way

home

Now, 25 years later, at age 95, I have a body of poetry, one volume published, another on the way, with many treasured moments and many beloved friends to thank for the richness of these years. My life has led me to poetry, and my poems have come of all this.

A Nonagenarian Contemplates Her Future

As I am carried aloft on invisible wings:

Will I see again the webbed lights of Boston,

Chicago, of Tucson, Nogales, of Great Falls, Montana?

Will I see again maples redden, oaks turn brown, birches

yellow, wineberries ripening in hedgerow brambles?

Will I see again glacial rivers sweeping

around red granite cliffs? Will I soak again

in springs heated deep in the earth?

Will I see the night sky and its strew of stars,

planets, constellations, meteors and

meteorites, a hundred thousand galaxies?

Will I see double rainbows across the heavens?

Will I know him again? Will he know me?

Will I watch again the sun touch the snow-pocked Tetons,

slide down their eastern slopes to light the prairie

carpets of yellow sweet clover?

Will I hear trumpets and trombones, French

horns and tubas, Berlioz in Dixieland,

the viola in Beethoven's late-life quartet?

Will I hear the cadences of Shakespeare's

Fear No More when I need to hear them?

Will I meet troops of friends on the road, some

battered, wounded, helping each other along,

looking like a Civil War retreat?

Will I remember the pain?

Will I feel gratitude for a full life, darkened

by sorrows, but not eclipsed?

Once more will I see a hawk floating over

eight lanes of traffic, wings outstretched,

every feathered tip etched against the sky?

Reflections for Readers

1. How does knowing that life is transitory affect how one lives?
2. This writer characterizes birds as spirits. How would you characterize spirits, and how might belief in guiding spirits and spirituality affect your life?
3. Aging carries each of us closer to the end of our lives, and we tend to reflect on what has been, what will be, and what will continue without our presence. What life experiences will you especially miss? What might you do to make the experiences of today more meaningful?

CHAPTER 7

The 80s Are the New 60s

Nan Lincoln
Reporter and author
Bass Harbor, ME
Age 70

Here's a pleasant picture: Eighty-year-olds Ruth and Doug Hare, married for 58 years—sitting side by side on a comfy sofa in their charming, tidy log home, tucked into the woods of Hall Quarry, Maine. At their feet, a couple of cats prowl, looking for a pat, or perhaps lunch.

Tonight, the Hares are looking forward to their weekly bridge game with friends; tomorrow, Ruth may have to pick up her three grandchildren from school in Tremont and keep them entertained until their daughter, Jen, gets out of work. Later in the week, some friends from Canada will be arriving for a three-day visit.

That all sounds like a pretty complete agenda for a pair of octogenarians—home, grandchildren, friends, bridge—and in another century, it would have been. But the Hares are perfect examples of a new twenty-first-century phenomenon, in which the 80s have become the new 60s.

In a few minutes, Doug will be going upstairs to work on the sermon he is writing on his computer for the service that he will be officiating over at the Islesford United Church of Christ next Sunday.

An ordained minister and theological scholar, Doug and his wife, Ruth, who provides the piano accompaniment for the hymns, travel by mailboat to Little Cranberry Island every Sunday in the summer, and every other Sunday in winter, to attend to a flock of congregants that ranges in size from about a dozen in the depths of winter to around 50 at the height of summer.

He and Ruth have been making the trip out to Cranberry for about 12 years now, and Doug says the gig came about in what one might call a *deus ex machina* moment, while he and his wife were taking friends out on the ferry to Islesford for a day of sightseeing.

"I just happened to overhear one of the women on the ferry talking to another and asking if she knew anyone who would be interested in being a part-time minister for their church," he recalls. "I had just retired that year, and hadn't planned on going back to work. But how often does one overhear something like that? I had to respond. I've never had a single regret."

While her husband is busy with his sermons, Ruth does not spend her days knitting and baking cookies for impending grandchildren's visits (although she does plenty of this, too).

At some point this week, she will drive to Bar Harbor to get a start on the account books that she is keeping for five area restaurants. Some of them haven't opened for the season yet, but she is looking forward to another busy summer. Until then, she is also doing the books for several other small businesses on Mount Desert Island.

"I wasn't trained in bookkeeping," Ruth says. "I was a teacher for most of my life. But I love working with numbers—balancing things out. I get a real sense of accomplishment when I've finished the task at hand and it all comes out the way it should."

The office where she works with her numbers is above two very lively clubs on Main Street in Bar Harbor, Maine, which she accesses by a set of narrow, steep stairs, starting in the interior of one of the bars. "Last year, they had a new bartender who would see me coming and going, coming and going," Ruth gleefully recalls. "And finally, she asked one of the other staff people, 'Who's that old lady who lives in the attic?'"

If the Hares lived the sort of quiet life that one might expect of a couple in their 80s, they probably could live comfortably on their savings, pensions, and Social Security. But they have places to go, people to see, and things to do.

Once a year, they make an extended trip to Europe to visit old friends that they first met 45 years ago, when Doug was a young minister on a traveling fellowship in Germany. At least once a year, they drive to Maryland to visit their oldest daughter, Laurie and her family, and every two years, they make a road trip to Toronto, where both of them have family. In fact, they have just recently returned from this biannual trip.

"It was a lot of driving and I got pretty tired of it," Ruth confesses—but she then admits that she made the trip a little longer when she took a wrong turn while crossing the border and mistakenly got on a road that passed through Quebec.

"I just hate Quebec City!" she exclaims. "I refuse to drive through it, so I turned around and recrossed the border, so we could enter somewhere else."

"Shortest visit we ever made to Canada," Doug adds with the wry laugh of someone who is long accustomed to his wife's strong opinions and still marvels at her audacity.

Ruth and Doug met as undergrads at Victoria College—part of the University of Toronto—and anyone knowing the two as individuals at that time would probably not have imagined them as a couple.

Doug, who was raised in northern Ontario, was the son of two doctors (his mother was the first female doctor in the province) and had been a sickly child, suffering from bovine tuberculosis, a form of the disease caused from drinking unpasteurized milk. "So I spent most of my grammar school days at home in bed while other boys my age were out there making friends and being active," he says.

He acknowledges that this quiet childhood may have contributed to making him the contemplative, scholarly sort of man that he would become. But, he insists, he was not interested at all in becoming a man of the church.

However, it turned out that the church was interested in him.

"I had been studying the Bible with our local pastor, who made it all into an interesting, lively discussion," Doug recalls. "Then one day, he came to my house, which really surprised me—and asked if I had ever considered the ministry. I said no, I was planning to be a doctor like my parents. He nodded and then just asked me to pray on it, which I did."

He says that mostly he prayed that God would understand why he could do so much more for the world as a doctor than he could as a minister. But at age 16, during an Easter church retreat, Doug says that he received his unequivocal calling and knew that he would have to answer it.

"The hard part was telling my father, who hoped, and had been led to expect, I would become a physician." But he cleared that hurdle smoothly and headed off to Victoria College to start on his path to the ministry, leaving his girlfriend at the time at home in Ontario.

That summer, while working at his first job as a temporary minister in Saskatchewan, he got a "Dear John" letter from his girl. Although he was heartbroken at the time, this did leave him unattached the following fall, when a friend suggested that Doug join him and his date, Ruth, another undergrad, on a double date.

"It was a dance, and halfway through the evening I switched dates and danced only with Ruth," he says. "She was just as feisty and fun as she is now. I fell in love that night, and I've never wavered since."

"I didn't know about that 'Dear John' letter," Ruth interjects, only half-joking. "I would have liked it better if I heard *you'd* sent that letter."

"Oh, but Ruth, you know how loyal I am," Doug responds. "I never could have done it, even if she was the wrong one for me. So I'm glad she sent the letter."

In any case, Doug wasn't the only one who fell in love that night. Much to her own surprise, Ruth found herself falling for the earnest, boyish-looking young minister. "My father was a minister," she says. "And I swore I would never marry a minister." She says that she just couldn't picture herself in the role of the quiet, docile clergyman's wife.

But she became a minister's wife on June 8, 1951, the very same day that Doug graduated from college. However, the qualities of quietude and docility are not something Ruth has been bringing to the job description all these years. While she has attended just about every church service that her husband has presided over in the last 50 or so years and has often provided the music, as she does on Islesford, she has refused to bend to the will of certain congregations that found it unseemly for their pastor's wife to be a working mother—and what's worse, a working mother who wore shorts!

In the first years of their marriage, Ruth *had* to work while Doug completed seminary school in New York. While she was mostly employed as a preschool teacher, she also had a memorable stint as the girl behind the ribbons-and-handkerchief counter at Bloomingdale's in Manhattan. "I'll never forget this one lady who came in and said she was having a birthday party for her little dog and wanted velvet ribbons for all the doggy guests," Ruth says. "I found her the ribbons she wanted, but I couldn't wait to get home and tell Doug."

Ruth says that she loved living in New York City and was sad when Doug was transferred to a parish in Pittsburgh—a city she never did cotton to. But both she and her husband were delighted when Doug went into teaching, rather than preaching, at the Pittsburgh Theological Seminary as a professor of the New Testament.

"Teaching best suits my nature," he says. "While I try to keep my sermons current and relevant, I am basically an historian, and religious history is often the source of my ideas." And, as the wife of a professor, who eventually was dean of the seminary, Ruth didn't have anyone telling her not to wear shorts.

In 1986, the couple bought a woodsy little plot of land in Hall Quarry on Mount Desert Island in Maine, which Doug cleared and prepared for the log home that they designed and had built. They planned to move there year round when Doug retired from the seminary in 1993.

Since that so-called retirement, in addition to his preaching job on Islesford, Doug has published several scholarly books on the New Testament—*Matthew: Interpretation, a Bible Commentary for Teaching and Preaching* (1993), *The Son of Man Tradition* (1990), *Mark* (1996), and *Chapters in a Life of Paul* (2000) and now writes occasional articles and essays for theological publications.

One might assume that this active working couple is unusually blessed with good health, which is why they are able to do as much as they do. But in truth, Doug has been plagued with scoliosis and chronic pain in his left leg from an unresolved case of the shingles, which has him both doubled over and listing alarmingly to port when he walks; and Ruth has had her fair share of aches and pains, including recent surgery on her elbow.

But they do consider themselves fortunate that their minds are still in good working order, and they both strongly believe that, for them, working is both fulfilling and one of the things that keeps them going.

Addendum

About three years after I wrote this, Ruth and Doug did retire. The couple made a final trip to Germany, and Ruth died a few months later of lung cancer. Despite being the wife of a minister, her faith was always peppered with doubt. But at least her fervent prayer that she be the first to go was answered. Doug suffered a stroke and followed a year later.

Reflections for Readers

1. Many people retire in their 60s or 70s. What are the costs and benefits of continuing to work beyond that?
2. How might continuing to work in your 80s keep you young?
3. How might physical health issues affect decisions about working or not working as you age? How are such decisions affected by the kind of work that you want to do?

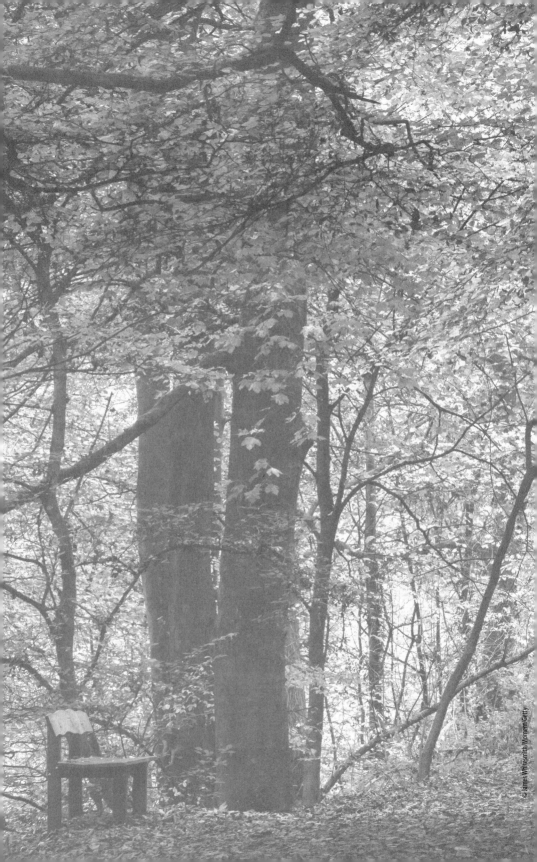

PART **II**

The Biology of Aging

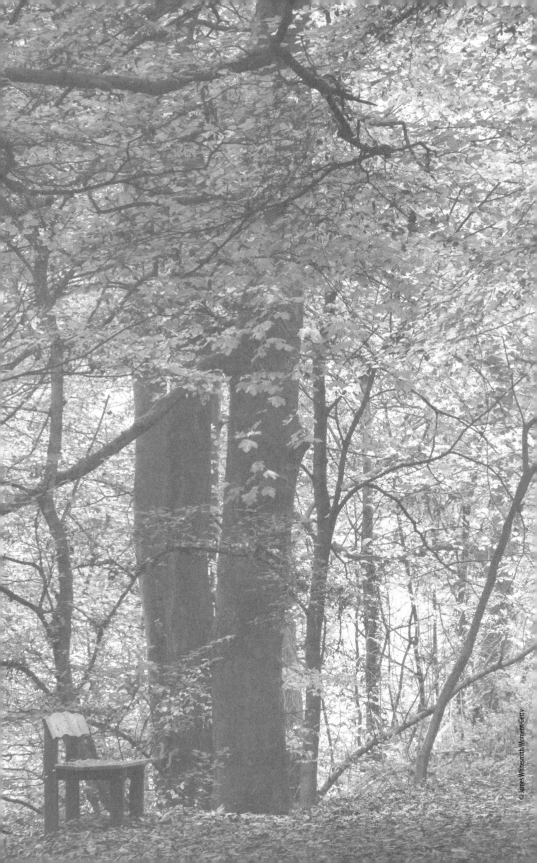

CHAPTER 8

The Second Fifty: Successful Aging

Glorianne Wittes, LICSW
Social Worker (retired) and artist
Dedham, MA

"It is not true that people stop pursuing dreams because they grow old, they grow old because they stop pursuing dreams."

—Gabriel Garcia Marquez

The percentage of Americans age 65 and older has more than tripled in the last 100 years, now representing 13% of the population. Not only are more people living into the second 50 years of life, 70,000 centenarians have entered their third 50 years. And by 2050, the U.S. Census Bureau estimates the number of centenarians will be 834,000.

The urgency of these numbers has begun to shift the emphasis from that of medically prolonging life to ensuring that a prolonged life is worth living. The concept of successful aging can be traced back to the 1950s and was popularized in the 1980s. It reflected changing views on aging in Western countries, where a stigma associated with old age (i.e., ageism) had led to considering older people as a burden on society. Consequently, most research had focused on negative aspects of growing older or preventing the decline of youth.

Research on successful aging, however, acknowledged the fact that there is a growing number of older adults functioning at a very high level and contributing to society. Scientists working in this area have sought to define what differentiates successful from unsuccessful aging in order to design effective strategies and medical interventions to protect health and well-being in aging. Many researchers became critical of the very term "successful aging" as it implies failure on the part of those who do not meet arbitrary criteria derived from neoliberal or biomedical definitions.

In the year 2000, as the world contemplated the potential of a new century, the eminent geriatric psychiatrist Gene Cohen published the results of a two-year, multisite study that he conducted for the National Endowment for the Arts, entitled "The Creative Age: Awakening Human Potential in the Second Half of Life." His results showed that creativity has a powerful anti-aging effect on the mind and body. He heralded a new juncture in the field of aging—one in which we move beyond studies of what aging is to what is possible, not despite aging but because of it.

"What has universally been denied is the potential of aging, and the ultimate expression of that potential, which is Creativity," wrote Dr. Cohen. He believed that the capacity for creativity in older adults went unnoticed in society due to negative attitudes toward later life. To Cohen, creativity was more than a simple artistic ability. He believed it to be the spark that illuminates the human spirit and ignites the desire to grow. This quality, he believed, was innate and something that we can use to shape our lives, especially as we age, to unleash new potentials for personal growth and expression.

In his study, Dr. Cohen proved that creativity has a powerful anti-aging effect on the mind and body. The study examined a number of healthy adults over the age of 65, many ranging between 80 and 100, who participated in twice-weekly programs of painting, writing, jewelry-making, or choral singing. In contrast to a control group, the participants showed better overall health and fewer health problems. They made fewer visits to the doctor and used less medication. They also had better morale and reported less loneliness thanks to feelings of self-control, mastery, and a sense of community with other participants.

Dr. Cohen's explanation of creativity is simple. The creative spirit thrives on being confronted with limited resources and the challenges that such limitations bring. These limitations force the brain to meet a challenge, to develop a "workaround ethic," and to come up with a solution born of necessity and creative exertion. To bring into existence something that we create leads to a feeling of personal mastery and contribution. This not only promotes self-esteem as we age, but importantly, it brings about a compensating regeneration of anatomical brain capacity. Even the weight and mass of the brain may increase as a result of regular creative exertion, a phenomenon that scientists call "neurogenesis."

Cohen describes an "if not now, when?" phenomenon, which has its beginnings as we enter our 40s and 50s. Around that time, our brains start firing on all cylinders and we begin to use both sides of the brain (the logical, analytical left and the artistic, intuitive right) together in lieu of a reliance on one side (typically the left). This stimulates us to be more creative in order to accomplish this integration and to grow in self-confidence and comfort with ourselves. This psychological liberation stage, prominent from midlife to late life, is characterized by an increasing sense of freedom to do the things that we've always wanted. Their prompt is an inner voice that asks us, "If not now, then when?" This in turn motivates us, giving us the courage to try something entirely new and self-expressive.

The old model of the aging brain portrayed a no-growth rigidity and a dying-off of neurons, especially after the age of 50. The new medical model and the science of the neuroplasticity of the brain see continued growth and flexibility in the brain when we engage in new and challenging activities, especially novel, creative ones.

Research into aging and the brain also stresses the necessity for elders to do things that challenge and engage our minds because they are different from what we normally do, or because they have the element of fun. Successful aging also requires that we stay connected with other people. We age better when we continue to engage with life and maintain close relationships. Those who do so have been found to eat better, exercise more, and smoke and drink less.

In many ways, we have to redefine ourselves in the face of many changes in ourselves and in the world. Successful or positive living, as it is more accurately known now, is no longer based on ego or endeavors. Life becomes different. Erik Erikson refers to this stage of life as "Integrity," when people come to terms with the meaning of life, have adjusted to their respective ailments or diseases, and have gained a resiliency that allows them to function in productive ways. Such resiliency is needed when we enter that period from about age 60 onward, when we may encounter significant upheavals in virtually every sector of life: social, professional, geographical, personal, and familial; and when the loss of loved ones is often an inescapable part of growing older. In the face of this inevitability, having a social support network in place in older adulthood is critical. Sadly, our friendship circles tend to grow ever smaller as we age, and the successive passing of each friend brings a sense of loneliness that impinges on our resilience.

Turning now to my own life for examples of all that I have written here, I have led a very full life, rich in loving relationships, diverse experiences and creativity. Now in my mid-80s, I have survived the loss of my beloved husband (nine years ago) and many friends and family members since his death, as well as health problems (some serious, others just annoying, such as failing eyesight and hearing). Few of my lifelong friends are still alive, and many of the friends that I have made here at NewBridge have died. My memory for people's names stinks. My mobility is very limited, and I dare not move without my walker. With (and despite) all that, I have maintained my creativity, making art and writing; I am adapting to all these technological advances that I find so hard; I am appreciating my wonderful children and granddaughters; and I still wake up to wonderful days, despite many sleepless nights. I feel, most of the time, like I am engaging in the trials of aging with some success and feel blessed that this is the case. When my time comes, it will be with no regrets.

Reflections for Readers

1. How can we define "successful aging" other than in terms of loss or decline?
2. In terms of successful aging, what priority would you put on each of the following:
   a. Good health
   b. Creativity
   c. Connection with other people
   d. Other values
3. How can creative expression support successful aging?
4. What holds some older adults back from expressing their creativity?

CHAPTER 9

Health Changes in Older Age

Stephanie S. Batista, MA

Third-year Doctoral student in Clinical Psychology
William James College
Newton, MA

When we are young, we cannot wait to be older. We beg our parents for independence, to go out with friends and to be on our own. We want the respect that comes with older age and are sure that the responsibilities are all worth it. But once we reach a certain age, we no longer wish to be older. Instead, we stop looking forward to the road ahead and wish to revert to our younger days. But why are we so apprehensive about older age? This is in great part reflective of negative stereotypes that are associated with aging. We have heard them all before; older adults are sick, fragile, and dependent on others (Abeles et al., 1998). They are weak and in poor health. They are incapable of learning anything new or living on their own. Although it is hard to ignore the negative beliefs related to older age, research shows a different, more positive view associated with aging.

The stage of "older age" is not all rosy. Some of the negative anticipations we hold as we become older are realistic and expectable. Although we might try our hardest to prevent the signs of aging, some changes and declines are inevitable. As we age, mild cognitive changes are likely to occur. We may experience a change in the way we process information and develop problems with our memory (Salzman, 2006). We may experience changes in vision and develop issues with our hearing. Our skin will likely lose elasticity and our hair may become thin. Our metabolism and sleep patterns may change and we may experience a decrease in energy (Segal et al., 2011).

While it may seem discouraging to grow old and experience these changes, there is some good news supported by current research. Although mild changes in cognition and one's physical ability are likely to occur, these changes do not generally impact one's daily function (Salzman, 2006). The majority of older adults do not experience cognitive impairment sufficient to interfere with their ability to live independently or make important life choices for themselves (Knight, 2004).

For many people, the idea of growing old is associated with poor physical health, illness, dependency, and living in nursing homes. But contrary to popular belief, the majority of older adults view themselves as being in good physical health (McGoran, 1995). Most older adults live on their own, and only about 5% of those aged 65 and older live in nursing homes (Segal et al., 2011). Are you surprised by this information? That is because the negative views related to older age have led us to believe the exact opposite. Despite the inevitable declines linked to aging, most older adults are healthy enough to carry out their normal, everyday activities (Robbins, 2015). They adapt to the necessary changes and continue to lead satisfying and productive lives.

Although challenges certainly do arise as one gets older, the majority of older adults are able to adjust successfully and live a healthy life because of the choices that they make and what they have learned as they have gotten older. We know that diet, exercise, and lifestyle choices are an important part of our health (Van Romer & Duggal, 2007). For this reason, it is important to stay on track with appropriate medical attention. It is also important to continue to exercise, eat healthy, get enough sleep, and stay hydrated (Segal et al., 2011). If you do not eat healthy or exercise regularly, it is not too late to change your habits. Adjusting your eating habits and exercise routine can help your mobility and overall health (Van Romer & Duggal, 2007). These maintenance measures can reduce your risk of illness and help you age positively.

Keeping our bodies healthy is an important factor in aging positively. Like our health and well-being, keeping our brains healthy is important as well. How do we do this? Talk to friends and spend time with loved ones on a regular basis. Maintaining relationships and staying connected are important parts of how we sustain our physical and emotional health (Rowe & Kahn, 2015). Many older adults help care for younger family members and provide support for their friends and loved ones. If friends are hard to find, there are groups and social activities in your community. Read a book, play games, or work on jigsaws or crossword puzzles (Abeles et al., 1998). Doing these activities and continuing to use your skills can help maintain your mental capacities as you age (Knight, 2004). While you may not be able to run as fast as you used to, or to dance like when you were a teenager, you can continue to participate in the activities you enjoy. You can also develop new activities to enjoy. Doing what you love to do will make you happier and healthier.

We all know the saying, "You can't teach an old dog new tricks." But that is not always the case. Another common misconception associated with old age is the inability to learn. Although learning patterns and tempos do change with age, the basic capacity for learning is maintained (McGoran, 1995). When it comes to older age, it is not too late to try a new activity or pick up a new hobby. Learn about the latest technologies to stay in touch with friends and up to date about health-related news. Travel to a new country or state, learn to play an instrument, or take a dance class. Join a social group or volunteer your time. You can still find something that you have always wanted to do and try it out. Your creativity is not lost, and there is still so much you can do. Participating in new activities will not only help you to enjoy your life, but it will also stimulate your brain.

Like fashion, the reality of old age has evolved, and society is slow to catch up with the latest trends. And while negative stereotypes exist, we must try to see past them and change perceptions based on emerging information. Although getting older can feel like a major change, much of how we experience the change is up to us. For this reason, it is important to look at our lives in a positive light and with high regard. If we focus on what is important now and appreciate what we have, we can acknowledge how far we have come. If we do our best to keep our bodies and minds healthy, we increase our chances of aging positively. Don't buy into the negative stereotypes and myths associated with aging; welcome this chapter of our lives with gratitude and positivity.

Reflections for Readers

1. How do "negative stereotypes" affect the way we think about our aging?
2. What can we reasonably do to maintain our health and vigor while we are aging?
3. Can new health habits be established in older age?
4. In what ways does cognitive processing change as we age?
5. What steps can seniors take to preserve cognitive functions such as memory and processing ability?

References

Abeles, N., Cooley, S., Deitch, I. M., Hinrichsen, G., Lopez, M. A., & Molinari, V. A. (1998). What practitioners should know about working with older adults. *Professional Psychology: Research and Practice, 29*(5), 413–427. doi:10.1037/0735-7028.29.5.413

Knight, B. (2004). *Psychotherapy with older adults.* (3rd ed.). Thousand Oaks, CA: Sage.

McGoran, J. (1995). Facts about ageing—myth and reality. *Social Alternatives, 14*(2), 40.

Robbins, L. A. (2015). Gauging aging: How does the American public truly perceive older age—and older people? *Generations, 39*(3), 17–21.

Rowe, J. W., & Kahn, R. L. (2015). Successful aging 2.0: Conceptual expansions for the 21st century. *The Journals of Gerontology: Series B: Psychological Sciences and Social Sciences, 70B*(4), 593–596. doi:10.1093/geronb/gbv025

Salzman, B. (2006). Myths and realities of aging. *Care Management Journals: Journal of Case Management; The Journal of Long-Term Home Health Care, 7*(3), 141–150.

Segal, D., Qualls, S., & Smyer, M. (2011). *Aging and mental health.* (2nd ed.). Malden, MA: Wiley-Blackwell.

Van Romer, L., & Duggal, N. (2007). Five aging myths. *Personal Excellence Essentials,* October, p. 6.

CHAPTER 10

Brain Health: Twenty-First Century Science on Sustaining Memory and Thinking as We Age

Aladdin Ossorio, PsyD

Coordinator, SageMind Program, Brenner Assessment Center
William James College
Newton, MA

I was inspired to study the relationship of aging, health, and the brain by my grandparents, Hy and Annie Whittman. Lifelong learners, they lived active, social lives. A young man at the time, I naïvely believed that everyone's grandparents aged with such passion and curiosity.

I distinctly recall, however, a moment when my grandfather wasn't in his typical good cheer. I'd picked him up from a doctor's visit. Settling into the old Ford, he turned to me, "These *guys*," he grumbled, referring to his physicians (who, at the time, were all men), "they keep changing their minds! Last year they told me to eat eggs. So I eat eggs. Now they say, 'Don't eat eggs—eggs are bad!' I tell them, 'What am I supposed to do with all the eggs I just ate?'" My grandfather shook his head in disgust, "I'm telling you, they change their minds every year. I don't think they know what the heck they're talking about."

My grandfather's frustration was understandable: scientific flip-flopping on basic questions like "What's good for my health?" has left many people uncertain, and maybe a bit cynical. Do "*these guys*," as my grandfather put it, know what the heck they're talking about? And if they don't, does anyone?

I've spent a good deal of time pursuing my grandfather's question—what's good for our health? It turns out that twenty-first century psychology is an ideal platform for seeking answers: psychologists today can synthesize knowledge across the sciences, bridging the biomedical and behavioral health fields. My own work focuses on integrating biology, neurology, neuropsychology, and health, all with the goal of understanding how to sustain and enhance thinking and memory as we age.

So what does science today tell us about optimal brain health?

First, a caveat: our knowledge remains incomplete. If there is one thing we've learned, it's this: the science of health rarely deals in absolutes. Rather, we learn by carefully compiling an increasingly accurate body of information.

With this caveat in mind, I invite you into a twenty-first century exploration of the science of the healthy aging brain.

What Makes for a Healthy Brain?

I'm often asked: "How do I sustain my memory? How do I stay at my best? What do I do if my thinking or memory is getting worse?" These are profound, potentially even life-changing, questions. Thankfully, we've begun making progress toward clear answers, and I'll begin with two recent realizations:

1. Your brain is simply a part of your body, and what is good for your body is virtually always good for your brain.
2. You have real control over the health of your brain as you age—you can take direct actions to decrease your chance of getting dementia and increase your chance of remaining sharp and vital.

Historically, we've thought of the diseases of aging, including dementia, as "a part of life" that comes with age; as what *happened to us* as we grew older. Today, we've begun to understand that we are, in fact, not just the passive victims of our brains. Indeed, how we live, what we do, and the choices we make can dramatically improve the health of our brains as we age. And there's more good news: most folks reading this *already know* what is good for our health, and what is good for our health is good for our brain.

What I will outline next is precisely *how and why* what is good for your health is also good for your brain. Let's get to it!

EXERCISE

Exercise is good for your heart. You know that. It's also good for your muscles and balance (in fact, older adults who are physically fit are less likely to fall and, when they do suffer health setbacks, they tend to recover more quickly and with fewer complications).

But did you know that exercise helps preserve a youthful, healthy brain? For example, using imaging technologies,[1] we can now "visualize" (make visible) your brain as you think. What we have found is that adults who exercise have brains that *look and behave* more like a young person's brain. Indeed, the brains of middle-aged and older adults who exercise solve problems more efficiently and react more quickly than the brains of older adults who are sedentary. Remarkably, exercise is one of the only activities known to science that can *generate healthy new brain cells.*

I should also mention this: exercise improves your mood. In fact, for many, exercise is a more effective tonic for depression and sadness than any pill or medication that your doctor can prescribe. Need I mention: I prescribe exercise!

So, what else sustains our memory and thinking—what else makes for a healthy aging brain?

SOCIALIZE

Curmudgeons unite—human beings are *social beings,* and we need each other's company. In fact, research suggests that *we need each other just as much as we need food, clothing, or water.*

Engaging with other people provides what I call "social nourishment," and social nourishment is as essential to our survival as any other nutrient: we need it to live and thrive.

Consider this: Infants who are not held and loved by others usually suffer profound cognitive and emotional problems. No man is an island and no woman stands alone. We do not flourish without each other. Rates of sadness and depression are higher for older adults who are socially isolated. Worse, troubling problems like Alzheimer's disease are more common in people who are isolated and alone.

The solution is simple: *reach out!* Be in contact! Engage in activities with other people. *Social nourishment is essential for your brain's well-being.*

---

[1] We now have many technologies to help us "see" the brain in action—thinking, feeling, acting. For a review of this science, I recommend Rita Carter's *The Brain Book.*

SLEEP

Most older adults need between seven and eight hours of sleep. Sadly, chronic poor sleep is associated with problems in thinking and memory, and even with dementia.

When you sleep well, your brain is cleansed—toxins are efficiently carried out of your brain and body. Moreover, sleep helps us develop and sustain our memories. From your brain's perspective, sleep is an *active process* that helps us remember tomorrow what we've learned today.

Perhaps the best news about sleep is this: you *can* improve your sleep. I often meet folks who feel discouraged about their sleep—who wake easily or often, who don't feel rested when rising, and who feel helpless to change their situation. Fortunately, psychologists can help: you can "relearn" good sleep habits and reclaim the restorative power of sleep. Better yet, it takes only a month or two.

I should also mention this: when we exercise, we sleep better. And, when we sleep well, we make better food choices! *It's all connected* . . . Which reminds me:

EAT WELL AND WISELY

Most everyone has tried a diet. Diets promise every possible benefit, from bliss to great sex to unencumbered longevity.

But what does science honestly tell us about the relationship between what we eat and our memory and thinking as we age?

Much, it turns out. *Good nutrition is associated with better memory and better overall cognition.* Fortunately, despite the myriad diets available and the many panderers of nutritional advice, good nutrition is not particularly complicated: as writer Michael Pollen said: "Eat food, not too much, mostly plants."

Notably, by "food," Pollen meant edibles found in the produce or meat section of your grocery. Western-style "processed foods"—products that are laden with additives (read the label!), fried foods, foods created by machine, bought in bags, or saturated with fats—are simply not "food."

Unfortunately, nutritional advice has become a political battleground: the financial stakes in the food industry are high. Rather than engage in the politics, I offer two scientifically validated approaches to promote healthy aging: Mediterranean eating patterns,[2] and the

---

[2] Details of Mediterranean eating can be found here: http://oldwayspt.org//

"MIND Diet."[3] Notably, these "diets" are not weight loss plans or short-term solutions—think of them as nutritional lifestyles, as ways of living and eating.

Incidentally, I should mention: when we eat well, we sleep better, and when we sleep better, our mood and our memory improve! Remember: we are integrated beings, and the relationship between our moods, minds, brains, and bodies is one of connection!

Final Thoughts

I think of exercise, socializing, sleep, and nutrition as the "first four" that promote positive health for our minds, brains, and bodies as we age. But there is more—far too much to review in this short chapter!

As a guidepost, I leave you with this: *We tend to age well when we have a reason to live.* When we have a meaning and purpose, we're motivated to make good choices. Find and pursue your passion, and your brain will join you!

Reflections for Readers

1. What does the term "body/brain connection" mean? And how might this connection change in older age?
2. What are "normal" memory changes that accompany advancing age? Are there ways that older adults can limit or reduce these changes?
3. How does socialization contribute to brain health?

---

[3] Details of the Mind Diet can be found here: https://www.rush.edu/news/diet-may-help-prevent-alzheimers

CHAPTER 11

Cognitive Skills: What to Expect as We Get Older

Ruth Kandel, MD

Gerontologist, NewBridge on the Charles (retired)
Dedham, MA

What happens when you meet an acquaintance on the street and can't remember his name? Do you become embarrassed? How about walking into a room and completely forgetting why you are there. Do you feel like this might be the beginning of dementia? Or, during a casual conversation with a friend, you suddenly cannot come up with a particular word that feels like it is on the tip of your tongue. Do you get anxious? These are just a few examples of changes we may experience as we get older. But how do we know which changes are normal and which signify something more serious, like dementia?

Let's start with memory. Can we have problems with our memory and not have dementia? To answer this question, we need to understand that there are different types of memory. Much of our modern understanding of how we form memories comes from one man known as H.M. (1926–2008) and the tragic surgery he had. H.M. had epilepsy that was severe enough to interfere with his everyday life. Although he was treated with antiseizure medications, back then, the doctors did not have the many options we now have with drugs. At the age of 27, unable to work because of his seizures, H.M. went with his family to see a doctor who performed experimental surgery.

The surgeon, William B. Scoville, removed a small part of his brain within the middle temporal lobe on both sides. What we learned from this unfortunate surgery transformed our knowledge of memory and the brain. H.M.'s seizures did improve, but he developed a profound memory loss such that he was unable to form new memories. His attention, speech, and behavior were unaffected, and if you walked into the room and introduced yourself, he would respond appropriately. But if he became momentarily distracted and shifted his attention to something else for a short period of time, he would have forgotten who you were.

The ability to form new memories is dependent on the very small part of the brain that was removed, within the middle temporal lobe, which includes the hippocampus and surrounding structures. H.M. could no longer form new memories. For example, he was not able to remember what he just read, or activities that he might have recently participated in, or even what he ate at his last meal.

So here is a question for you. After H.M. had the surgery, when his parents came to visit, did he remember them? The answer is yes! What we learned from this surgery is that older memories are stored in different parts of the brain not connected to the hippocampus. H.M. remembered his family and information that he had learned prior to the surgery. He would know that George Washington was the first President of the United States, but he would not be able to remember any new presidents elected after his surgery.

Another question for you. Now that H.M. could not form new memories, did his IQ drop? Was he angry and hostile? Could he do crossword puzzles? The answer is no to all the questions except for the last. There are several important points here. To lose one's ability to form new memories does not rob one of intellect. H.M.'s IQ remained above average. His personality did not change radically, and he kept his great sense of humor and had a positive outlook on life. He lived in the moment, however, and was dependent for the remainder of his life on other people. He lived with his parents while they were alive and eventually moved to a nursing home.

What we now know is that the hippocampus is usually the first part of the brain that is affected by Alzheimer's disease. What happened to H.M. overnight is similar to what happens, more gradually and usually less severely, to people with Alzheimer's. The earliest symptom seen in Alzheimer's disease, in many instances, is an inability to learn and remember new information. This is often accompanied by a rapid rate of forgetting. Someone with dementia may forget what they ate for dinner the night before or what their plans are for the day. They may get lost in familiar places or ask the same question repeatedly. These are all examples of the ability to form new memories. But older memories are more resilient and less likely to be forgotten, especially in the early stages of the disease. That is why someone with Alzheimer's disease may not recall what happened two days ago, but will still remember events from 20 years ago.

With normal aging, people can be forgetful, but the symptoms are much milder. Examples might include forgetting someone's name or where the car is parked. The Alzheimer's Association often says not to worry if you lose your keys, but finding them and not knowing what to do with them suggests something more serious. The main point with normal aging is that these symptoms, although frustrating, do not interfere with one's everyday activities. From a cognitive point of view, a person can continue shopping, cooking, managing finances, working, and essentially continuing with life.

There is another type of memory, known as "semantic memory," that includes our general fund of information or practical knowledge, such as knowing the capital of Massachusetts. This is affected in Alzheimer's disease, although a little later in the disease process. With normal aging, older individuals usually do not have significant impairment with semantic memory; however, it may take a longer time to access the information. The fact that we need more time to do things as we age led to some inaccurate conclusions years ago, when researchers studying aging would administer the same tests to the young and old. Because they did not give older individuals more time to complete these exams, elders had lower scores. This led to the erroneous conclusion that cognitive impairment is inevitable in older age. We now know that this is not correct, and if you give older people more time to complete the test, they can perform the same as younger individuals.

Let's now turn our attention to attention. What about going into a room and then forgetting why you are even there? There could be many reasons for this, including problems with attention. We live in a very busy world with many distractions. With age, these distractions may increasingly get in our way. We need more time to process things, especially complex tasks. In this fast-paced world, it is not always easy to slow down. There are deadlines, both professional and personal. But doing one task at a time without dividing our attention will actually help get things done faster.

Wait—we are not done with attention yet. In addition to dementia, there are several changes with aging that may contribute to problems with driving, including visual and hearing loss, arthritis limiting range of motion of the neck, the need for more time to process information, and, yes, attention. When you think about it, driving requires us to be able to divide our attention to respond to a changing environment in a timely fashion. Given that tasks involving divided attention are more difficult with age, it is important for older individuals to be aware of any problems while driving. There are a number of places that offer training with driving simulation to help both assess and improve performance on the road.

Another attentional problem often mentioned with aging is the reduced capacity to inhibit irrelevant stimuli. In other words, as we age, we take in more information, discriminating less about what is essential. Interestingly, this also can be a strength and, at least in part, may explain why wisdom appears to increase with age. For example, in studies cited by in the New York Times (Reistad-Long, 2008) where young and old people were asked to read material that included unexpected words or phrases, older adults took much more time completing the task than college students. The assumption was that they paid attention to all the words, including the so-called irrelevant ones. Later, when asked questions that were focused on these unexpected words, older individuals scored much better. In the real world, taking in everything including possibly irrelevant information can be advantageous. People often do not know ahead of time what facts may later become very important. Older individuals, by taking in more information, may be in a better position to handle future problems or make more informed decisions. Some believe this is one of the many characteristics that contribute to increasing wisdom in old age.

So what about language? The good news is that language remains relatively stable with age. In fact, vocabulary may even improve over time, as does depth of comprehension. A common problem that people may experience has to do with the process of getting words out. In conversation, it might take longer and be more difficult to find the right words. The information is there, but retrieving it may take some time. Older individuals still have the ability to tell a good story—and probably even better than a younger counterpart because of the added experiences with age.

Let's go back to the situation where a person does not remember the name of an acquaintance. This is not uncommon and nothing to worry about. Feeling anxious only makes it more difficult to recall the name (or any information). Remember to be gentle with yourself; you are not alone. Strategies to help remember someone's name include repeating it several times or making an association with that name. For example, try to connect the person's name with someone else who has the same name (who can be a celebrity); or make some other connection with the name based on some physical feature or personality characteristic.

There is another problem that can get in the way and limit communication, making a person appear more impaired. That problem is hearing loss. This is often complicated by embarrassment or denial about the loss that can be frustrating for all involved. There are now a variety of hearing aids available that can greatly help with communication—but first this often-hidden problem needs to come out in the open.

Let's talk about executive function. This is considered a higher-order cognitive skill that allows people to plan and organize their lives. Executive function is dependent on the integrity of the frontal lobes, the most highly evolved part of our brain, and helps with decision-making and problem-solving. It plays a key role in helping us deal with novel situations, abstract thinking, and mental flexibility. Executive function helps us monitor inappropriate responses. And the list goes on. While there can be age-related decline in executive function (e.g., problems with mental flexibility or abstract thinking), there is great variability in how these functions change with age, with many areas remaining stable over time. Executive function is compromised in a variety of conditions, especially frontotemporal dementia, Alzheimer's disease, and vascular dementia.

Here again we find another example of how an age-related change may turn out to be a strength. In this case, the age-related change is a decline in executive function resulting in a decreased capacity to inhibit responses. A study by Apfelbaum, Krendl, and Ambady (2010) found that this decline in normal aging may allow the older person to provide better advice in uncomfortable situations. In their study, they divided older individuals into two groups: those with high executive function and those with low executive function. They then had both groups of older individuals, along with young adults, provide critical advice to troubled obese teenagers. Those older adults with lower executive function provided more open and empathetic advice than did the other two groups. And doctors specializing in treating obese individuals rated this same group (those with lower executive function) as providing the kind of advice to these teens that had the greatest potential to promote change.

Having touched upon some general cognitive changes that we see with normal aging, probably what is most compelling is the great variability we see among people. We do know that cognitive decline is not inevitable, and there are some older individuals who exhibit no change at all with age. Also, the changes that are seen are not necessarily uniform. Some people might have more problems with their memory, and others with their language skills. One important unifying characteristic is that no matter what the change, in normal aging, the extent is much less than what you see in dementia. This means that with normal aging, one remains functionally independent. So despite mild memory loss or difficulty with language, the changes are not severe enough to cause a problem in how one functions every day. You can still manage your checkbook, cook, go grocery shopping, or do your job. This is a critical distinction between changes in cognition with age and dementia.

Okay! Now that we know about some cognitive changes that can occur as we age, here are some suggestions to help maintain cognitive health:

Treat hypertension in midlife. A number of studies suggest a relationship between midlife hypertension and later cognitive decline.

Treat risk factors for the heart. This includes hypertension, smoking, obesity, diabetes, and elevated cholesterol. What is good for the heart is good for the brain.

Be socially engaged. Have an active social life and remain connected with others. People who are socially isolated are at risk for cognitive decline.

Remain intellectually active. Engage in a variety of activities. Playing bridge and taking classes are good examples. Try learning something new, like a musical instrument or another language. Continue to do things you love, like reading or doing crossword puzzles.

Be physically active. This is as good for the brain as it is for your heart. Studies reveal that a wide range of physical activity helps prevent cognitive decline. And the activities can be fun. In fact, one study (Verghese et al., 2003). showed that dancing could reduce the risk of dementia. The important thing is to keep moving.

Review medications. Have a talk with your clinician about medications. There are a number of drugs that may have an adverse effect on your cognition. Even over-the-counter medications like antihistamines can increase confusion.

Avoid sensory deprivation. Check out your hearing and vision. It is difficult to learn anything if you can't hear what is being said. Diminished vision can lead to increased falls and potentially to head trauma. Problems with hearing and vision may both contribute to difficulty completing tasks and to social isolation.

Treat depression. Depression is associated with difficulty concentrating and remembering, worse performance on tests of cognition, and decreased motivation. It also has a negative impact on quality of life.

Eat a healthy diet. This includes eating fruits and vegetables, legumes, whole grains, and nuts. Have less red meat and increase fish and poultry. There are a variety of diets that appear to diminish cognitive decline, including the Mediterranean diet.

Sleep. Make sure to get enough sleep. It is amazing how much better you feel with a good night's rest, and this can also help with cognition, mood, and health.

Active strategies. Some studies suggest that using strategies to better encode new information may help us with our memory. And while you are at it, remember to give yourself more time.

Purpose in life. Yes, some research suggests having a meaningful purpose in life may decrease mortality, disability, and even dementia.

And one final point. You are never too old to do something amazing. Frank Lloyd Wright designed the Guggenheim Museum during the last 16 years of his life, starting at age 75. Giuseppe Verdi composed *Falstaff,* his incredible opera, when he was nearly 80 years old. And let us not forget the many writers who are well into their 90s, including the primary author of this book!

Reflections for Readers

1. Why is it that "old memories" stay intact longer than more recent ones?
2. Why is multitasking not "elder-friendly"?
3. What is meant by "executive functioning," and what is it responsible for?
4. What should elders and family members look for to distinguish between cognitive changes that are normal in the aging process and those—such as symptoms of dementia—that require medical intervention?
5. What is the difference between an inability to learn new information and an inability to remember old information?
6. What tasks are involved in safe driving? Are elders capable of driving safely? What can elders do to ensure that their driving remains safe?

References

Apfelbaum, E. P., Krendl, A. C., & Ambady, N. (2010). Age-related decline in executive function predicts better advice-giving in uncomfortable social contexts. *Journal of Experimental Social Psychology, 46,* 1074–1077.

Reistad-Long, S. (2008, May 20). Older brain really may be a wiser brain. *The New York Times,* p. 5.

Verghese, J., Lipton, R. B., Katz, M. J., Hall, C. B., Derby, C. A., Kuslansky, G., . . . Buschke, H. (2003). Leisure activities and the risk of dementia in the elderly. *New England Journal of Medicine, 348*(25), 2508–2516.

CHAPTER 12

Will I Be in Good Health in My 70s, 80s, 90s, 100s?

Genevieve Geller Wyner, EdM, LMHC
Licensed Mental Health Counselor and
Vice President of Human Resources (retired)
Shawmut Corporation
Dedham, MA
Age 86

Wouldn't we all like to know! Well, here is the answer: YES!

Of course, no one can really predict the future. Yet here's why the question in the title of this chapter challenges us and invites us to answer it for ourselves. The reason the answer is "yes" is that we can, in fact, achieve good health and happiness for ourselves in our older age. Whether you're currently getting around using a cane or a walker, don't need any support to go places by foot, are being pushed in a wheelchair, or something else, the answer lies within you.

I had always pictured myself as being a very active grandmother: teaching my grandchildren tennis, taking them out to lunch and to the theater, playing catch with them, having fun with them. Yet gradually, over the years, things changed; I had a knee replacement, then another one, followed by a hip replacement, then a spinal fusion. Then I slipped and broke my neck, had a laminectomy, and was diagnosed with heart failure. There's more—but you get the picture, I'm sure.

I was lucky. We were financially secure, and I was able to buy helpful aids for myself—a walker, a cane, a battery-operated scooter, whatever I needed. But that really didn't matter. The most important resources to be healthy, to feel healthy, to think healthy were inside me. It really didn't matter, rich or poor.

It was how I began to look at life; my attitude changed and I changed. I didn't do this all by myself. I sought guidance and support from people who had been through this kind of experience. I began to realize that I was not the center of the universe.

I began practicing "thinking of other people" and their needs before focusing on myself. It was a relief to take the focus off myself.

And perhaps most importantly, I tried not to let myself start feeling sorry for myself—"poor me! Why did this happen to me?" Even if you're in very good health with no mobility problems at all, thinking of others first and having the humility to recognize that you're not the center of the universe are important steps toward achieving happiness, as well as good health.

One more suggestion to help put things in perspective and block feelings of self-pity that might be lurking in the shadows: try thinking of three things to be grateful for today. Even if you're mad at the world, you can come up with three. (The blue sky is a good one if you're stuck.) And so it seems we do have choices to find happiness and good health, today, tomorrow, and in the years ahead.

Many people today are living to 100-plus years in good health, both mentally and physically. Suggestions for staying healthy and happy in your older age abound on the Internet or in books full of advice and guidance found in your local library. You're familiar with most of these recommendations, but here are some things you should do and be to give yourself the chance for your healthiest older years:

1. Get a good night's sleep! It wouldn't hurt to talk this over with your doctor to determine what that would be.
2. Exercise regularly. Keep active.
3. Make sure that your home and bathroom are arranged with safety in mind to help prevent falls.
4. Mark all your medications clearly—and take them as prescribed.
5. Be sure that you have a primary care doctor and that he or she knows you, and see him or her for regular checkups. If there is a geriatrician available, consider getting a referral and going to him or her for a consultation.
6. Be sure that your immunizations and screenings are up to date.
7. Eat nutritious food; follow a sensible diet. Decide on a healthy weight and maintain it.
8. If you drive . . . consider getting a driving checkup once a year. Your senior center can refer you.

9. Have your primary care physician refer you, as appropriate, for vision, dental, and hearing checkups. Also, ask your doctor for a referral to a podiatrist if you have any foot problems, especially if you are diabetic.

Reflections for Readers

1. How can attitude affect "the hand we're dealt" with respect to our health?
2. Can a "good attitude" be developed by choice? Can it be taught?
3. This author suggests that a "good attitude" consists of recognizing that one is not "the center of the universe" and of not thinking of oneself first. Do you agree with this definition of a "good attitude"? Do you have other suggestions?
4. If in fact someone is not in good health in later life, how might that person adjust to the situation without feeling sorry for himself or herself?
5. What do you think of practicing gratitude? Would it lead to a better attitude? To better health?

13

Vision and Hearing Loss in the Elderly

Scott Mankowitz, MD

Emergency Department, East Orange General Hospital
East Orange, NJ

Approximately 20% of persons older than 70 have impaired vision, and nearly a third have hearing loss. These sensory deficits make it harder for elders to communicate with others and make it more difficult for them to get around. This can lead to cognitive decline, social isolation, and depression. More ominously, visual impairment increases the risk of falls and fractures, sometimes leading to premature death.

Visual Impairment

Visual impairment, defined as vision that cannot be corrected with glasses, is highly prevalent among elders. **Figure 13-1** shows the extent of visual impairment among different population groups in the United States and how such impairment increases with age. Even in those without visual impairment, more than 9 of 10 elders wear corrective lenses. There are four main causes of visual impairment and blindness: cataracts, macular degeneration, glaucoma, and diabetic retinopathy.

CATARACTS

In patients with cataracts, the lens of the eye (called the *crystalline lens*) becomes cloudy. Symptoms include blurry or hazy vision, reduced intensity of colors, and increased glare from lights, especially when driving at night. People often describe the sensation of looking through frosted

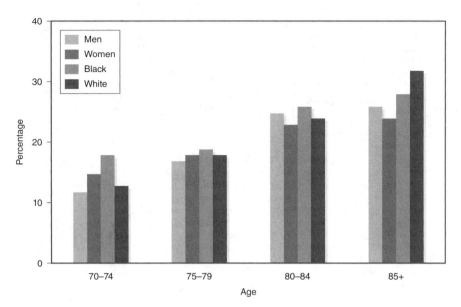

FIGURE 13-1   Visual impairment in the United States by age

Data from Desai, M., Pratt, L. A., Lentzner, H., & Robinson, K. N. (2001). Trends in vision and hearing among older Americans. *Aging Trends, 2.* Hyattsville, MD: National Center for Health Statistics.

glass or fog. Cataracts are quite common. A total of 6 out of 10 people over age 60, and almost everyone over age 80, has at least one cataract.

For some patients, changing the prescription of their eyeglasses may temporarily improve vision. Using an antiglare coating on eyeglasses can help reduce the glare for night driving, and increasing ambient light may help with reading. Ultimately, however, the definitive treatment is surgery.

One common operation is called *phacoemulsification.* A small incision is made in the cornea, and an ultrasound probe is inserted into the eye. The sound waves break down the cloudy crystalline lens so it can be suctioned out. Since this results in loss of refractive power, the patient will need stronger glasses. With correction, however, visual acuity tends to improve dramatically.

Another option is extracapsular surgery. In this procedure, the crystalline lens is surgically removed and replaced with a plastic disc called an *intraocular lens (IOL).* Interestingly, while Medicare normally will not pay for glasses or contact lenses, it does cover these items in patients who have an IOL placed.

In some cases, it is even possible to place an IOL that corrects presbyopia or astigmatism, so that postoperatively, up to 70% of patients do not need glasses at all. Unfortunately, Medicare does not pay for "premium" corrective IOLs.

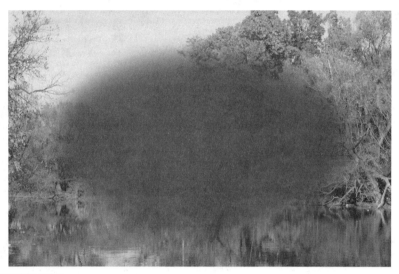

FIGURE 13-2

Courtesy of Scott Mankowitz, MD

MACULAR DEGENERATION

As we age, the cells in the center of the retina degrade and fail in a process called age-related macular degeneration (AMD). Since only the central cells are affected, people tend to lose central vision, while peripheral vision is preserved. It is not clear what causes AMD, but age, smoking, and family history appear to be the most common risk factors. AMD is quite common and affects approximately one-fourth of persons over age 70. Blacks and whites, men and women are affected equally. Unlike cataracts, there are no medications or treatments for AMD.

An example of what a person with macular degeneration sees is shown in **Figure 13-2**. The central vision is blurry or lacks color, while peripheral vision is intact.

GLAUCOMA

In patients with glaucoma, increased intraocular pressure causes progressive damage to the optic nerve, eventually resulting in permanent blindness. Like high blood pressure, the disease is insidious and usually goes unnoticed until it causes complications. By that point, the damage is irreversible. Approximately half the people with glaucoma don't know they have it.

The course of the disease is not unalterable. An ophthalmologist or optometrist can measure intraocular pressure in the office with a machine called a *tonometer*. If the pressure is high, there are many different kinds of eyedrops that can be used to treat glaucoma and keep the pressure under control.

Glaucoma shows an alarming racial preference. A total of 15% of older blacks and only 7% of whites have glaucoma. Men and women are affected equally.

DIABETIC RETINOPATHY

Diabetic retinopathy (DR) is a gradual destruction of the retina as a complication of diabetes mellitus. The retinal blood vessels become rigid, which makes them bleed or leak fluid, which in turn can result in edema (swelling) of the macula, causing vision loss.

Unlike the other diseases, DR is more common in younger adults and is the most common cause of blindness among people with diabetes. Treatment of all diabetic complications, including DR, involves tight control of the diabetes itself. Taking medications, having a healthy diet, and staying active can all prevent the progression of DR. Because DR has a very slow course, it is particularly important for diabetics to have yearly ophthalmological exams to detect DR.

If the DR has progressed, there are some newer therapies that may be useful. Vascular endothelial growth factor (VEGF) is a protein that causes blood vessels to grow and leak in a way very similar to DR. When a drug is administered to block this protein, it can reverse the abnormal blood vessel growth and decrease fluid in the retina. Anti-VEGF drugs like Avastin, Lucentis, and Eylea are injected into the eye monthly. Lasers can also be used to cauterize leaking blood vessels and are often used in conjunction with anti-VEGF to prevent blindness.

Hearing Loss

Hearing loss afflicts approximately one-third of persons over age 70, and up to one-half of patients over 85. There are stark race and gender differences, with blacks and women affected significantly less than men and whites. **Figure 13-3** presents data on hearing loss for different population groups in the United States and shows how hearing losses increase with advancing age. Patients with hearing loss are somewhat less likely to seek medical care. While up to 98% of people with visual loss talk to their doctor about it, only 74% of people with hearing loss do so.

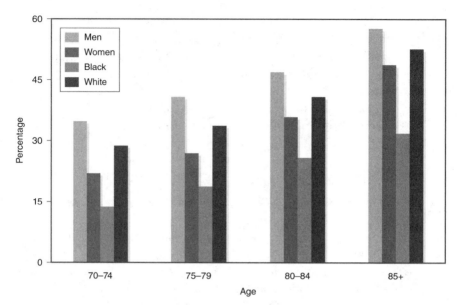

FIGURE 13-3 Hearing loss in the United States by age and race

Data from Desai, M., Pratt, L. A., Lentzner, H., & Robinson, K. N. (2001). Trends in vision and hearing among older Americans. *Aging Trends, 2.* Hyattsville, MD: National Center for Health Statistics.

The cause or causes of hearing loss has not been identified. Some risk factors include exposure to loud noises, smoking, repeated ear infections, and certain chemicals. There are no treatments for most forms of hearing loss. Some assistive technologies include hearing aids, amplified telephones, and subtitles on televisions.

Sensory Loss and Quality of Life

Exchange of information with others, an important aspect of everyday life, can be seriously impaired in individuals with hearing loss. In a study by Dalton et al. (2003), patients with hearing loss reported trouble in several of the following situations: talking with a cashier at a store, understanding dialogue in a movie or at the theater, being able to follow conversations when at a physician's office, understanding conversations when several people are talking, and understanding the conversation when talking on the telephone. These deficits were associated with lower vitality, social functioning, emotional availability, mental health, physical availability, and physical functioning. Surprisingly, people with hearing loss tend to under-report hearing-related difficulties. In this study, only 22% of people with a mild hearing loss and 56% of people with moderate to severe hearing loss reported any deficit. Even among those with hearing loss, only 15% used a hearing aid, despite evidence that hearing aids can reverse the adverse effects on quality of life in elderly adults living with hearing loss.

Reduced visual acuity significantly reduces participation in social or religious activities, mobility, activities of daily living, and visually intensive tasks. It increases the risk of having hip fractures, nursing home placement, being functionally impaired or having depressive symptoms; it also increases the need for community and/or family support. In patients with other significant medical problems, such as stroke or severe rheumatoid arthritis, patients with visual impairment tend to have lower self-reported quality of life than those with normal vision. Patients with visual impairment require more formal and informal, paid and unpaid, support, such as rehabilitation and counseling and physical aids. However, unlike hearing loss, much visual loss can be improved or prevented through careful medical treatment.

Reflections for Readers

1. How can you explain the fact that people are more reluctant to seek medical care for hearing losses than they are for vision losses?
2. What are the emotional impediments to wearing hearing aids? What are the emotional impediments to wearing glasses?
3. How do deficits in sensory input—vision or hearing—affect quality of life?

References

Desai M., Pratt, L. A., Lentzner, H., Robinson, K. N. (2001). Trends in vision and hearing among older Americans. *Aging Trends*, No. 2. Hyattsville, MD: National Center for Health Statistics.

Dalton, D. S., Cruickshanks, K. J., Klein, B. E. K., Klein, R., Wiley, T. L., & Nondahl, D. M. (2003). The impact of hearing loss on quality of life in older adults. *The Gerontologist, 43*(5), 661–668.

Further Reading

Park, S. J., Ahn, S., Woo, S. J., & Park, K. H. (2015). Extent of exacerbation of chronic health conditions by visual impairment in terms of health-related quality of life. *JAMA Ophthalmology, 133*(11), 1267–1275.

Vu, H. T. V., Keeffe, J. E., McCarty, C. A., & Taylor, H. R. (2005). Impact of unilateral and bilateral vision loss on quality of life. *British Journal of Ophthalmology, 89*(3), 360–363.

CHAPTER 14

©James Whitesmith/Moment/Getty

Stroke

(for Lillian)

Ellen Beth Siegel, JD, PsyD
Clinical Psychologist
Cambridge, MA

Her pink-polished nails grab

the wheelchair's arm,

her scrabbling feet

clench the iron bars.

She's grown thin, weak, old,

though the days haven't draped

her soft-skinned face with age.

Hot, hot means water. *The girl, the girl*

means anyone at all. Her jaws clamp,

and spit, word-salad.

She is fed by patient hands,

bathed by gentle wrists,

held by firm brown thumbs.

TV flickers past her.

She cannot click a change

and she stares, dully,

or calls *hello, hello*

for someone,

waiting somewhere,

to hear her.

Peanut butter crackers—

their paper wrappings snap.

She hunts her gaping maw, chewing

greedy bites of cellophane. The day-nurse

pulls a cracker out, puts it in her hand,

pats her smooth pink skin . . .

brown-sugar voice lifting:

Come, baby, let's fix your hair nice.

Soft stroke on stroke.

And her smile gleams, but only

on the left side of her face.

Reflections for Readers

1. If you have ever met or worked with a person who has suffered a stroke, does the description in this poem ring true to you?
2. What emotions does this poem bring up for you? What do you think the characters in the poem—the patient and the caregiver—were feeling?
3. What strikes you about the attitude and the behavior of the caregiver in this poem? If you were the caregiver, would you have done anything differently?
4. What should be the goals of a caregiver dealing with someone who has had a stroke?

CHAPTER 15

Everything You Would Like to Know About Medications and Their Effect on Aging

Carolyn Arnish, PharmD, RPh and Leanne Jasset, RPh
Manager and Owner
Dedham Pharmacy & Medical Supply
Dedham, MA

We're living in a pharmaceutical era, with about 100 new FDA-approved prescription and nonprescription medications coming to market annually. As aging adults, it's our chore and choice to know which of these drugs may improve our quality of life and whether any of them can prolong our lives.

From a pharmacist's perspective, not only are we seeking to find medication treatment options for our patients, but we also strive to find solutions without side effects. When I first thought about this title, my initial medical training led me to think: "Shouldn't it be how aging affects medications?" but upon further consideration, I think this was a rather glass-half-full approach. Medications truly have an impact on aging—they can make you feel better *or* worse. It is how you use them that can change the outcome.

Pharmacy school teaches us to think of a baseline patient as a 25-year-old, 154-pound male, and then extrapolate medications to children, pregnant women, and the elderly (especially since it is also most ethical to try new medications on these healthy volunteers). Not surprisingly, there are fewer variables in this "ideal" healthy male that could affect the expected outcome of a given drug, as opposed to someone who is smaller, has different hormones, or has confounding disease states. Variables that could change the effect of the drug in your body include percentage of muscle and fat, bodily water content, liver function, and kidney function, as well as genetics, which uniquely influences enzymes in our body to break down drugs that we take, either quickly or slowly. Some drugs are attracted to water and some to fat; this changes how they distribute into our body and how long they stay around before they are eliminated. Drugs are cleaned out from our bodies in two main ways: some through the liver and others through the kidneys, so should anything go wrong with these organs, medications may build up and cause additive and subsequently adverse effects. It is important to be aware that every body is unique, and with age, muscle mass is lower and organ function is often slowed, making medication metabolism change. Anatomically as we age, our bodies undergo many changes, so Drug "X" at Dose "Y" gives a wide array of results—which can be either good or bad.

Getting past the complicated calculations of right-and-wrong doses for individual patients, aging poses a whole host of other challenges to achieve the optimal benefit from the treatment plan our prescribers have decided upon. Perhaps the most important and difficult of these is "medication compliance." Professors recited constantly: "A drug that was prescribed and not taken, is as good as no drug prescribed." I won't bore you with statistics on how many patients take their medications the way the physician prescribed, but I would like to outline why it is not an easy task to "take what the doctor ordered." Physical challenges, such as vision and dexterity, are the first hurdles. Prescription bottles are written in notoriously small writing, and even for those with slightly abnormal vision, they can be a challenge to read. Needless to say, the vast majority of seniors face vision and dexterity issues, making it difficult simply to select the right pill bottle and open it. For dexterity issues, some pharmacies carry an "easy-open" or "non-childproof cap" for ease of opening the bottle, but it is important to remember that if you have young children or pets visiting or living with you, this could be a safety hazard. Vision is far more challenging since the solutions are not quite as economical or easy—Braille works for some, and other options include magnifying glasses, color-coded bottles, and bar-code technology to scan a bottle and have it read the name to you. Always ask your pharmacist if you have any physical challenges that may prevent you from taking your medication; I'm sure they would be happy to help you think of creative solutions!

Memory is perhaps the most frustrating hurdle for both patients and caregivers to achieve medication adherence. For some of us, it can be challenging to give up our autonomy with regard to health care and medication management. Fortunately, there are many options for those with memory deficiencies to either manage medications themselves, if appropriate and safe, or to have a pharmacy or caregiver manage them. Almost all pharmacies have the capacity to "autofill" your medications so you don't have to remember to fill them, but if you forget to pick up your medication or to take it, you end up with a stockpile of expired drugs sitting around your house, which could be a safety hazard for you and others living with you, as well as a financial and environmental waste. I always encourage patients to have a list of their medications (with dose and indication) on hand at all times, especially if they have trouble saying drug names or remembering them (which even includes medical professionals!). It is important to note that even if you know a few letters of the drug name, many medications are what we call "look-alike/sound-alike drugs" and if you know that "hyd" are the first three letters, that can apply to five different pharmaceutical products!

Knowing what the medication is being used to treat (or the "indication") is also crucial to practicing safe medication management. You are your own best advocate, and you know your body better than any physician because you live in it, whether you are 18 years old or 118! I want all of my patients to know what they are taking and why they are taking it because this has been shown to increase people's willingness and effort to comply with their medication schedules and thus improve their health condition. There are pill organizers, medication reminder alarms, phone applications, routine triggers, and family members to remind us to take our medicine, but sometimes these things aren't enough. Companies like Medicine-on-Time and PillPack have designed their whole business model on simplifying medication schedules and automating them as a service. Many retail pharmacies also have systems to prepack medications into simpler formats so that memory, vision, and dexterity become less of an obstacle to taking your pills.

Safety is the primary teaching point for everything pharmacy-related in the geriatric population. As we age, we tend to have multiple disease states, medications, and a doctor for each issue, which creates a perfect storm for medication errors and interactions. The American Geriatrics Society has created a list of potentially inappropriate medications for those not on hospice or palliative care called the "Beers Criteria." This list is used primarily by healthcare professionals to help guide selection of medications to create a safer lineup of medications that, for example, are less likely to harm your kidneys or increase risk of falling. Pharmacies have software to help run drug interaction profiles and can easily enter a list of your medications and tell you instantly if there are any interactions to be concerned about, even with food, alcohol, vitamins, or supplements. Drugs can interact with many substances, like milk or grapefruit juice, not just other drugs or alcohol! It can be challenging for doctors and pharmacists to accurately run these interactions, especially if you take over-the-counter drugs or herbals, vitamins, or supplements that are not listed on your medical history or medication profile list; therefore, it is extremely important that you tell your doctor and pharmacist about everything you take, even if you just take them as needed. Some prescription drugs contain the same or similar ingredients found in over-the-counter drugs, which could cause therapeutic duplication and perhaps overdose of these medications. Again, the tiny print on over-the-counter products can hide ingredients that you may not even know are in the product.

Having multiple specialty doctors is wonderful to get expert knowledge on specific medical issues, but unfortunately, not all doctors share the same medical record system, which may cause redundancies in your care. It is important to note, also, that retail pharmacies do not have any access to your medical records. Because of this, you may find yourself answering the same questions over and over again about your medications, history, and allergies. In this case, the best thing you can do is give consistent answers to all your physicians (unless things with your health have changed, of course) and let them all know about the other doctors you are seeing in case they need to consult with one another so that no duplications are made.

Lastly, if you believe that you are experiencing side effects from a new medication, contact the physician who prescribed it. Pharmacists are always able to counsel you on the possible side effects or teach you about how the drug works, but remember: they are unable to adjust your dose or change your medication without prescriber approval. Good pharmacies will take the time to answer any questions you may have when starting a new medication, or if you have concerns about current therapy. The ultimate goal is to have your doctors working in concert, with open communication lines to your pharmacy, which should provide you with knowledge and the prescribed medications to prevent illness or treat your medical issues.

It is important to be prepared for all scenarios. Doctors don't always pick the right medicine, pharmacies don't always dispense the right medicine, and sometimes you forget to take your pills. When errors happen, as they inevitably do, have a plan! For example, if you notice that the pills you received are a different color, shape, or design from what you are used to, always ask a question. You can either look up pills online in pill-identifier databases or call your pharmacy to find out exactly what was dispensed to you. Oftentimes it is a false alarm—the manufacturer changed or the design is new—but it is better to confirm that than to take the wrong medication. If you forget to take your medication when you are supposed to, know whom to call or whether you can take it late.

If your pharmacy or doctor's office is closed, have a planned contact should you have emergent questions or health issues.

With the right support network, doctors, and pharmacy, aging with health issues can be a positive experience. Know that the health professionals that you work with want your health to improve, and if you need help organizing your pills, remembering to take them, or managing side effects, we can always offer solutions if you ask. When you have a list in your head or on paper and keep track of your medications, your health providers will take note of your diligence and respect your effort in taking responsibility for managing your health care. With so many moving parts in health care, it is imperative that all patients and/or caretakers have a basic understanding of all prescription medications, over-the-counter products, and herbals/supplements that you take. Knowing your medications will help reduce errors, increase compliance, and ultimately improve your overall health.

As older citizens, we strive to have the best healthcare provided to us as our bodily functions slowly decline. The best we can do is to identify our struggles with our medication management, and ask for help to come up with solutions. Pharmacies and patients are constantly striving for better solutions to challenges seniors face to manage the drugs prescribed to them and new ideas are always in the pipeline. Pharmacists are there to help you and are generally much more easily accessible than physicians. Pharmacies are your gateway to understanding your medications and achieving your health management goals. If you have physical, mental, or financial challenges that come with your medication management, there is always someone in a pharmacy to help or explain complicated situations. You are never alone in managing your health!

Reflections for Readers

1. What factors interfere with a person's medication compliance, and how can compliance be increased?
2. How might financial issues affect a person's medication compliance? Can you suggest ways for medical professionals to raise this issue with patients? What steps can medical professionals take to help patients with financial difficulties obtain the medications they need?
3. What is the patient's responsibility in communicating to doctors and pharmacies about medications? How might society better educate consumers in this regard?
4. Why is it important for individuals to maintain current lists of medications?

PART III

Emotional Responses to Aging

© James Whitesmith/Moment/Getty

CHAPTER 16

Aging: From Aging to Adolescence and Back Again

Judith S. Goldstein, PhD

Author and Founder/Executive Director, Humanity in Action

New York, NY

Age 76

There are those of us who are lucky and those who are not. Some people age—or whatever that means and whenever it takes place—with spunk, style, and little pain. Others suffer severe losses in body, mind, and spirit. The first case is the better way to go. But not much is in our control. We hardly know if aging relates to our genes or good fortune.

What is clear is that all of our lives will change as we age: depletion will take on the beat of regularity. Losing friends and family members will become routine. Those who died young or in middle age were regarded as the unlucky exceptions. But as we age, loss becomes routine. We expect to feel constant pain as we separate from those whose love, friendship, and histories are entwined with ours. We stake our lives on entwining with family and friends—whether those relationships are close or distant. They provide the markers of our lives. It takes courage to stay on the field of living as the numbers of our families and friends diminish by the month and year.

Aging is a crapshoot and challenge. So were our adolescent years—but with such different expectations. Then, a long time ago, everything was possible—from the good to the feared. Everything was future-based. When we navigated the years from being children to adults, we had our own high expectations of what was ahead—or others projected them onto us. We thought about the future with hope, uncertainty, and a wide range of expectations: building new families and/or making careers. We knew what the expectations were in the natural cycle of growth and responsibilities. We didn't always meet them, but we knew what was ahead as we watched our parents and siblings. (For those of us who were born in the 1930s and 1940s, the expectations were socially fixed and far different from today, when gender issues are more progressive and flexible.)

And yet aging and adolescence have something in common: there are wide physical differences affecting both groups. Adolescence is more fun and promising, looking toward a future that is unknown. There are problems, of course. Obviously, boys and girls have different rates of development in their teen years. A group of 13-year-olds consists of all different sizes and signs of physical maturation. Some girls make it fast: almost overnight, they take on the face and body that will define them for decades until signs of old age set in. Some boys will be short, some tall, some with baby voices, some with deep resonance, some waiting longingly with smooth skin to look like men while their peers have already started to shave. A high school football game or a bar mitzvah will produce a mixed bag of adolescents who might all act the same but present a hundred varieties of unfinished forms. All is expectation. All is comparison with one's peers. All is insecurity about bodies and attractiveness to others.

At the other end of the cycle of physical change—the aging that sets in now in our 60s or 70s—the differences are equally striking. The varieties of aging are as great as those experienced in adolescence. Some people remain active and erect; some sadly are bent over with physical impairments. Some are subject to awful diseases. The hair, gone or getting less robust, turns gray or white. One loses inches. And when in a group, at a reunion or funeral, we look at each other with a comparative eye that is tinged with sympathy and often sadness, and often with poignant surprise. Sometimes we don't even recognize old friends because so much has changed. The vigor is gone, the physical strength is diminished, the ears and eyes are less dependable, the memory is often a mystery of uncertain dependability, and a wife or husband has already passed away or is infirm.

It is clear that when we see our aging peers, we feel like survivors in a losing battle against inevitable weakness and decline. It is a social matter, as were the changes in adolescence. Back then, we shared with friends and family the wild bursts of energy, maturing, and hopes—and confusions. Today, we share in a different way. We are part of a diminishing group of people who measure their own changes in comparison to others. And the changes are as pronounced, leading toward the unmistakable, inevitable, irreversible, and unalterable change.

Reflections for Readers

1. In adolescence, "everything seems possible." Is there a way to preserve that attitude in later years—and if so, would it be desirable to do so?

2. In both adolescence and aging, great physical changes occur. What is it about the changes inherent in aging that makes them seem so much more negative than the difficulties of adolescence?

3. To what extent are we able to regulate how we age? How much of the aging process is simply a matter of luck?

4. If we maintain a positive attitude toward aging, will we be better able to age "with spunk, style, and little pain"? How does attitude affect or interact with the physical changes of aging?

CHAPTER 17

Notes from the Far North

Geraldine Zetzel, MEd
Poet, teacher, and meditation practice leader
Lexington, MA
Age 89

Here on our ice floe

we drift in amiable harmony

admiring on winter nights

the pale-green crackling curtains

of the Aurora Borealis.

Beside the whale-oil lanterns

some of us hold hands, others

hunker down hooded, solitary.

By sputtering light we tell

each other the stories

of our previous lives—

our histories keep us warm.

From time to time, of course,

someone slips off the edge

into the black water. It happens.

Then we sew their names into

sealskin boats, float them out

into the waves, chanting the old words.

On clear nights we sometimes can see

the mainland, its fires star-blue

across the sheet ice between us.

From time to time they send us

parcels—used blankets, biscuits,

pemmican wrapped in old newspaper.

In summertime cargo ships

steam past in the distance, busily

steering away southwards.

Do we mind? Of course.

They say we are content,

resigned—don't believe it.

First published in *Traveling Light* by Geraldine Zetzel (2016)

Reflections for Readers

1. What is the author referring to by saying "the far north"?
2. How do you understand the phrase "our histories keep us warm"?
3. What in this poem addresses our memories of those who have passed on?
4. The author writes of a ritual—sewing the names of those who are lost into sealskin boats and floating them out into the waves. What do you see as the role of the ritual? How might rituals console survivors?
5. Elders see their lives as having ongoing value. Do younger people agree? What stereotypes consign elders to a metaphorical version of being set adrift on an ice floe?

Time Caught Up on Me

(Dedicated to my wife, Liane)

Sherwin (Sam) Lehrer, PhD

Muscle Biophysics, Boston Biomedical Research Institute;
Principal Research Associate, Harvard Medical School (retired)
Dedham, MA
Age 82

Whose arms are these? I ask.

Time says: "They are the arms of all

who have aged."

Why did I suddenly notice?

Time says: "Because you had time."

The spots on my arms and face

are freckles, I told my grandson.

The others know but say:

"My, how well you look."

Why can't she remember?

Time says: "Time clumps our brains."

All that is left now is a cheerful child

with little talk, so different from times past.

Do I have time to finish?

Time asks: "What?"

I have much to do.

Time says: "Keep doing

though you may not finish,

for time does not wait."

What good is time?

Time says: "To see the new.

With time you may

watch the short cycles of seasons,

the longer cycle of growth,

and be gone before the sadness

of the end of cycles."

Time says: "Let time pass."

Reflections for Readers

1. Why are changes in our physical appearance often experienced as "startling"?
2. How does the decline of one spouse affect the spousal relationship in a long-term marriage/partnership? Are there special considerations that apply when one spouse has advanced dementia? When one spouse has a debilitating physical illness?
3. Does the perception of the passage of time contract or expand with advancing age?
4. Which changes in aging are "minor annoyances"? Which are major problems? And which are advantages?
5. We will probably all agree that it can be difficult to accept our own aging. Are the issues the same or different when it comes to accepting the aging of a loved one?

The Other Side of Time

Liane Reif-Lehrer, PhD
Retina Research, Eye Research Institute;
Associate Professor, Harvard Medical School;
Grants Consultant (retired)
Dedham, MA
Age 82

I.

Once when the sky hung low over life,

I looked beyond the sun, and saw there

what the days to come might bring.

The mirrored clouds showed even beyond that

into the thoughts of tomorrow

and the hauntings of the years before nights began.

II.

On borrowed grass and borrowed time

the moon seeped in

and wound around me,

entwining my hair

in its golden streams.

In the valley before morning

there dance before my eyes

images of the might-have-been,

in the shadow of myself,

and the wishing of the me

inside the me, inside the me.

III.

When the darkness of day descended

upon my dreams and turned them into reality,

I cried, for they were gone,

and suddenly the world was cold again:

friends, who existed only in my mind,

disappeared, and unfamiliar phantoms

who could not feel, inherited my life,

with their own qualms, and my questions,

and scars which did not match mine.

I cried for the green days of dreaming,

untouched by the world of now—

so gentle and perfect in all their innocence

and raptures of the will.

IV.

The dew and the secrecy of the trees

hid our youthful fancies from the world

that had already learned it was all just a lie.

In the center of our universe

the perfection seemed real

and the real seemed real

and the real seemed grotesque, but oh so far away,

in a time that would surely never come—

and if it came indeed, would not touch us—not me!

But it came, in fact, rolling in on a billowing wave,

as quickly as it does for every man;

and though I tried to run away,

it found me, nonetheless, in the end.

First published in *Poems Unremembered* by Liane Reif-Lehrer (2017)

Reflections for Readers

1. What does this poem suggest about the concept of time from an aging person's perspective? About aging?
2. What emotions are expressed here?
3. To what extent do you believe such feelings are typical or unique for older people?
4. In normal aging, the person remains himself or herself, just older, but for a person with dementia, the predisease person begins to disappear as the disease takes root. How are the changes of dementia manifested? In what ways does the person change and in what ways does she or he stay the same?
5. The poet appears to regard the future and her aged self with foreboding. Is this generally true for younger people? What about as people move into middle age? How do elders regard themselves?

CHAPTER 20

From Generation to Generation

Diana Hope Bronner, MEd
Special needs Teacher Educator (retired)
Dedham, MA
Age 78

There she sits, her back to me, and all I can recognize is her puff of white hair.

Her body in the chair looks so small, like that of a child; the shoulders are rounded and almost seem to meet in front of her; her chest is hollowed out, not hollowed in.

She is my mother. I know because her face lights up when she sees me and she calls me "honey."

She walks bent over her walker, her "Cadillac"; she walks slowly as in a dream, talking all the while about this and that, oblivious to oncoming cars, to people. I think if I walk just a little faster, she'll somehow keep up with me, and then I feel guilty.

She is my mother. I know, because she calls me "honey."

She stands in the grocery checkout line, fumbling for her card, what button to press. People waiting in line behind watch impatiently—she is beautifully oblivious. She tells me and her friends that I am the Mommy now and that she listens to me.

She dresses in her pressed white pants and pressed embroidered blouse, but meatloaf from the afternoon meal leaves its stain and ruins the image. She tucks in her blouse to hide the evidence.

She tries to please me by saying that she turned off the water faucet; she thanks me for helping her. She so wants to be independent . . . but it's so hard to be.

She is my mother. I know, because she says "I love you."

What happened to my Mother, the tall strong woman who could so easily cast off anyone who didn't meet her expectations? What happened to the tall, strong woman who dressed to the nines, proudly walked New York's Fifth Avenue showing off herself and her handsome Dalmatian dog? What happened to those dark, defiant eyes that could be so angry? What happened to the mother I didn't see for years because she was too tough for me? What happened to that woman who was the life of the party, with her dirty jokes told with a put-on Jewish accent?

Why am I having so much trouble adjusting to this new mother/child of mine?

"No!" my shout turns inward, "*this* isn't my mother! Where is she?"

I too will reach this same stage, old, frail, dependent. Will my son recognize *me?* Will he also be impatient, as I am with my mother? Will he too live in denial, as I am?

What is this end of life? It seems truly to take us right back to the beginning of life, a full circle, and if you believe so, into a new beginning.

Yes, I am aging, as did my mother, as does everyone and everything. It is inevitable—but do I really believe this? After all, I am "only" 78 and I have many years ahead of me . . . or do I? Hey, someone could be in their 60s or 50s and get hit by a car or die from a disease; being deceased is not necessarily a function of age. Who knows? But here I am, living in a retirement community. What a shock, going to the theater as a group and getting on and off a bus in full view of the public, a bus that advertises "NewBridge on the Charles Retirement Community," i.e., an aging community! Am I one of the people who belong on that bus? Can't be! Who would have ever thought this could be me, announcing I am getting old?

Actually, I love my retirement cottage, where I live with my also-aging husband and my also-aging dog. We all enjoy the many opportunities to graciously and gratefully age in place. I get to do things I never did before, like run a photography club, lead a meditation group, hang art exhibits, participate in the Yom Hashoah[1] observance, the memorial service for our deceased members, and the life-giving tree planting ceremony for the Sylvia Band Memorial Grove. I have more friends here than I've had in my whole life, friends I love and care about, opportunities to be there for those friends as they go through the vicissitudes of their lives. I go

---

[1] Yom Hashoah, the Hebrew term for "Holocaust Remembrance Day," is the day commemorating the approximately six million Jews who perished in the Holocaust as a result of the actions carried out by Nazi Germany.

to Chorus, where I can sing off-key, but nobody can hear well enough to know who it is and even if they did, they couldn't care less. The programs, the classes—oh my, it's like being at a university. And the exercise programs to keep me young and fit. Along with my aging dog, beloved companion that he is, I still trudge up the hill, perhaps not as fast as we used to go, but the goal of getting to the top has to be reached if we want to get home to biscuits and hot chocolate or whatever.

Yes, it is all wonderful and life-giving. But in spite of it, I am still aging. I ask myself whether I am able to do those exotic trips we used to take, even in recent years—Mongolia, riding a camel, sleeping in yurts; Namibia, learning its history, experiencing its culture, climbing those sand dunes. My eyes water, my nose runs, my body is shrinking in one way and expanding in another. The lines on my face look like road maps; hair—well, we won't talk about that! I guess the good news is that with my diminishing memory, I won't remember what used to be and will just accept what is in the present moment. Who knows what the future will bring, but whatever it is, I will age as gracefully as possible.

Will I be as I wrote about my mother? Will my son see in me what I saw in my mother? I don't know . . . I only know I will do my aging in my own way.

Reflections for Readers

1. What concerns about the aging process are expressed in this essay?
2. How can the aging process assist or interfere with intergenerational rapprochements?
3. What do this author's words suggest about the importance of aging in place and living independently?
4. After reading about this author's experiences, how would you feel about living in a senior community? Is this different from how you felt previously? If so, why?

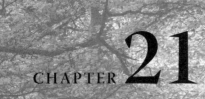

21

©James Whitesmith/Moment/Getty

My Thickest File

Ben Slomoff, MA
Business Executive, Mediator, and Arbitrator (retired)
Walnut Creek, CA
Age 103

It's my thickest file—

Sad: it makes me smile.

Try being sentimental

About Medicare supplemental,

Try sorting your healthcare file

And dealing with this paper pile.

Oh! How I hate maturity, yet

Thank God for Social Security.

As I lose bodily functions,

There's less income, few deductions.

Each blue bruise on my arm

Sets off an inner alarm.

98

To keep my pace quicker

My pillbox keeps getting thicker.

Sure I am nervous, every week

Another memorial service.

To preserve my youth

I'm in a horrible stew

What can I do?

My choices are so few.

My mind still works,

I'm still in style,

I think I'll hang around awhile.

First published in *A Stalwart Bends: Poems and Reflections* by Ben Slomoff

Reflections for Readers

1. How can humor aid in the aging process?
2. What aids do seniors need to keep track of their often-complicated medical situations?
3. What are the emotional impediments to keeping track of medical needs, and how can seniors be helped to address those impediments?

PART **IV**

Coming to Terms with the Changes Caused by Aging

CHAPTER 22

Aging Easier

Erlene Rosowsky, PsyD
Director, Geropsychology Concentration
Core Faculty, William James College
Newton, MA

There are truly some important, and quite wonderful, positive occurrences as we become older. We have a broader, deeper view of the world and of how to make our way through it. We are more comfortable and accepting of who we are, of the person we have become. We feel less pressure to achieve major, life-defining goals. We can graciously decline or relinquish membership in the "gotta run" generation. (Sigh of relief.) And yet, we can still be amazed. We can still learn and grow. We can still feel passion.

As a geropsychologist, I am frequently asked what I think contributes to a sense of well-being and good mental health in older age. I offer these thoughts in response.

Self-Acceptance

Reminiscence, life review, is a universal and stage-appropriate activity as we become older. Reminiscence is not simply a collection of passive musings, but rather a purposeful process that serves an important function. That is, despite fits and starts, bumps and peaks, in healthy old age, we become able to see the whole picture of our life and who we are, and come to accept this person as "me."

There comes then in old age, a moment of reconciliation, a convergence, between who we had hoped the "me" would be, the life we had expected to live, and who we are and the life we actually have lived. Self-acceptance embraces both the reality and the joy and the disappointment and the sadness of that reality.

However, there is still time to create changes in yourself or your life. You remain a powerful agent of change even when old; perhaps especially

103

when old. Review and reenjoy the good times. Recall how problems were met and addressed in the past. No one gets to be a certain age without having lived and survived that certain number of years!

Positive Relations with Others

In older age, we are able to exercise some choice of others with whom we want to spend our time, to choose with whom to importantly populate our world. Who will we spend time with when time itself becomes an increasingly precious commodity? Much attention gets paid to the loss of others in older age, but it is also an opportune time to make a new friend, especially one who is different from yourself and your other friends.

We can become more others-oriented, and this is good and stage-appropriate, indeed necessary. In old age, no one can make it alone. Mutual interdependence becomes the coin of the realm. We must recognize when we need help, be willing to engage help, and appreciate help received. When we offer help we feel appreciated. So do others. It is wise to express appreciation liberally and criticism parsimoniously. Think of this in terms of "exchange theory," with the added benefits of connection and possibly love.

Respect of "Uniqueness" (Others' and Our Own)

Recall how during adolescence, everyone had to be pretty much the same: wear the same clothes, read the same books, enjoy the same movies, and think and act just the same as everyone else in the group. Older age offers an opportunity to accept one's uniqueness.

One of the delightful perks of becoming an older adult is in being increasingly freed from the judgment of others and even able to shed some of the social demands and proprieties that have often felt constraining. Consider the emergence of the Red Hat Society reflected in the poem, "Warning," encouraging aspiring elders to "wear purple with a red hat which doesn't go, and doesn't suit me" (Joseph, 1961). A little eccentricity can serve to introduce a bit of passion and enliven life. And a slightly new way of being might keep those who think they know us well on their toes!

Personal Growth

"Becoming" who we are does not end in older age. We continue to grow (not just the waistline) and develop throughout sentient life. In older age, we can foster our capacity to grow as we have the time to attend to "becoming" rather than "achieving." We know that a genuine openness to experience enables us to become more flexible in our ways of thinking and acting; to be able to cope in different ways when we experience different things and different roles, gains and losses, such as grandparenthood or widowhood. Older age is a good time to learn something new. You don't have to be "good" at it. Take chances. Guess. You might be right.

Purpose and Meaning

With so many changes in life during older age, and losses of roles and relationships, our very reasons for being here, understandably, can become strained. Having a purpose helps us get out of bed in the morning and get going, even when the going is tough. Most important, having meaning in our lives enables us to continue to feel like ourselves; the same "me," only older. Our life history is dynamic. It does not end until we do. And our history, our ongoing story, needs to be cultivated and lived and savored. Savor most what you most value.

Reconciliation

Forgive what you can, and appreciate the liberation you feel. Remorse and bitterness are heavy and can weigh us down. I often share with folks the image of the aging process as akin to being in a small boat, traversing frequently choppy waters while navigating an uncharted course. It is wise to lighten one's load and be selective of what heavy baggage is important at this stage to carry along.

Generativity

You've learned a lot through your life so far. You have much to share, to pass along. This is often best achieved through doing and modeling. Each semester in my Geropsychology course, the class wrestles through discussion to achieve consensus for a definition of wisdom in older adults. How do we identify the "wise elder"? The students inevitably come to address the concept of generativity and the product of legacy. One especially thoughtful contribution to the definition was offered in the voice of the younger adults, the recipients of the bequeathed wisdom:

> "The wise older adult might leave an externally recognizable legacy, or might not. It may be that the legacy is what is within *us*."

Commitment

Meaning and purpose require the commitment of our resources, including time, energy, and focus, as well as fiscal resources. As we age, the amount, availability, and apportionment of our resources change. However, authentic commitment continues to mean a mindful choice of where and how we invest these resources.

Optimism

Optimism allows openness to experience, without looking at experiences through a "gray lens" and maladaptive cognitions. The openness can be a thought, an intention, or a plan and has a future orientation, whether immediate or further into the future. Optimism can be in response to "futures" generated by others: their thoughts, plans, and intentions. Optimism can be a response to events that just happen, not having been under our control or anyone else's.

Optimism is not magical thinking (although a little magic sometimes helps), but rather a more future-oriented, positive attitude. Optimism is nurtured when we recall things that turned out well, rather than focusing excessively on those that did not. Try feeding your mind with thoughts that reflect a positive attitude. Catch yourself when you say (to yourself or aloud) "It will never work out." "This always happens to me." "Why bother? Nothing good will come of it!"

Practice a bit of optimism every day. And just like practicing the piano (remember that?), start on middle-C: CAN do!

Altruism

Something else to practice is to be more other-focused and concerned about the well-being of others. This does not require a grand, expansive gesture. It means, rather, to allow ourselves to see another's point of view and hold it as respectfully as we do our own, even if we don't agree. It means understanding that another's way of thinking and being is as essential to them, as unique, as our own. Sometimes a kind word, a gesture of acceptance, can provide an opportunity for change and healing in a fellow being. Think of the community as a group of fellow beings, worthy of our focus and concern.

Humor

According to Freud, humor is a highly mature defense mechanism theorized as helping to protect or limit what is painful for us to bear. And

Freud was a pretty funny guy, so he should know. What we do know is that life can have its rough edges, and that the ability to see its surreal qualities and splash these with humor can help. The process of aging, becoming old, affords many changes and challenges that are well addressed with humor, as Hallmark delights in letting us know. Laughing together can gentle the process.

Concluding Thoughts

I heard somewhere that "the wisest guru," when asked what words of advice he would bequeath his seekers, offered the following:

> *Rest when you are tired.*
>
> *Eat when you are hungry.*

I might add:

> *Move to the extent that you are able.*
>
> *Smile often; start now.*

Reflections for Readers

1. What are some ways that one can create change in later life?
2. What does it mean "to grow" as we become old?
3. How is maintaining a sense of purpose in later life important to our mental health?
4. How can you apply reminiscence or memory to enrich your life as you age? How can you use it to add to the experience of your family and friends?
5. How can elders express their individuality and uniqueness in growthful ways?
6. What constitutes a "wise elder"?
7. How can someone working with elders foster optimism?
8. Why is altruism important? Is it a value of importance only to elders, or to everyone?

Reference

Joseph, J. (1961). "Warning." *Poetry archive*. Retrieved from http://www.poetryarchive.org/poet/jenny-joseph

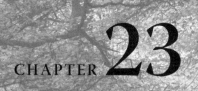

Eldercare Strategies: Useful Thoughts and Actions When You Are the "Elder," When You Are the "Care," When You Are Both

Lynne Sherman, MA, LMFT
Licensed Marriage and Family Therapist (retired)
Santa Barbara, CA
Age 71

There is no one-size-fits-all strategy when it comes to eldercare. Here are some things to consider as you prepare for this journey. There are things you can do, ways you can decide to think, attitudes you can decide to have, that may make eldercare a better experience for you. Notice I am not providing Pollyanna gloss here about the "wonderful adventure of eldercare." We all know how this story ends: somebody dies. That is a sad thing, and to suggest that you can get through the experience without some measure of grief is really unfair to you. If I set that up as a norm, you might be under the additional load of going through the experience and trying to be smiley and optimistic all the time, even though your heart may at times feel like it is breaking. But we can be realistic without being tragic.

I have had personal experience with eldercare: my great uncle, my grandmother, my husband's Mom, my Mom and, most recently, my Dad. My parents were the "front line" caregivers for my Gram and my great-uncle. My husband's mother lived with my husband and me for the last years of her life, right through to the end. My Dad was the primary caregiver for my Mom, and I was very involved. I was the primary caretaker of his enormous grief when she died. I was my Dad's primary caregiver as his own self-sufficiency waned. In each situation, when we needed it, we hired some help. I met some amazing people, good and bad, along the way, and I learned from all of them. In my professional life as a counselor in private practice, I have helped clients think through their eldercare dilemmas and I taught free classes in eldercare issues to employees as part of a corporate wellness program. All of these experiences provided me with ideas that I hope will be helpful to you.

My psychotherapy was influenced by a philosophy that advised, "If you are unhappy, do what you can to change the situation, then try to change your attitudes about the parts of the situation you can't change." Yes, we *can* decide what we think. We each have some self-determination about that. For instance, I could have chosen to think my Dad's death was the worst crisis I would ever suffer and I would never recover from it. Had I done that, I would be likely to feel despondent for the rest of my life. I decided instead to think that my Dad's death was a really bad but inevitable situation, one I had been bracing against for many years. I decided to think that while I would never "get over" it, I would adapt to the loss; and the good memories and gratitude for his love would be an inspiration and a comfort to me for the rest of my life. I feel sad that he is not here with me, and I feel glad that I have the memories of a lifetime of great experiences with him.

You are not stuck with what you happen to be thinking. You can question it and tweak it to provide a more balanced and realistic way of looking at your situation. A popular adage among cognitive therapists is "Don't believe everything you think!" So I can feel sad and feel glad at the same time? Yes. We rarely feel just one feeling about a major situation. I think we have feeling "bouquets," made up of fragrant flowers and some thistles, too. Check in with your own feelings about the situation that caused you to read my chapter. Perhaps you feel sad, and anxious, and tired, and grateful, and hopeful, and angry, and determined. In my practice, I used a "feelings list." This was a list of positive and negative feelings. My client would tape it to the fridge and periodically scan the list and touch all the feelings that resonated with the current mood. Doing this reveals that you are having a mix of feelings. This is the depth and richness of your emotional state. Each different feeling in the bouquet can be the basis of a self-statement about your situation. You are not locked into one negative way of seeing yourself in any moment. The story you decide to tell yourself about your situation can provide you with strength and solace. This includes honoring your negative emotions, such as "I am feeling really sad and exhausted; I forgive myself for my absentmindedness and my short temper today." It may take a little practice to deliberately modify your self-statements. Getting a few sessions with a cognitive behavioral counselor can be really helpful. There are also many self-help articles and books about "self-talk," emotional IQ, and self-affirming statements. Your library and the Internet are two free sources for this type of ready wisdom.

When you are the Elder, there are several factors that will influence how your eldercare scenario might unfold: your current level of ability, your relationship with your caregiver, and your personal and community resources. You can evaluate the degree of care you need at this point. You can anticipate that whatever degree of assistance you now need, you are likely to need a greater degree of help later. We all know this. We have seen our friends and acquaintances go through this. Did we honestly think it would never happen to us?

Think about your situation with your caregiver. What is the relationship? Is this an adult child, sibling, or other relative? Is the caregiver a professional? The character of the relationship is going to influence the degree and type of care you can realistically expect. For instance, if you are relying on your son or daughter and the relationship has always been difficult, it is not going to transform itself into some fantasy ideal because of the drama of your impending end of life. In fact, the stresses and strains of the situation could make things worse. Be realistic. Can you really move in with the daughter you typically fight with? Is that fair to either of you? I truly hope that you have a child you have a good enough relationship with to rely on him or her for caregiving. But if your relationship is fraught with tension, give yourself some breathing room.

I have spoken with many Elders who feel that their children should be their sole caregivers: "I took care of my kids, now they should take care of me." That is a nice ideal, but it may not work. As the Elder who needs care, keep an open mind about yourself. Try to be realistic about what your children or other caregivers can realistically provide emotionally or logistically. Inventory your feelings about staying in your own home, living with your kids, or moving to assisted living. Everyone is different. It was of paramount importance for my Dad to remain in his own home. My mother-in-law was relieved to move in with us. Our neighbor was delighted to move to assisted living and be free of the burdens of meal preparation and social isolation. Keep your autonomy and do it your way.

Many of us do-it-yourself types love our feeling of self-sufficiency. As we age, our pride in being able to keep our own homes can become a suspicion about having strangers come into our homes for homemaking tasks that we once could manage with ease. I have consoled so many guilt-ridden children who could not provide the home care their parent needed and watched as their parent's nutrition and safety slipped into disarray. I advise you not to be that stubborn parent. You still are the king or queen of your castle. You are the one hiring and firing and writing the paychecks. If you are so worried that the help will steal the jewelry, give it to your heirs now. We get old. We get feeble. When it comes to accepting help, we can still act like jerks; let's not. We can adjust to having help by phasing in assistance for the heavier housekeeping while we still have the physical and mental ability to adapt to "having strangers come in."

Fear about being "ripped off" by the help is really about the need to establish financial boundaries. I advise you to think about ways in which you can keep yourself and your assets safe. You might establish an estate plan that sets forth how you want your finances managed when you are unable to write checks yourself. Your spendthrift child may not be the best person to manage your money. Hiring a professional fiduciary may be a good way to make sure that your money stays in your account. All states have laws against financial abuse of an elder. When abuse happens, boundaries were not set up in the first place, and by the time the law steps in, the damage is done.

When you are the Care, you need to balance your needs with your Elder's needs. Will your Elder continue to live in his or her own home, move in with you, downsize to another home (perhaps near you), or go to assisted living? It will be so much easier on you if you support your Elder in doing what he or she wants to do. Whenever possible, the Elder's wishes come first. Check in with your own feelings about what you had always thought should be your proper role. An exception might be in the case of advanced dementia, in which your Elder has an unrealistic idea of his or her abilities to remain safely at home. Work with the Elder you have, not the person you want your Elder to be.

Whichever living situation your Elder chooses, your life has entered a time and space dimension that requires your vigilance and attention. Yes, your life is on hold. You won't be making any travel plans unless you arrange coverage by people you can trust and whom your Elder accepts. Fortunately and unfortunately, this situation won't go on forever.

As a caregiver, your chief concerns are around preventing the physical and social isolation of your Elder. This will be time-consuming whether you live near or far from your Elder. This will require you to be organized and resourceful and to manage your time well. Projects will remain unfinished, your home may be a bit messy, and you may miss out on some of the activities you enjoyed. You will need help. Help comes in many forms. Do you have a sibling who lives far from your Elder? Use their occasional visit as a bit of a respite for yourself. Let them know what to expect and let them know what you are doing on a daily basis. If you are the "local" child, you are doing most of the day-to-day work. Out-of-town siblings can provide emotional, financial, and social support with their visits and phone or video calls with your Elder. They can provide a fresh perspective and new ideas when they come to visit. Hire help when you can. Your parent may not accept a housekeeper; so maybe *you* should get a housekeeper so you can clean your Mom's house.

If you need to vent about your frustrations, and there will be many, I advise you to choose someone outside your family whom you can trust. A close friend who does not gossip is one good choice. A family counselor will have a kind ear and resourceful ideas. You can find one through your insurance coverage. Venting is important. Venting is sometimes about "unloading" on a sympathetic ear. Sometimes a good laugh will serve the purpose. This is a time when you need to take care of your heart, emotionally. Let other folks solve the world's problems in endless debates. Skip the heavy movies and downer novels.

I advise you to maintain good financial boundaries. I am assuming that you are honest and trustworthy, but others in your family may not be as generous as I. Keep good records. Save all your receipts. As bitter thanks for all your hard work, you may be called to account. You may want to give your siblings periodic reports on the income and expenses for your Elder. If you are charging for your time, keep excellent time records.

When you are both the Elder and the Care, you are typical among those caregiving. With our longer life spans, we are often seniors taking care of seniors. It is doubly important to take care of ourselves by getting help, emotionally, physically, and financially. We have a double load of dealing with our own waning physical stamina and our Elder's growing need for our support. We have an advantage, though. We typically have a long and close emotional connection with our Elder. As seniors ourselves, we have both sympathy and empathy for our Elder. We have some wisdom because we have been on the planet awhile. We have the shared experiences of friends and family who have gone before us.

As a society, ours is far less than ideal in supporting us in our elder-care. You may be wondering, where will you find all this "help" I keep mentioning? Every county in the United States has an Area Agency on Aging. You can look yours up online or at your local library. They all maintain directories of organizations and resources for services. It is kind of a Sears catalog for us elders. Ideally, you will find people you can meet with to help you find and plan and hire the resources you need at a level you can afford.

If you have health insurance through your employer, or if you are a member of AARP, ask them about senior services. For instance, Raytheon has an Employee Assistance Program, and one of the benefits involves providing a local social worker to do an in-home assessment of your Elder and recommend services that are realistic and attuned to the Elder's wishes. Be brave. Ask around. I hope that your search is rewarded with the help you need.

Reflections for Readers

1. What attitudes about aging and eldercare can we modify in ourselves as we, our parents, or our clients consider the inevitable end of the aging process?
2. What difference will it make to think, "My Dad's death was a really bad but inevitable situation long prepared for," as opposed to thinking, "My Dad's death was the worst crisis I will ever suffer and I will never recover from it"?
3. What strategies can we use to adapt to a loss? Where can we look for comfort or inspiration in the face of a loss?
4. What guidance would you offer to an elder deciding what kind of care he or she needs and what kind of caregiver can best provide it?
5. What factors should be considered in choosing a professional caregiver? Will this be different if the person making the choice is a child or other family member, rather than the elder himself or herself?
6. How might a family deal with a situation in which what an elder wants for care differs from what the family thinks the elder needs? This could relate to the level of care, or to who should provide the care.

CHAPTER 24

Dealing with Hearing and Vision Loss as We Age

Nancy Lelewer Sonnabend
Associate in Neurology, Harvard Medical
School (retired), and nonfiction writer
Boston, MA
Age 82

I am in my early 80s and continue to enjoy life, despite having significant hearing and vision problems. They represent challenges, but I have never let them define who I am, nor do I let them restrict my life. I enjoy life, and my hearing and vision problems are not going to change that.

It really wasn't a surprise when my hearing started to go. My mom began to lose her hearing in her 40s, and, as she aged, it got progressively worse. What was shocking to me was how I discovered the hearing loss in my left ear.

I was in my 60s when it happened. I was talking on the phone, which I had cradled between the right side of my head and my shoulder while I was writing with my right hand. I was getting a stiff neck, so I transferred the phone to my left side, where I heard nothing. I figured I must have been disconnected. I went to hang up the phone, but, as it passed in front of me, I heard a voice speaking, so I put the phone to my right ear and I had not been disconnected. Then I put the phone to my left ear, and there was total silence. I moved the phone from one ear to the other a couple of times because I could not believe it.

A few weeks later, a truck advertising free hearing screenings appeared on my street. I decided to enter. The tester asked me how my hearing was, and I said, "Fine."

After about 20 minutes, he came out and said, "You said your hearing is fine. Do you know you are practically deaf in your left ear?"

"I wasn't sure," I said.

It was a very lonely night. Then I said to myself, *You still have one good ear, so be happy about that,* and I was.

After my parents died, I went through a very stressful period and lost much of my hearing in my right ear, which up until this point was my "good" ear. I went to a well-known hospital for a hearing aid and a cochlear implant. I got the hearing aid, but for 15 years, I asked for a cochlear implant and was told I was not a candidate. I was never given a reason why. In fact, the head of the department told me he hoped I'd never get a cochlear implant.

Then I was elected to the national board of the Hearing Loss Association of America (HLAA). After my first board meeting, several board members took me aside and said, "You don't hear. Why have you never gotten a cochlear implant?" When I told them I wasn't a candidate, and the names of the doctors who were telling me that, they told me to go to Dr. Roland at NYU Cochlear Implant Center. Two months later, I had a cochlear implant and got my life back.

I was lucky that someone recommended Geoff Plant as the person to go to after having a cochlear implant. I knew he was from Australia, so I was worried about his accent. Thus, I signed up with him and with two others for auditory rehab. The other two I dropped within a month. Geoff I'm still seeing. He is, without question, the best in the world. And he is in Somerville, 10 minutes from my home. Sometimes one just gets lucky!

I'm still going to New York for my cochlear implant mapping (fine-tuning the electrodes), but instead of going once a month, which I did for the first year and a half, and then every three months, I'm now on six-month recall.

During the 15 years before I received my cochlear implant, I never stopped going to parties, lectures, musicals, and out to noisy restaurants. Often I would understand two words out of every paragraph, but I was not going to stay home and feel sorry for myself. I have tried to educate everyone I come in contact with of the need to face people with hearing loss and to speak a bit slower and more distinctly to us. Yelling doesn't help. On the contrary, it makes matters worse.

I have also been active in getting hearing loops (sometimes called *induction loops*) installed in major facilities in Boston: the City Council Room, the balconies at Boston's Symphony Hall, a room at the TD

Garden, a large room at Lesley University, a common room at Harvard Institute for Learning in Retirement, and several common rooms at retirement villages. A hearing loop system consists of a copper wire usually laid around the base of the room or in different configurations, depending on the area to be covered. The ends of the loop are connected to an amplifier, which takes the signal from a microphone or other sound input and creates a weak magnetic field with the signal superimposed on it. This signal in a looped room can be picked up wirelessly by people with T-coils (telecoils) on their hearing aids and/ or cochlear implants. The signal goes directly into their ears and eliminates background noise and/or reverberation. With a simple "flick of a switch," the person with hearing aids and/or cochlear implants gets rid of interfering noise and receives a clear signal. This makes listening so much easier. I have a loop system in my home, and it allows me much better access to my television, radio, and CD player. I can't imagine life without it.

For those with hearing loss, I recommend joining HLAA. It has a plethora of information on its website about ways to help people hear. Also, HLAA's local chapters around the country provide support for people with hearing loss and their families too. HLAA publishes an award-winning bimonthly magazine that is included with membership. Additionally, HLAA hosts a fantastic conference once a year for people with hearing loss, their families, and friends.

After several years of dealing with hearing loss, I was quite surprised when my ophthalmologist sent me to a retinal specialist in 2005. I was told I needed retinal surgery on my left eye. In the prior two months, I had lost both my parents; Dad at just short of 99, and Mom at 94. Although Mom had cataract surgery and my Dad had begun to develop macular degeneration in his mid-90s, I did not consider that they had eye problems. Having just turned 70, I was not about to have someone dig in my eye, knowing that during the surgery, I could lose my macula. Finally, after five years, I went to another retinal surgeon in Boston, and then one in New York. The latter recommended that I use the surgeon I'd just been to in Boston, whom she regarded highly.

I had the surgery, which has prevented the retina, thus far, from covering my macula. The surgery was not fun. I had to lie on my back for 45 minutes, without moving, while the surgeon scraped and then sutured my eye. In two-thirds of the cases, the anesthesia puts your eye and your optic nerve to sleep. I was part of the one-third, in which my optic nerve stayed awake, so I watched everything she did.

With my left eye, I have little central vision, but my peripheral vision is still good. I wear glasses with a prism on the left side, so that I don't see two different parts of the text when I read. It's an inconvenience, not a life-changing condition, and I still am able to maintain an active lifestyle.

My message, to those of us who are aging with hearing loss and/or vision problems, is to count your blessings. You can still walk, eat, enjoy the company of others, exercise, and learn about all the wonders of the world in which we live. Don't give up, and don't feel sorry for yourself, as there are many people our age unable to enjoy their lives because of extensive health and other challenges. Greet each day with a smile, and make the most of it.

Reflections for Readers

1. What unique difficulties do older adults with hearing and vision problems face?
2. What kind of psychological and social impact might hearing and vision problems have in older adulthood?
3. What resources are available to seniors to compensate for declines in hearing and vision? What psychological adjustments are required to accommodate to these sensory declines?
4. What does this author's narrative suggest about the most productive ways to approach hearing and vision problems in older age?

CHAPTER 25

Adaptations

Irving I. Silverman
Business Manager, Publication Division,
National Knitwear Association and
Proprietor of the Kosher Food and Jewish Life Expo (retired)
Dedham, MA
Age 97

I was born with very poor vision—and my parents got me glasses. All of a sudden, the world that had existed in a blur became clearer.

As I have aged, my hearing has gone from bad to worse—and after some internal struggle, I agreed to try hearing aids. Amazing: I could interact so much better with those around me when I could hear what they were saying!

After I underwent surgery for a brain tumor at age 89, my children encouraged me to move from the two homes I maintained to a retirement community. In their opinion, going from one home to the other was too much wear and tear on me, and neither home was near any of them. I said NO!—but after thinking it over, I began to realize the advantages for me of taking their advice. In my own houses, I was alone much of the time, and depended on others to take me places (I don't drive). In a retirement community, I would be surrounded by peers, with cultural and educational programs right there in the community, no need to go anywhere else. Though moving took me away from many friends and familiar institutions, I have still been able to stay in contact through email and phone, and the move introduced me to a new circle of people and institutions to care about. I ended up with *more* people in my life!

In my 90s, my balance has become precarious. At first, I rejected the idea of using a cane—I didn't want to "look like an invalid"—but the cane did help me keep steady . . . and when the cane was not enough, after initial protests on my part, I progressed to a walker. Now I can get around wherever I need to go . . . and isn't that the point, that getting around is more important than what mechanisms we use to do it?

Aging can bring changes in your energy level, tiredness, and physical endurance; it certainly has for me. My recourse has been to consult with my doctor. When she recommended a physical therapy evaluation and an occupational therapy checkup, I took advantage of those resources, especially since I knew they could help me avoid falls. (As you age, fall occurrences are more prevalent. You may need to make changes in your home environment, such as removing loose rugs and clutter, to prevent yourself from falling; most falls take place in the home.) And another resource I found on my own: when I am tired, I take a nap!

Instead of focusing on the "poor me" of what I can no longer do (or, in the case of my vision, what I could never do), I have shifted my focus to how I can adapt. There is nothing wrong with improving vision or hearing with eyeglasses or hearing aids; there is nothing wrong with improving mobility via a cane, walker, wheelchair, or scooter. Many people use these aids.

And that brings me to the subject of aides, people who can help us function better. Like many, I initially resisted the idea of employing an aide. What would that person *do* all day; how would I keep an aide busy? After I tried it, I found that many of the annoying little tasks that had filled my time could be done by someone else—often, more efficiently than by me—freeing me up for things I like more. I also found that having someone around can be a comfort and a pleasure.

I try to think about "how can I *best* function?" and look for tools that help me do just that. What I want others to understand here is that the overriding "tool" for adapting to aging is maintaining a positive attitude. That's not always easy to do. Along with glasses, hearing aids, canes, and the like, I have learned to turn to others, both friends and professionals, for help in dealing with the sadnesses that life sometimes brings. We seniors want to—and can—live full and rewarding lives. Using all the tools available to us, and maintaining positivity, are the best ways for us to do that.

Reflections for Readers

1. Why might an older adult initially resist aids for walking, vision, or hearing?

2. What does this author's story suggest about the best way to introduce such aids in seniors' lives?

3. How might keeping a positive attitude help someone to cope with physical limitations? How can one foster such an attitude, even in the face of stress and hardship?

4. How can one avoid blaming oneself for nonexistent or lost capacities, and how can others help one deal with such feelings?

CHAPTER 26

Brooding

Monica McAlpine, PhD

Professor Emerita of English, University of Massachusetts, Boston

Brighton, MA

Age 76

Would it suck the marrow

out of my porous bones?

But I am not so leathery

I couldn't balloon up.

I could lug it around, too.

I've got the back muscles.

Would I go natural?

No sense risking a stroke.

Let them cut it out.

Then the milk would flow.

At seventy, to breed—

a state of pure desire.

Only the eggs are old.

First published in *Poetry Quarterly*, Spring 2015, #22

Reflections for Readers

1. What feelings are conveyed in this poem?
2. What does this poem suggest about growing older?

3. Pregnancy is not an experience that one associates with elders, but how might you use the loss of the ability to become pregnant as a metaphor for other losses that occur in one's later life?

4. The author suggests that, despite aging, one retains important capacities, but one still needs to be careful. How might you apply those two opposing factors, continuing capacity and carefulness, to other situations more typical of the aging population?

5. To what extent can you relate to themes expressed in this poem?

PART V

Using Internal Strengths

CHAPTER 27

Becoming a Good Listener

Stephen Colwell, MBA
Executive Director, NewBridge on the Charles
Dedham, MA

When teaching classes on communication, I often ask, "Who here doesn't know how to listen?" The class giggles a little nervously, and, of course, no one raises a hand.

The simple fact is that we all know how to listen, but we often fail to realize that hearing is not the same as listening. Hearing involves receiving sound, whereas listening involves *understanding.* Merriam-Webster defines the word *listen* as "to hear something with thoughtful attention."

What makes a person a good listener? I've seen many decent suggestions, such as "Stop talking," "Remove distractions," etc. Learning to understand what is being said is obviously very important as well. But I think the most distinctive attribute for a good listener is the ability to empathize with the speaker—to *connect* with the speaker.

Too often, one listens to respond. One lives with the hope that an interesting *bon mot* will convince the other of the weakness of their position. Many listen like the other person is an opponent on the other side of a chessboard. Every move will create a countermove to place an opinion on the defensive. In a debate, some defend well; others are aggressive, but the goal is to never lose, and in rare cases, to actually pummel the opponent into submission. To secure victory, in a sense, is to stave off being wrong for another time. For me, I get a nice little adrenaline rush, as I am very good at debates.

But I found there was a cost for me—a cost so great that I wept when I realized what it was. For every submissive opponent, there was an abandonment of the conversation. It wasn't that I was right so much as the other person was saying, "Enough already, I don't want to do this anymore. It's not fun and *you are not listening anyway.*"

My compelling arguments, my *need* to be right, were no longer being heard. I could have been speaking to a wall for all of the effect I was creating. My adrenaline rush would be inadequate to satisfy my junkielike need to win the debate. I would press on, harder, more determined. Some would walk away, while others would fully engage, testing my tenacity. My needs trumped all.

I lost friendships and family members from this drive. And when I realized that *I* was the only reason this had happened, I cried. My habit of winning was costing me everything I held dear. I knew if I continued, I might lose my wife and my kids. No one wishes to be the submissive one in any conversation. Yet, I was insisting on it with everyone around me. I know I wouldn't put up with it; why should they?

Good listening, particularly when the stakes are high, is heavy lifting. Anyone can give voice to their opinions, but it takes special skill to listen when what is being said runs contrary to one's beliefs. To actually suspend your views in order to stay connected with the speaker is very difficult.

After the tears, I don't know if I got lucky or if I was finally in a place where I could actually listen, but I started to recognize that the greater goal of communication was to create a connection. I knew that I didn't need to agree with other people to learn and grow from what they were saying. I realized that others could contribute to me if I gave them space to do so. Ironically, in creating that space, I also found that I could be heard. When another speaker can sense that I listen with true empathy and connection, he/she will *feel* the relationship and will be capable of listening better to my views.

The most ironic part of this journey is that the very pain I inflicted on others and the pain I received from their subsequent indifference to me allow me to be compassionate and present to anyone who struggles with listening. Been there, done that—and regretted it deeply. I choose to make it a practice to listen to those I used to leave unheard, regardless of their views, no matter how difficult it may be for me to hear what they have to say.

I've come to learn how to listen behind what is being said, to glean the core of one's views. I've become an explorer of others' worlds, deeply curious about what makes a person who he or she is. As someone once said to me, a complaint is never about what is being complained about, it's about a deeper need. I try to listen into that.

I have had people open up to me in ways that I never thought possible. I had one woman sitting next to me on an airplane talk about the baby she gave up for adoption. A man told me about his failing business.

Another, a divorce. Still another person described the agonizing pain she felt when her husband died prematurely, and suddenly she needed to support her two young kids. In every case, I didn't state my views, give advice, or even say, "I know how you feel" (not that anyone can ever know how another person feels). I simply listened in silence and awe of the person sitting next to me, recognizing the sacred moment I was experiencing.

Every person I've ever met longs to be heard, to be understood . . . to be loved unconditionally. Listening is one of the most intimate gifts one can ever give another. I say that it is the true source of love. Listening can heal wounds. Listening can bring comfort to the distressed. Listening determines the quality of every relationship.

Reflections for Readers

1. What is the difference between hearing and listening?
2. What is the role of empathic connection in becoming a good listener? What can someone do to increase the ability to listen empathically?
3. What is difficult about being a good listener?
4. How might you become a better listener in your professional and personal life?
5. How might being a good listener contribute to positive aging?

28

Developing the Skill of Optimism

Nicholas A. Covino, PsyD
President, William James College
Newton, MA

Does the perspective that you have on the world matter? If it does, what are some of the consequences of a predominantly positive or negative point of view? If there are advantages to a particular outlook, can that perspective be altered and improved?

Psychology is a complex discipline, with theories that regularly change and empirical research that continues to expand our fund of information. A prevalent model of stress and illness, for example, was developed by the research team of Thomas Holmes and Richard Rahe (1967), who assigned a numerical value to a list of positive (e.g., holiday) and negative (e.g., death of a spouse) stressful events that they called Life Change Units (LCUs). In their investigations, they found that individuals with medical illnesses often had experienced one or more LCUs prior to the onset of illness.

The researchers created a rating scale that posited the likelihood of developing a subsequent medical illness based on the number of LCUs experienced from a low of below 150 to a high of above 300. Later, the cognitive psychologist Richard Lazarus and his colleague Susan Folkman (1984) made the important distinction that it is not the kind or even the degree of adversity in the life event, but the meaning that the person gives to it (appraisal) that determines its impact.

The birth of a child, a promotion at work, or filing for a divorce could each be the best life experience for someone—or it could be the worst. The assessment that the person attributes to the event, not the apparent severity of it, will determine whether any psychological stress is experienced by the individual, and if so, how much.

For quite some time, psychologists believed that the individual's perspective on the world was universal and, mostly, fixed. They gave the name "traits" to these supposedly immutable aspects of personality that would influence the person's thoughts and behaviors, independent of circumstances. Those who, for example, held that they and others can influence most of life's outcomes were described by Julian Rotter (1954) as believers in *internal locus of control.*

When life events are judged to determine the human being's state of mind and quality of life, people believe in *external locus of control.* A positive outcome for the former group is considered to be the end product of careful study, practice, talent, or preparation. On the other hand, subscribers to external locus of control attribute success to factors such as good fortune or team effort.

Research finds that people fall along a continuum between these two poles, and that emotional, behavioral, and health consequences are associated with the position that they hold. For example, those with internal locus of control tend to be achievement oriented, overly prepared, and perform better when they are allowed to work at their own pace. Their mood is more optimistic, and they are prone to take care of their physical condition. External-locus-of-control individuals are more tentative, are more easily influenced by others, and tend to blame others or circumstances for their failures. Pessimism is a regular partner for these people.

It is not only beauty that is in the eye of the beholder, but threat, danger, and adversity; embracing one or more of these perspectives will lead to predictable physiological responses and expectable mood and health consequences. Whether the person sees the glass as half-full (optimism) or half-empty (pessimism) has an impact upon health and psychological well-being. Physically healthy individuals who have an angry, pessimistic perspective are prone to develop heart disease in relation to the degree of their negative emotions (Jenkins, 1971; Tindle et al., 2009; Williams et al., 2000).

The research on the contribution of anger to the occurrence of heart disease has been so compelling, in fact, that health care professionals now view the risk factors associated with negative emotions at the same level as smoking and obesity (APA, 2003).

Early work in psychosomatic medicine established the link between perceived danger, sustained physiological arousal, and physical illness. Patients who see danger, whether real or imagined, trigger a complex autonomic nervous system process involving hormones and neurotransmitters (i.e., fight/flight response) that alarms and activates the cardiovascular, respiratory, genitourinary, and digestive systems (Cannon, 1932; Selye, 1956). Among patients who already have medical disorders such as asthma, irritable bowel syndrome, and pain, stress adds to the symptom picture. Among those without chronic medical illness, the perception of threat can lead to problems such as insomnia, chest pain, functional gastrointestinal pain, and shortness of breath (Covino, 2008). When people are chronically frustrated in their effort to escape or master threat or pain, they learn to become helpless and develop depression (Seligman, 1972).

Cognitive psychologists assert that the cart before the horse known as depression is the manner in which the individual views self and circumstances; depression doesn't lead to low self-esteem, they believe; it is created by the thinking style of the person. Pessimistic views of one's worth (e.g., "I am an unlovable failure") or the outcomes that one can expect from the world ("The world is unfair") or the future ("Things are unlikely to get better") serve as the interpretive lenses for people that can lead to self-fulfilling prophesies. This triad of dysfunctional beliefs about self, the environment, and the future produce automatic thoughts within the individual who come to catastrophize, personalize, and overgeneralize adverse life-events (Beck, Rush, Shaw, & Emery, 1979).

Fortunately, a good deal of research finds that people can be helped to revise these negative perspectives and ameliorate their adverse consequences. Cognitive behavioral therapy (CBT) includes a number of interventions that can lessen the "automatic" quality of a patient's dysfunctional beliefs, teach people to confront and revise their thinking, and encourage them to experiment with new behaviors (Beck, 1995). This is not an exercise in exhortation, but it is an educational process in which errors in logic are identified, challenged, tested, and reconstructed. Patients are asked to record their thoughts and beliefs, examine the evidence in support or in opposition to them, consider alternative explanations to their dysfunctional beliefs, and experiment with holding and conducting alternate conclusions and behaviors. Tendencies of thinking toward using overgeneralization, catastrophic evaluation, and self-criticism are identified, and the individual learns to reframe his or her perspective on self, the environment, and the future in a more positive fashion.

The research and writing of M. E. P. Seligman and his colleagues extend this work on cognition and behavior change. They label perspective and perception as "explanatory style" (Seligman & Nolen-Hoeksema,

1987). Similar to other theorists, they propose that people who see adverse events as caused by their action or inaction ("My driving is terrible") as opposed to the environment ("Boy, those Boston drivers are maniacs"), or as stable (enduring) versus rare and unlikely to be repeated in the future, commonly experience depression and develop physical illnesses.

They propose that people identify the weaknesses in their attributional style and take corrective action by challenging and changing their perspectives and analysis. However, Seligman takes this work on cognitive restructuring further to propose that people can be taught to develop optimism (Seligman, 2004) and to develop a more positive psychology (Seligman & Csikszentmihalyi, 2000).

Since their research finds that those who "quit trying" tend to believe that adverse events are due to their shortcomings or are likely to be permanent, positive psychologists encourage people to continue to argue with their pessimistic thoughts. In addition, in classrooms, workshops, and writings, positive psychologists help their students to identify their signature strengths (what one is good at or enjoys doing) and exhort them to live an engaged and productive life. These are not intellectual exercises, but planned events. "Gratitude visits," for example, are opportunities to thank others for the positive contributions that they have made in one's life.

Signature strengths and personal values can be derived from self-reflection or a questionnaire, and they become vehicles for the individual's intentional acts. Pleasure, which is an end point that can be derived from passive pursuits like alcohol or daydreaming, is distinguished from the target goal of gratification that is the result of an investment of oneself in a productive activity. Optimists seek opportunities to practice their personal strengths in noble pursuits. As they develop a real sense of mastery over their environment, a sense of gratitude, and the gratification from making the lives of others and the world a better place, they build their capacity for optimism.

As optimism grows, it serves to protect the individual against episodes of depression and the adverse physical conditions associated with discordant mood (Seligman, 2004; Seligman & Csikszentmihalyi, 2000). Seligman and the positive psychologists are currently celebrated for recalibrating the focus of clinical psychology from that of pathology to positivism.

The perspective that one has about personal value or ability, the individual's sense of permanence and fairness in the environment and belief in the likelihood that the future will bring opportunity and reward are all shaped by parents, family life, and personal experience. Negative thinking along these lines can lead to depression and physical illness. An optimistic point of view is not achieved by acquiring a pair of rose-colored glasses, but by a life of dedication to correcting dysfunctional thinking, identifying one's strengths, practicing gratitude and respect, and working to improve the world. This kind of a noble life brings emotional, health, and social benefits for the individual and for the community. Students of most religious traditions have seen these ideas before!

Reflections for Readers

1. How might the aging process of an optimist differ from that of a pessimist?
2. Why might some older adults have difficulty maintaining a positive attitude?
3. How might you begin to develop or strengthen the skill of optimism in your life?
4. What key factors determine whether a given life event creates or relieves stress?
5. Do you believe "gratitude visits" can have a positive impact on one's life? How?

References

American Psychological Association. (2003). Hostility is among best predictors of heart disease in men. *Monitor on Psychology, 34,* 15.

Beck, A. T., Rush, A. J., Shaw, B. F., & Emery, G. (1979). *Cognitive therapy of depression.* New York, NY: Guilford Press.

Beck, J. S. (1995). *Cognitive therapy: Basics and beyond.* New York, NY: Guilford Press.

Cannon, W. B. (1932). *The wisdom of the body.* New York, NY: Norton.

Covino, N. A. (2008). Medical illnesses, conditions, and procedures. In M. R. Nash & A. Barnier (Eds.), *Oxford handbook of hypnosis; Theory, research and practice.* Oxford, UK: Oxford University Press.

Holmes, T. H., & Rahe, R. H. (1967). The social readjustment rating scale. *Journal of Psychosomatic Research, 11*(2), 213–218.

Jenkins, C. D. (1971). Psychologic and social precursors of coronary disease (first of two parts). *New England Journal of Medicine, 284*(5), 244–255.

Lazarus, R. S., & Folkman, S. (1984). *Stress, appraisal, and coping.* New York, NY: Springer.

Rotter, J. B. (1954). *Social learning and clinical psychology.* New York: Prentice-Hall.

Seligman, M. E. P. (1972). Learned helplessness. *Annual Review of Medicine, 23*(1): 407–412.

Seligman, M. E. P. (2004). Can happiness be taught? *Daedalus, 133,* 80–87.

Seligman, M. E. P., & Csikszentmihalyi, M. (2000). Positive psychology: An introduction. *American Psychologist, 55*(1), 5–14.

Seligman, M. E. P., & Nolen-Hoeksema, S. (1987). Explanatory style and depression. In D. Magnusson & A. Ohman, *Psychopathology: An interactional perspective* (pp. 125–139). New York, NY: Academic Press.

Selye, H. (1956). *The stress of life.* New York, NY: McGraw-Hill.

Tindle, H. A., Chang, Y. F., Kuller, L. H., Manson, J. E., Robinson, J. G., Rosal, M. C., . . ., Matthews, K. A. (2009). Optimism, cynical hostility, and incident coronary heart disease and mortality in the Women's Health Initiative. *Circulation, 120*(8), 656–662.

Williams, J. E., Paton, C. C., Siegler, I. C., Eigenbrodt, M. L., Nieto, F. J., & Tyroler, H. A. (2000). Anger proneness predicts coronary heart disease risk prospective analysis from the Atherosclerosis Risk In Communities (ARIC) study. *Circulation, 101,* 2034–2039.

CHAPTER 29

Making Each Day Count

Justin L. Wyner, MBA

Chairman Emeritus, Shawmut Corporation

Dedham, MA

Age 91

A few years before my father passed away at the age of 89, in 1984, I had the occasion to be with him when he felt an unfamiliar pain. Over the telephone, his doctor suggested that he go by ambulance to the hospital. When we arrived in the ER, the doctor attending asked me, "Your father is 87, Mr. Wyner, does he understand everything you say to him?" I responded with some annoyance that of course my father understood everything he would say to him; he could still recite every play of Shakespeare's.

The doctor went into the examining room and, leaning over my father, who was still lying on a gurney, he asked in a condescending way, "What do you want me to do, Mr. Wyner, make you younger?" and my father responded with words that will always be with me: "Younger I have been, Doctor. Make me older."

My father made every hour of every day worthy of enjoyment or experiencing. When he finally died, two years later, it was of lymphoma. We did things together to the end. Two weeks before he passed away, we had been fly fishing for trout. And my father was only following the example of *his* father, who died early one morning in his 80s while preparing to go fishing at 5 a.m., before making his daily trip to his office at 18 Tremont Street in Boston.

And so I have had those examples to follow. As one gets older, I believe that it is necessary to continue to look for new challenges that will give you a reason to get up and out of bed every morning, as the old challenges are often picked up by those who are younger and more in a position to take them on. Better yet, if at all possible, don't give way to the younger generation—just allow them in. I find working side by side with younger people keeps me more active and more open to the amazing discoveries and developments that are happening every day and then able to apply them, perhaps in some way that will be helpful to others who might be in need.

Some 40 years ago, when digital watches were in their infancy, Citizens Watch, a Japanese digital watch company, came out with a special watch designed for sailboat racing. At the time, Genevieve and I had a sailboat that we kept at the New Bedford Yacht Club in Padanaram, Massachusetts, and were participating in the club's weekly informal races. I thought that this new watch would be of great assistance to us on those Wednesday afternoons, and was about to purchase one, when I noticed in the specifications that it was not waterproof. "Who needs a sailboat racing watch that will die the first time we take in a bit of water?" reasoned I. I started calling the U.S. telephone numbers of the Japanese company to ask when and if they would have a waterproof version. I finally received a return call from the U.S. Vice President of Citizens, who said to me, "Of course, we will eventually have a waterproof version, but Mr. Wyner, if you keep looking ahead at the possible future version of watches that might be better for you, you will die before you buy your next watch."

And with that, I had an epiphany that has guided me ever since. When there is a new version of an Apple phone, iPad, watch, or what have you, I am up at 3 a.m. on the opening day of sales and on the Internet when it becomes 12:01 a.m. in Apple's headquarters in Cupertino, California, to put in the first order and get the first delivery . . . and so it has gone with the first Segway in Boston, Tesla model S number 805 (almost the first in Boston), and all sorts of other things that continue to challenge me to understand and get with every day. It has certainly made each day promise to be more exciting than the day before. And it gives me another reason to do my very best to keep the physical gift that God has given me—my body—in the best condition that a commitment to daily exercise and sensible eating can provide.

Some of us are more fortunate than others, but I have been blessed to know people who are very physically challenged and have led wonderful and full lives, pushing what gifts and abilities they have every day. I must confess, I really hate my morning workouts, but I continue them every day because I believe that doing them is the difference between life and death . . . and every day when I come home from those exercises, I actually find myself much more alert and energized to face the day and enjoy the opportunities it offers, a sharp contrast to the way I feel on the occasional day that I miss my workout. So, for me, when I wake up to begin a new day, it is with much gratitude and anticipation as to what new challenge this new day will bring to me. Life can continue to be exciting as long as we live! But *we* have to make it happen!

Reflections for Readers

1. Why do you think it is so important to this author to stay current with the latest technology?
2. Why might it be important for an older adult to maintain contact with younger generations?
3. What can others do to help seniors live fully and experience optimism?
4. How can you work to make every day in your life count?
5. Is it possible to enjoy the experience of getting older? Why or why not?

CHAPTER 30

Mastering the Art of Aging

Irving I. Silverman
Business Manager, Publication Division,
National Knitwear Association and
Proprietor of the Kosher Food and Jewish Life Expo (retired)
Dedham, MA
Age 97

It's easy—just decide you want to accomplish it. You'll need the will and determination. Wake up each morning after a good night's sleep and think how fortunate you are to be alive and well. Then think about all the wonderful things you can do today. What new things are you ready to explore? If the weather is acceptable, put on an outer jacket, a hat, and a pair of sunglasses and you're ready for a pleasant hike or walk. If you planned ahead yesterday and invited a friend to accompany you, you're set to enjoy the bounty of nature and a spirited conversation on any topic of your mutual choice.

Then, visit the fitness center or gym for a brisk 40 minutes of exercise to awaken your muscles and joints. A cup of coffee, tea, or hot chocolate, with or without any accompaniment, alone or with a companion, might be a pleasant wake-up treat. What else is your pleasure? A half-hour with the morning newspaper or listening to the news on radio or TV might bring you up to date on the morning news to keep abreast of what interests you.

I haven't mentioned your choice of a healthy breakfast in a café or your home, depending on your choice of company or solitude. Either one will please you and will gladden your appetite. Then, look at the list of available activities you have recorded as possible events to enjoy today. Here, we go back to the need to plan some things to occupy you for mental or physical stimulation.

Let me interject a thought here to overcome the possibility of having nothing to do and being unhappy or bored. The key here is planning. You need to accept the responsibility of *planning* to do the things that interest and please you. That's not to say that you have to be busy every minute of every day, but to avoid boredom and lethargy and to avoid missing out on programs that would interest you, you need to plan ahead.

If you have access to a daily, weekly, or monthly schedule of activities, take advantage of this schedule. Avoid the possibility of overscheduling yourself to be like a whirling dervish and tiring yourself. There's a difference between intelligently scheduling yourself and imposing unwelcome stress on yourself. That wouldn't be fun, and it actually might be harmful, creating exhaustion rather than a positive living experience.

Now that we have covered the advantage of planning, let's move on to "doing." What interests you, what activities do you enjoy most? Attending music programs, lectures, field trips, social interaction, engaging in political discussions, reading, watching movies, attending concerts, doing any kind of crafts, hobbies—make your own list. Include some things you've never done and want to try out, such as playing bridge or other games or trying a sport. That's mastering the art of aging.

So are meeting new friends, trying new foods, exploring new experiences. These are all parts of the jigsaw puzzle of enriching your life. A word of caution: don't overburden yourself by trying too many things at the same time. There is joy in trying new things and being with new people. Slow down; you have a rich lifetime ahead of you, and if you will it, it can happen.

Mastering the art of aging is a challenging concept. Consider some of the suggestions of your peers, and even your children. You may have always told them how to live their lives. Good ideas can come from many people and sources; listen to them and benefit from them. You may also benefit from some of the ideas in this book, coming from those who are already in their older years, from psychologists who work with seniors, and from others who are in a position to know and help. Take advantage of the professionals available to you. We're all living in an era of positive change and growth.

That's not to say that all is well and worth absorbing in our society, but fortunately we can benefit from the dynamic improvements provided by medical technology. We may get confused at times by the conflicting stream of advice and information that envelops us, but rest assured we will survive. Sort out the pluses and minuses of living. Choose the path of positive psychology and you, your children, and your grandchildren will forge a new future. And we may be afforded a longer life span than our parents and ancestors; believe it, it's true!

Living longer is certainly on the horizon. Now comes the challenge to live better, healthier, and more productively. We can and must accomplish it! Mastering aging is the goal toward which each of us must aspire.

Tomorrow is only a few years away, and you, the readers of this book, will make yesterday only a remembrance. Onward!

Reflections for Readers

1. What additional "keys" might you suggest to mastering the art of aging?
2. How might simple pleasures be incorporated throughout the day to enrich one's life?
3. What is the risk of overburdening oneself with activities?
4. How does one sort between the value of "living well" and "living long"? What do you believe constitutes a good life?

CHAPTER 31

Accepting Rejection: Finding Meaningful Replacement of What One Doesn't or Can't Have

Caryn B. Finard

Stay-at-home mom (retired)
Dedham, MA

Webster's Dictionary defines *rejection* as "to refuse affection or recognition to a person." It is a long and arduous journey to accepting rejection, and it takes many paths along the way.

It can be difficult to trust people when they are hurting or rejecting us. We have to start by setting boundaries and holding people accountable for their behavior. We have to set limits and let people know that it is not acceptable to cast us off or cause us pain. Dealing with someone who denies us our right to be treated with respect and dignity, we need to put that person in his or her place. Asserting ourselves—having a voice—gives us a sense of power and a feeling of well-being.

We all should have the privilege to think of ourselves as whole and complete just the way we are. We don't have to justify our existence or behavior. What we *do* have to do is step up to the plate, continue on and *believe* that we are worthy of being loved, all while being cognizant that we belong in a world that challenges us and sometimes makes us doubt and blame ourselves for others' injustices and callousness. We often feel that we are not valued. It is then that we have to take a long and hard look at ourselves and maintain our confidence that we are able and competent beings. Self-confidence is a powerful tool for "rejecting" rejection.

We need connections with people to grow and flourish. Connection affects our experiences. The more connected we are with others, the better we feel about ourselves—and them. Connection contributes to a better life.

It is simpler to accept rejection when we learn that we have some control over those who attempt to reject us. Then, when we take a stand and are refused affection or recognition, we can still rely on our own self-worth to continue to feel valuable.

Taking another look at what we experience when rejected, we feel *hurt*. This emotion can be paralyzing. It is painful and unrelenting. We wonder, "What did I do wrong?" "What did I do to cause this person to rebuff me?" What often follows is the "blame game." This is when the recipient feels it is his or her fault and problem that a rejection occurred.

Some of these reactions to rejection are coping mechanisms that aid the griever to survive and find eventual acceptance to rejection.

As we grow older, we often find that we are more tolerant of others not agreeing with us, not liking every decision we make, or not showing interest in us. Age frequently brings the wisdom that not everyone will like us or be interested in us. In essence, though we are "rejected," we have developed the strength and—yes—the wisdom to realize that *we* don't like or enjoy everyone either, and that does not make those others bad or worthless individuals. It just makes for a situation where we all have our preferences and move in the direction of what pleases us.

Rejection hurts more at younger ages because everything seems "life or death." As we get older, one advantage is that we worry less about the world loving us and focus more on the people and activities that really matter; and if someone does not like or love us, that is not a problem worth worrying about.

Rejection is okay! It gives us more room to pursue those who truly love us and situations that matter to us. Rejection frees us up for better things and better relationships.

When we reach out to someone who doesn't reach back, it's time to go on with our lives and tell ourselves we are okay. There'll be others who appreciate us just as we are.

Finding replacements for what we don't have or can't have offers many options. Look for ways to plug the hole of pain.

When rejected, take time for yourself. Weeping is therapeutic. It provides an outlet for your emotions.

Concentrate on positive relationships: people who value and appreciate you. Take the time to do things with those with whom you can share joy and fulfillment. Enjoy a movie together, go to a concert, or share a book reading. When you let the person you're with know that he or she counts, you are making a difference.

Animals can be a source of comfort and balance. They make us feel needed and exude unconditional love. Go to a shelter, adopt a pet, and nurture it. Often a pet and its owner bond and become loyal "pals." Taking walks in the park with your dog, going to the beach together, dodging the waves, feeling the surf trickling between your toes; all these contribute to feelings of pleasure and joy.

See the beauty in each and every day! Enjoy, count your blessings. There's a lot to be grateful for!

Revel at the gift of a majestic sunset. Feel the sun's rays permeating the air. Listen to the balmy whistling wind penetrating your soul.

Have fun. Throw caution to the wind. Celebrate your life and be self-indulgent. Go out and buy something luxurious and outrageous.

No one likes to feel unimportant, uncared for, or invisible. Do something for someone else that contributes to his or her happiness and your self-esteem. Help others experience *joie de vivre*. You will get back more than you give.

Music soothes the soul. Go to a concert, sing in the shower, play your favorite tunes. Feel enriched. These are all life enrichers that help us come out the other side. It is not about making things the same, but rather adventures that help us move forward with life.

Reflections for Readers

1. How might one's experience of rejection differ in older versus younger adulthood? Does our tolerance for handling rejections change as we age?
2. What might we learn from rejection?
3. What resources are key to handling rejection?
4. What is the relationship between how others see us and how we see ourselves?
5. What can we do to strengthen our self-image?

PART **VI**

Broadening Horizons

© James Whitesmith/Moment/Getty

CHAPTER 32

The Benefits of Volunteering as an Older Person

John Averell, PhD
Physicist, Polaroid Corporation (retired)
Dedham, MA
Age 82

When I retired from my job in 2000 as a computer software developer, life changed dramatically, as it does for most. I wasn't getting paid for doing anything anymore!

Most of my life, I did a lot of volunteering. Sang in the church choir, played my French horn, first in church, then in symphonies and bands up until 2015. I volunteered my time on a senior website (created by the MIT Media Lab) from 2001 until 2014 as an editor and technical computer support person. When I moved to NewBridge on the Charles in 2010, other opportunities opened up as editor-in-chief of *The Bridge Journal,* and in several capacities as expert computer support in various organizations.

So the questions arise: Why volunteer, what do I get from it, does this really help me as I grow older, with the health and memory problems that seem to accompany just about everyone? What are the benefits, and to whom? What does it cost me to volunteer?

The concept of volunteering is that you are giving your time to work for an individual or organization without direct financial compensation. There are some positions, notably "internships," that do have longer-term compensations for the volunteer: experience and professional contacts that in future may result in a better job. As you grow "older," into the over-70 range, it seems unlikely that this motivation dominates.

A primary benefit to a volunteer is personal satisfaction in helping others. Perhaps you are motivated from a religious "commandment" or *mitzvah.*[1] The so-called Golden Rule is apparently a universal principle in all major religions and ethical societies—namely, to do for others what you would have them do for you.

At this point, I refer to my own religious background as a Christian on this principle. When Jesus is asked by a lawyer, "Who is my neighbor?" he replies with the well-known parable of the Good Samaritan. After the instructive story illustrating the point, the answer is clear: Your neighbor is whomever you are able to help. Wherever you are, whatever your religion, your time, effort, or money can be volunteered to help someone in need.

Accompanying this commandment often is a reminder that you should not do good expecting either a reward or public recognition for the deed. This seems to me an excellent basis for volunteering, one that can continue from youth through very old age. It can be manifested in different ways at different ages, as ability and opportunities arise.

Being part of a large retirement community opens one's eyes to finding ways to volunteer your time for the good of others, as well as your own satisfaction. We become aware that any troubles of our own are almost invariably similar to others around us. There are opportunities to make new friends, eat dinner with them, commiserate with their problems, and offer help in many ways. These are volunteer activities that mean a great deal not only to others, but also to yourself.

But what does it cost to be a volunteer? *Commitment* is the requirement. Once having started on a good deed, you need to continue on as long as needed or promised to finish your job. This turns out to be harder and harder as you enter and progress through older years. After all, you want to relax, to enjoy the fruits of your labor (hopefully there are some), and to do what you planned to do "when I have time." So be careful what you volunteer for!

Consider the reference above to the Good Samaritan. He took the trouble to cross the street to care for the injured man, took him to an inn, and paid the innkeeper to feed and house him. He came back the next day to pay the bill and said he would return later to pay any additional charges. In returning, he demonstrated commitment.

Commitment also means giving up some of your own time for a promised obligation. As you grow older, although time is more available

---

[1]In Jewish law, "mitzvah" is translated both as "commandment" and "good deed."

(barring medical appointments), the desire to stick to a volunteer job may be hard. Again, I refer to a New Testament comment from the Apostle Paul to the church in Galatia that he founded: "And let us not be weary in well doing: for in due season we shall reap, if we faint not."

What additional benefits accrue to us older volunteers? By nature and evolution, we are a social species. We tend to wither away and become depressed when cut off from others. It can become too easy to simply sit in our room on our favorite chairs, watch TV, read a book, eat alone. These are good things in moderation, but seriously debilitating if that is all of life as we age.

Volunteering usually guarantees that we get out and interact with other people. We have to think about someone else. Having personal goals that are larger than personal comfort, or even personal education, is part of staying human. Everyone I see or hear of who is in their 90s or 100s is participating in group efforts. They may be just dancing or singing together, organized or not, but it involves them with other people.

Last is a concern that many people face, or should face but don't. Sometimes it is *better to pass the torch.* This comes from my own experiences.

I was a musician almost all my life. After retirement, I stepped down from the Melrose Symphony Orchestra, simply because I could no longer play my horn well enough. So I joined the Wakefield Retired Men's Club Band. Perfect! I played an alto horn well enough. I became a co-conductor of the band in 2002. I really loved conducting. But after entering NewBridge, I had to drive 27 miles to a 9:30 a.m. rehearsal in Wakefield along Rte. 128—a brutal drive in commuter traffic. Finally, with new eye trouble, I had to leave this volunteer group. But I had been careful to help recruit and train new co-conductors.

I loved being part of the *Melrose Mirror,* a senior monthly website magazine. The underlying software to run this (still) successful site is now very outdated, but so well constructed by MIT that it can be run by members with minimal technical expertise. Unfortunately, I became the only person who really understood the code and how it all works. I moved from Melrose in 2004, but continued to participate remotely from wherever I lived until about 2014. I realized that unless one of the local Melrose volunteers could continue running the site, it would fail at some point. I worked hard for years to educate successors, but finally have had to withdraw support so that someone will catch on, or the *Mirror* will gracefully cease.

The point is, if your successful volunteer work has made you indispensable to an organization that is meant to continue on without you, you must recognize that, at some point, a successor needs to be found and trained. It is hard to step away sometimes. After all, you feel that you know best how to do the job. It probably isn't true. In fact, it better not be true. Pass the torch and move on to a new volunteer task that you enjoy and can do.

The reasons for moving on can be multifold as we grow older. But there are always new ways to volunteer, and it is your job to find them and grow older gracefully.

Reflections for Readers

1. What do you see as the primary benefits of volunteering in older age?
2. What are some of the potential pitfalls of volunteer work?
3. How might such pitfalls be avoided?
4. How can seniors use volunteering to mentor younger generations?
5. Why is "passing the torch" important? How can a person continue to feel vital and engaged after passing the torch?

CHAPTER 33

Prolong Your Life—
Get in the Pool

Gerald Sands

Chairman Emeritus, CCS Companies

Dedham, MA

In 1966, l started my own business, and it took all my efforts to keep it afloat. Early morning to late evening, every chore was done by me until I could afford to hire an employee some two years later. Despite my young age, the stress was taking its toll on my sleep and causing me to develop fast-food-eating habits. An employee shamed me when she mentioned that my slim figure was not that slim anymore. In 1969, I joined a health club and forced myself to set aside four hours a week for exercising.

Working with a trainer, I was put through a series of weight lifting and cardiovascular routines. In addition, at the crack of dawn, I took a three-mile jog every other day. Before too long, I began to feel and see results. Unused muscles firmed up, my eating habits improved, and sleep came more naturally.

One day, a sign was posted that the gym would be closed for six weeks for renovations. The gym had become such an important part of my routine that I literally panicked. One of the trainers saw my distress and said that the swimming pool would be an excellent alternative, and he would show me some basic water aerobic routines. At first, I questioned how a swimming pool could provide the same strenuous workout as the combination of gymnastics and outside jogging.

He joined me in the pool and showed me the basics of water aerobics. Using the buoyancy of the water, we increased the intensity of the workouts. In addition, he introduced me to an array of weights and flotation devices. Motivated, I went online to get additional water aerobic materials. Using the various weights and flotation devices, I created

149

a 6-day/30-minute vigorous routine that was broken down into three components: cardiovascular, upper body, and lower body. These half-hour nonstop sessions more than equaled the intensity of previous one-hour gym workouts.

Moving to NewBridge was fabulous, with a swimming pool just an elevator ride away from my apartment. Since I still work, NewBridge's management was kind enough to change the opening hour to 5:00 a.m., so I could start my days in the pool.

About four years ago, I came down with a rare type of pneumonia. At first I thought this was a long-duration flu and I waited about a month before seeing my doctor. It was so unusual for me not to feel fabulous, I had assumed that this would leave me soon. Low-grade fever, weight loss, and coughing episodes, all more serious than I had thought, led to my primary care doctor sending me directly to the Pulmonary Department of Tufts Medical Center.

Apparently, I was so ill that they needed to do a series of lung biopsies to determine the source of my illness. The form of pneumonia I had contracted has over a 50% mortality rate and is treated with steroids.

The pulmonary staff told my wife that the extraordinary physical condition I was in was the reason for my survival. There is no question that this was due to my vigorous pool workouts.

After two weeks of hospitalization, I was released and sent to the NewBridge Rehabilitation Unit. For 15 days, though in a much weakened condition, I insisted that I be allowed to walk slowly to help get me back in shape as rapidly as possible. With an oxygen tank on wheels and my consumption at 10 liters, I went back and forth through the halls, resting every 5 minutes. Daily, I would add time and speed to my walking. This helped in my recuperation, and my need for oxygen went down to 2 liters. When I left rehab to return home, I no longer needed supplemental oxygen.

Let's fast forward to the present. My days start with a strong cup of black coffee and a trip to the pool. A 30-minute vigorous workout provides me with the energy and get-go to face the world. Neighbors often remark how fast I walk, which just comes naturally. My mood is always positive and upbeat, a direct result of the sense of well-being that comes from exercising. A few years back, my gerontologist said, without question, I had to be his healthiest patient.

The beauty of the swimming pool is that regardless of your age or physical condition, you can achieve great benefits by just "walking laps." Even if you are using a walker, you will find the water will give you stability. Your immediate goal should be feeling comfortable and safe as you slowly walk from side to side. There may be a reluctance to walk without any assistance, which is understandable. But the water will give you the balance you need. As you build up your confidence, you will take pride in knowing you are greatly enhancing your cardiovascular health. There is no need to know how to swim, as you will be on your feet during your pool time.

The goal is to build up your endurance and speed, with a sense of confidence that you are helping your heart, as well as your balance. Once you have built up your stamina, you can add weight lifting to your workouts. Start with the lightest weights, and then add a few more reps, until you go to heavier weights. This will help keep your muscles toned, and you will see and feel the results. As you progress, you might want to join a supervised weekly water aerobics program.

If you are retired, it will be easier to make time for the pool. If you are fortunate enough to have a pool where you live, my suggestion is to go to the pool shortly after you wake up. It's much easier to put on a bathing suit and robe first thing, rather than having to get dressed first, undress and put on your suit, and then get dressed yet once again. Doing your swim first will also stop you from making excuses *not* to go to the pool.

Since water aerobics allows you to be on your feet, an added pleasure is to get an iPod so you can work out with your favorite songs.

In closing, remember we all spent the first nine months in water, so follow my lead—you'll feel like a kid again. Good health and long life to you!!

Reflections for Readers

1. What are the benefits of pool exercises for seniors? How might such exercises be particularly well suited for older adults?
2. What might make it difficult to maintain regular exercise in older adulthood?
3. How might having a well-defined routine help someone maintain regular exercise?
4. Are there other types of exercise that would be appropriate for older adults?

CHAPTER 34

Exercise and Aging: But I Don't Wanna—How to Get Unstuck from That Easy Chair

Lynne Sherman, MA, LMFT
Licensed Marriage and Family Therapist (retired)
Santa Barbara, CA
Age 71

You know you need to exercise. You can list the benefits. You've heard the pleas from your doctor. Nothing's working. You still don't want to. That's OK. Really? Yes! Let me reassure you that most people first getting into exercise don't have much enthusiasm. But people still do begin and continue with exercise in their lives, and you can, too.

Here are some ways to overcome inertia. First, don't call yourself "lazy," even if you think it is true; describing yourself in negative terms is not going to help you. This is a time when you need to be your own best friend. Nobody wants to take a class from a punishing teacher. Instead, be sympathetic *and* encouraging to yourself. If we are going to talk you into exercise, you are going to need some constructive "self-talk."

Try some of these sympathetic *and* encouraging statements:

- "I know I feel achy and moving does not feel good so I will be careful and gentle with myself and bit by bit my body will feel better."
- "I am worried about losing my balance or injuring myself, so I will start exercise in a guided supported setting, like physical therapy or a class at the community center. Gradually my balance will improve."

- "I feel very self-conscious exercising so for now I will exercise at home, in private. Later, I will look for loose fitting clothing and choose the type of physical activity that won't embarrass me when I am with others."
- "I feel so tired all the time I don't know how I will find the energy to exercise so I will begin with five minutes at a time and work up the number of times I can exercise each day."

Take another look at the above examples. They reveal secrets to success:

> *Be careful and gentle with yourself.*

> *Don't push your body too much.* Gradually you will build up to more exercise.

Use physical therapy settings or stretch and movement classes to help you gain confidence.

If you feel self-conscious, it is OK to exercise at home. You can find appropriate instructional videos on YouTube.

Exercise every day. Start with five minutes. For some of us just putting on our walking shoes is a workout! So start with that. You are more likely to stick to your new lifestyle if you do it every day. It's like making your bed or brushing your teeth, an automatic habit.

Here are some more ways to outsmart your habit of inertia.

Make a "no cancel" contract with a friend. Arrange to meet an exercise pal at a certain location the same day and time every week. Agree that you can't call each other to cancel. That means if you don't show up, your walking friend will be standing there waiting for you and wondering if you stood her up. This method kept me jogging with a friend every Sunday at 9 AM for two years! We finally stopped when she moved away.

Break your exercise into small periods that can be over before they feel like a burden. Research has shown that thirty minutes of exercise each day is beneficial even if you do this in three 10-minute sessions.

Be inefficient. Make several trips when one would do. Finally! Our increasing problems with memory can help us get healthier. My Dad, Mel, would take paperwork to shred out to the garage. Instead of making one trip, he would make ten. Every time he finished with a piece of paper, he would walk it from his desk at one end of the house to his shredder at the other. He was 97 and limited his exercise to inside his home because of balance and vision challenges.

I agree exercise can be boring. While you are stretching or practicing balance exercises, you can listen to NPR radio or podcasts or talk to a friend on speakerphone. You can listen to an audiobook. You can concentrate more carefully on your posture and correct form when stretching, lifting and doing calisthenics. If you are walking outdoors, fine-tune your awareness to the little wonders you may overlook. Every day that I went for a walk when I had not wanted to, I was rewarded with an unexpected sight.

Vary your exercise. We are all familiar with the typical forms of exercise; walking, jogging, swimming, treadmill, etc. Exercise is not limited to the gym. Dancing, gardening, housework, washing and waxing the car can all be good forms of exercise. Think of exercise as just moving your body. Anything can be exercise.

Cleaning out all your closets could be part of your exercise routine next month. A closet a day is pretty good, especially if you are carrying items to the garage or the donation center. Needing to exercise may be a good incentive to wash some windows. Most household maintenance projects count as exercise.

Learn a new exercise by taking a class. Water aerobics, Tai Chi, Chi Gong, yoga, resistance training, bowling, table tennis, square dance, line dance, and hula hoop dance are all offered in classes. Look at listings by your local adult education school, YMCA, Jewish Community Center. There are also clubs that teach you when you join. I belonged to a square dance club when I was in high school. For those of you who like Facebook, you can find "meet ups" where local people gather at a certain time to practice. I often see a Tai Chi group at one of our local parks. Check your local Area Agency of Aging directory for listings of classes. Trying to get better at an activity will certainly tackle the boredom problem! This is very true with bowling, where you can keep score. Your classmates may become your friends.

Acquire a four-footed exercise buddy. Mine is a horse, but you don't have to go to that extreme. You may decide to buy a dog. If so, be careful to get one that won't grow up to pull you off your feet. If you don't want the responsibility of owning your own pet, ask around; you may have a neighbor who would be grateful if you would walk her dog while she is away at work. You can also volunteer as a dog walker at your local animal shelter.

Treat yourself to some data. Numbers can be very motivating. Get a pedometer and wear it all day. Every evening, write the day's steps on your wall calendar. If you are managing your weight, get a digital scale with tenth of pound gradations. I like to weigh every day and write my weight down on my calendar. Research shows that if you nip weight gain in the bud, before you have gained back four pounds, you can lose those few pounds easily and maintain your weight. The daily weigh-ins provide frequent data. The numbers motivate you to keep moving.

An exercise plan is a good deal you make with yourself. Tell your doctor of your plan. Write it down. Here are examples:

- I plan to lose twenty pounds in six months by eating better and by exercising thirty minutes every day. I will weigh in every day and mark my weight and the exercise I did on my wall calendar each day.
- I plan to walk thirty minutes every day. I can walk in ten-minute sessions if I need to. I will wear a pedometer and write my steps on my calendar every evening. My goal is to increase the number of steps each day over the next six weeks.

Reward yourself for sticking to your plan. Food is not a helpful reward. Treat yourself to a massage or a spa day. Brag to a supportive friend. Brag to yourself. Remember those sympathetic and encouraging statements? Now you can incorporate some of your accomplishments into your encouragement. Over time you will need less sympathy because if you stick with it, exercise gets to be more enjoyable. Meet a friend for a walk instead of a lunch.

Acquire some new exercise gear. There are all sorts of lovely gizmos. "Fitbit"-type wearables allow you to track your vitals and keep a training record. "Theraband" offers a variety of products for resistance training. Resistance bands or flexibility bands are very inexpensive. All types of equipment are on sale cheap at your local thrift store. Check Craigslist for bargains as well. (A tip: Meet your Craigslist seller at a public place. Don't go to a seller's home by yourself.)

Read self-help books. Reading when you already agree with the author feels motivating. It is like buying a paperback cheering squad. Check your local library for titles that give you encouragement.

My suggestions come from my thirty years of experience as a cognitive behavioral psychotherapist. As a licensed Marriage and Family Therapist in California I most enjoyed working with clients who needed to get in shape or lose weight. Some were recovering from auto accidents. Some were trying to recover from a lifetime of bad habits. Cognitive behavioral therapists work with your thoughts and your actions. We are pretty good at helping individuals unlock their motivation. Everyone has a different combination. I hope by trying a mix of these ideas you will be able to unlock the door and walk through to a lifestyle of better health.

Reflections for Readers

1. What are some of the best ways to overcome the inertia of staying on the couch and remaining inactive? What unique challenges might an older person face in this regard?
2. To what extent does attitude matter when it comes to exercising? After reading this essay, what do you believe is the best attitude to have when approaching exercise?
3. What are some of the best ways to reward oneself for exercising?

CHAPTER 35

The Importance of Travel

Sherwin (Sam) Lehrer, PhD

Muscle Biophysics, Boston Biomedical Research Institute;
Principal Research Associate, Harvard Medical School (retired)
Dedham, MA
Age 82

> Travel is fatal to prejudice, bigotry, and narrow-mindedness, and many of our people need it sorely on these accounts. Broad, wholesome, charitable views of men and things cannot be acquired by vegetating in one little corner of the earth all one's lifetime.
>
> —Mark Twain

What is wise? Several dictionaries define wise as "possessing good judgment and knowledge obtained by learning or experience." Clearly the older you get, the more experience you have, but you may not necessarily be wiser. So, I would change the definition to emphasize experience: possessing good judgment and knowledge, usually by learning *from* experience. However, some people have a great deal of experience, even traumatic experience, but are not wiser. Knowledge can come only if one is curious and maintains an open mind while experiencing, and it is easier to maintain an open mind when young, when opinions, prejudices, and judgments have not yet been solidified. Learning then will follow. Extrapolating Mark Twain's advice, the road to being wise is to eliminate prejudice, bigotry, and narrow-mindedness. One way to do this is to experience other cultures by traveling.

In 1956, when we were graduate students, Liane, my wife-to-be, and I lived at International House in Berkeley, California. It was there that we met each other and students from around the world, and it was there that I realized how little I knew about the rest of the world.

So, in 1960, just after finishing graduate school and marrying, Liane and I decided to travel around the world. Our goal was to take time off in order to refresh ourselves and better decide what we wanted to do before becoming more settled. So we worked in the Boston area for real wages for two years, saved money, and planned our trip.

Planning involved tentatively deciding where and how long to stay in a given place, deciding which guidebooks to take, and getting appropriate shots and visas. We had few responsibilities. Liane's mother was independent and healthy. My parents seemed fine, had each other, and had recently moved to Florida. We had no children or pets. We were young and healthy.

We bought "round-the-world" open airline tickets for $1,000 each and $3,000 in traveler's checks and spent nine months traveling. We told friends and family that we would pick up mail addressed to "American Express, [City, Country,] c/o us," after giving them a tentative itinerary, with corrections sent occasionally by mail. We were very flexible and were able to make reservations for the next flight just a few days before.

We tried to stick to our budget of $5/day each for room and food so that our savings would last the full nine months. Our travel in 1962–1963 took us to Hawaii, Japan, Hong Kong, Thailand, Rangoon, Burma (Myanmar today), India, Nepal, Iran, Beirut, Turkey, Egypt, Cyprus, Israel, and Germany. In Germany, we picked up a VW bug that we had previously ordered and traveled on through Austria, Yugoslavia, Greece, Italy, Switzerland, France, Holland, Belgium, Germany, Denmark, and England, and then shipped the car back home.

Arming ourselves with the around-the-world airplane tickets, our traveler's checks, two suitcases and two handbags, a couple of cameras, a couple of guidebooks, and some ideas of where to go, we were off. We did it and were back in the USA in nine months. How did we do it, what did we learn, and did we become wiser?

During our travels, many places were visually exciting, and we recorded the sights with our cameras; after arriving home, we found several hundred slides and many rolls of B&W negatives. But we were also stimulated by smells, sounds, and tastes. I will simply list some observations from notes and from photos that we made during our 1963 trip and then see if I can make generalizations.

Japan: Polite, reserved people. Personal space respected; for example, we chose two 6' × 3' tatamis next to each other on the floor in the hold of an overnight ship, wrapped ourselves up with clothes, and slept a few feet from others. Cleanliness: no handshaking during introductions, just bowing; no directly touching money in shops; money handed to and from on a tray. Pretty girls in department store greeting "Ohayou gozaimasu" (Good Morning), wiping the escalator handrail, and bowing. Street scenes: Geisha and Maiko girls walking wearing ancient garments; babies strapped on backs of women (never on men); men wear gray or black suits; many wearing surgical masks. Efficiency: trains. Restaurants: display food and prices outside, no bread—but rice. Pickles for breakfast. Entertainment: dance club—only male patrons—girls asking men to dance—taking them to the toilet, then waiting to escort them back—pachinko parlors for the addicted young. Ancient theater—Noh, Kabuki—flower arranging, bonsai. Ryokan (Japanese inn)—bedding on tatami, scroll, and flowers—shower before using communal *ofuro* (hot tub). Traditions: especially in Kyoto—festivals, castles, medieval clothing. Shrines: call the spirit with a gong. Go to the next shrine, collect colorful entrance ticket; family in-front-of photos for album, say a prayer, tie a paper wish to a tree.

Hiroshima—quiet—remembrance. Gardens, trees manicured, Ryōan-ji (Zen garden) with raked stones like waves for meditation. A sense of order, organization, neatness, simplicity, and beauty.

Hong Kong: Crowds. Bamboo scaffolding all over like decoration on top of old. Shops inside and outside. Tailor with a tape measure around his neck "make you a suit—take only two days." Camera shops, food. Very poor and very rich. Sampans in bay. Lantao island—a funeral, a wailing woman in white followed by musicians; an escapee from mainland China, scared and hungry, asks for food; we brought him to monastery. At Chinese border, barbed wire and soldiers on the other side like in Israel in divided Jerusalem.

Bangkok: city of canals (most gone now) and many Buddhas—old and new—upright and sleeping. Friendly people—beautiful women, colorful clothes. Giggling girls leading us to their house in Thonburi. Showing Liane how to Thai dance with pointed fingers. We said goodbye. They said "goodbye, I love you with the bottom of my heart" (American movie influence). Lizards in hotel room, keeping insects down. Hot, spicy food, great tastes. Young man takes us around knowing we had no money, just to have contact with Americans—he only wanted "the Radio Amateur's Handbook." (I sent it to him months later.)

Rangoon: Suspicious people—military rule. Shwe Dagon Pagoda. Hundreds of hot steps on bare feet to top. Jungle of small pagodas, private Buddhas, gilded, washed. Synagogue. Met a Jew from Bombay who invited us to stay when we get to Bombay—we did for a week—like Jews traveling in medieval times helped by a network of Jews in Middle East and Asia.

India and Nepal: Calcutta. Unbelievable numbers of street people living along road in huts made of pipes or discarded construction material. Empty lot used as communal toilet, squatting with gown drawn around legs. Katmandu. Airline pilot in hotel eating with fingers. Mix of cultures, Buddhist and Hindu, Nepali, Indian, Tibetan. Mangy dogs, surrounded by snowy mountains. Many people just watching. Sherpas, Anglo-dominated hotels, Edmund Hillary encircled. Friendly. Always run after by children, wanting to interact. Living Goddess. In Pokhara, Tibetan refugees surround us; curious, colorful skirts and boots, handsome smiling people, friendly without words.

India: Buses and trains, crowded, chickens, boxes with animals, etc. Caste system, chain of command. Moghul fortresses, medieval observatory Jantar Mantar, Jaipur. Agra, Taj Mahal at dawn. Boisterous New Year's Eve party at the Agra Club, Bombay, on the harbor—actors club—red light district—massage by boy—chicken we got to know eaten at last dinner. Ancient caves of Ajanta and Ellora, wall paintings of Buddhas. Elephants in Jaipur. Great food. Snake charmer with mongoose. Variety of people and dress. Jains, Parsees, Hindus, Buddhists. Young couple in shrine: they do pilgrimage each year at wedding anniversary—he holds my hand on way out.

Beirut: Ancient Byblos and Baalbek, Cedars of Lebanon. Saw Palestinian refugee camp from taxi. A postman invited us to his house that evening for tea and English speaking.

Iran: Tehran: Shah's palace after dark. Isfahan—Old town—Jewish school. Bought miniature painting—beautiful mosques. Shaking minaret mosque.

Egypt: Cairo—Big Souk—Giza pyramids—Liane on camel—Driver's hands wander while helping her off—Sphinx—son et lumière. Luxor. Carnak. Valley of Kings across Nile—tombs with wall paintings. Copt store man "good price for mummy bead necklace," because we were like him, Christian. Bought some—they could be fake.

Cyprus: Castles. Ancient Neolithic ruins. Beautiful sea and landscape. Easy travel between Turkish and Greek areas.

Israel: Jerusalem divided, soldiers guarding bridge. Tel Aviv, no queuing in post office, pushing to get to the front. Sephardi complaining about discrimination. Kibbutz Rivivim in desert: tomato sandwiches for breakfast, worked in field. Acco, Dead Sea swim, Eilat, Red Sea swim, Solomon's mines, walked to top of Masada. Kibbutz Am Yad, artist there.

Turkey: Ankara, Ataturk's tomb. Istanbul. Walking in rain and snow in sandals. Cold hotel room in Beyoglu—next-door covert business deals between Arabs and Israelis. Call to prayer. Misty waterfront, from

Galata Bridge—porters with wooden backpacks covered with rugs unloading ships. The Sook (market) teaming—coaxed into Jewish rug shop for tea—hoping for a sale before tea came. Hagia Sophia/Blue mosque. Dynamic covered market.

Europe: Munich. Got car. Dachau. Inn in Austria—framed award letter from Hitler on wall. Ski in Innsbruck, Austria. Vienna, Liane's childhood home—father's grave in Friedrichshof. Yugoslavia, Slivovitz for breakfast. Zagreb, Beograd. Liane fought paying parking ticket—went to police station and won. Skopje, strolling around square at dusk. Greece friendly. Mykonos, white; donkeys; yoghurt and bread. Italy: Naples, Todi, Florence, Milan, Turin. Switzerland; clean room, France; dirty room. Belgium: Bruxelles, Bruges. Holland, Denmark friendly—Tivoli—*smörrebröd.* Viking festival—met Danish princess. England. Home.

What did I learn from this travel experience? It is hard to reflect on this 53 years later, but I think that as a result of this trip, I have been able to interact better with people from a variety of different cultures. I realize that "rules of behavior" differ culturally, and I interact carefully with people, observing before acting. While traveling, I do not assume that locals can speak English; I speak slowly and avoid slang. At work, I have employed students from different countries and also easily collaborated with scientists from many other countries, particularly Japan. My interest in photography, stimulated by the trip, continues. Some of my B&W photographs from the trip can be seen at Newbridge on the Charles, Dedham, Massachusetts. We traveled with our children later, even when they were very young, which I know has had a positive influence on them. Am I wiser? Perhaps, but at a minimum I have the many memories of that trip to keep me company.

Reflections for Readers

1. How do you believe travels in one's youth affect later life?
2. How might travel and exposure to different cultures benefit an older adult?
3. What barriers might get in the way of traveling and interacting with people of different cultures? Are there special barriers related to older age?

CHAPTER 36

Accepting People with Different Backgrounds

Diana Hope Bronner, MEd
Special needs Teacher Educator (retired)
Dedham, MA
Age 78

As a child, I don't think I ever felt comfortable in my socioeconomic world. My sister did, though. Her friends all lived in upper-class neighborhoods and were as sophisticated as she was. I, on the other hand, loved wearing "dungarees" even when on a special train trip for the day into cosmopolitan New York City, with my mother and sister dressed to the nines.

My friends were different from my sister's. One girl was Mary Chen (Chinese), another, Gillian Clark (Australian), and another, Norma Jean Fitzgerald (Black). We were a happy group, comfortable with each other, though what we did together, I no longer remember. I wanted to invite Norma Jean to our home for a sleepover, but my parents discouraged that by putting into my young head that once Norma Jean saw our fine house, she would not be happy in her (implied) meager home. I was so very sad, for me as well as for her. I lost track of these friends and would love to find them again. They were a big influence on my life, although I didn't realize it at the time. But I think being exposed to them, with their different backgrounds and cultures, enabled me to be more open as I have gone through life.

One of my passions in life has been traveling. Upon reflection, I realized that I had two criteria for my destinations. One is the need to see and be with wildlife around the world. The other is to go to countries where the culture is different from mine. To this end, I have been to many countries on all continents. I have been to 10 countries in Africa, most recently to Namibia. Several years ago, I traveled to Mongolia. I've been seriously interested in Native American culture, as well as Buddhism. While traveling in Russia and Africa, I bonded with women in both areas and corresponded and gave financial aid for as long as possible.

One woman, Ba'Bushka (not meaning the scarf she was wearing, but rather an old woman), lived in Svirstroy, a small village in Russia. We met as she was trying to sell flowers to earn a little more money, which she desperately needed. I indicated that I did not want the flowers, but rather, her picture. I gave her the requested money and took her photograph. I later went back and gave her more money. She took my hand, pulling me down onto the bench where she was sitting. She put her arms around me and gave me a kiss like my Russian grandmother used to give.

She babbled away in Russian and I could understand none of it. I finally left her to find our guide, who interpreted what my Ba'Bushka was saying. When Ba'Bushka saw me, she again pulled me down next to her. The only thing I remember was that she said that "our hearts have touched," and I had to agree.

She gave me her address and thus began a correspondence between us that lasted for several years. I would send her money to buy firewood to get her through the cold winters. She painted and recaulked her meager little house. My U.S. dollars went a long way in her currency. She had a pension of $24 a month.

She wrote, among other things, that her happiest times in the world were having her grandchildren stay with her for the summer. She cared for them, fed them, and loved them. I was so touched because it told me that we are all the same under the skin, with the same need to love and be loved. Our cultures may be different, but that is secondary to basic human needs. If it were left to the "little" people, there would be no conflicts. One day, I got a letter from my Ba'Bushka's daughter that her mother had died at the age of 64.

Another beautiful memory from my travels is of a lovely young woman I met on a boat on Lake Victoria in Africa. She was a nun and wanted to become a nurse. I corresponded with her and sent money to help her buy books she needed for her studies. I no longer hear from her and think she must have died in the war between the Tutsis and the Hutus.

As I go through this process of aging, I realize how fortunate I have been to be exposed to such a variety of people and cultures! It is so important to be open to new ways of thinking. It fosters tolerance and acceptance of others, as well as being mind- and heart-expanding. I feel culturally enriched through my many interactions with those of different belief systems. And it has enabled me to see others without judgment—so important in this age of intolerance.

Reflections for Readers

1. What is the role of tolerance in older age? How does one develop tolerance? Does tolerance increase or decrease with age?
2. What do we stand to learn from people with backgrounds different from our own?
3. How might overseas experiences affect one's perspective on life and aging?
4. What might be hard about accepting people with different backgrounds? How might we avoid these pitfalls?

CHAPTER 37

Fitting In and Standing Out

Richard Payne Evans, EdM
Management Consultant and Teacher of
Organizational Behavior (retired)
North Chelmsford, MA
Age 80

Organizations are my meat, and moving in and out of them my sizzle. I have learned and profited from a lifetime of studying and reflecting on individuals and groups moving in and out of organizations, and how organizations behave as they choose whom to hire and fire. As I enter my ninth decade, I welcome this opportunity to set in print some of this experience and thought. I hope that you will find wisdom in my reflections. But, first I want to give you a little background on who I am and why I hold the beliefs I do.

My approach is colored by my having the good fortune of having been born an African American. I have faced fitting in and have had to overcome many prejudices and acts of discrimination. In no case did I plead to be spared the challenges of being an African American. I am proud to have had more than my share of triumphs over discrimination and prejudice.

One such challenge and triumph is worth mentioning here. It came early in my life, when I was entering grade school, and has been a continuing influence in my life to this day. I was six years old when I entered the Shady Hill School in Cambridge, Massachusetts. This was an unusual experience for the school, my family, me, and the private-school community in Greater Boston.

The head of the school and the parents of the first grade class decided that it was time to integrate the school. The country had officially joined World War II in a fight against fascism, and it was an appropriate time to make a statement about antidiscrimination and integration of the races closer to home.

Shady Hill was known to be a very strong academic school, highly selective, and very progressive in the character of John Dewey, the educator and philosopher. Several Shady Hill parents knew my father and knew that he had a child—me—who was entering first grade. So after some negotiation between the school and my parents, I entered this new world—into a unique experiment for all concerned.

My parents were more anxious than I realized at the time. My father had had a similar experience when he was young. He had graduated first in his class in a local high school and received a full scholarship to Harvard College, class of 1925. He was one of four members of his class who were Negroes (the term for people of color at the time), but if he had concerns about my entering Shady Hill, he did not voice them to me. My mother was much more expressive to me and talked about whatever concerned her, including my father's interests and anything else that crossed her excited mind. She had grown up in Canada and moved to the Boston area to get away from the racism she experienced in New Brunswick. Each of my parents was supportive of me.

The school was also very helpful to my parents and me, although as I think back 74 years or so, I realize that they were as inexperienced as we were as to what to expect. I was the first black student to be admitted and enter in the history of the school. Clearly to everyone, my first task was to fit in. Over the next nine years, I learned my academic and organizational lessons well. This was a triumph that pointed the way to standing out—not for what I looked like, but for what I did—and was based on my learning the fitting-in skills I will talk about below.

During the last year at Shady Hill, I had the opportunity to be in the senior play, *Princess Ida*, an operetta by Gilbert and Sullivan. I discovered that I loved being on stage, which I continued throughout my high school years at The Putney School in Vermont, where I acted in several plays. Theater became a major thrust of my interests, and I moved on to major in theater and fine arts at Boston University. As I honed my acting skills—performing in front of people, stepping outside of myself, standing in another's shoes—I realized that I had been learning how to stand out, which is as important as it is to fit in.

In those formative years and during the many years that followed, I had to learn to grow and to prosper from working hard and holding to standards that I could be proud of. It became increasingly important to stand out because of what I had accomplished. Standing out was quite easy as an African American studying and working in a white

Caucasian-dominated world, if only because of my skin color. But standing out because of the quality of my thinking or the quality of my deeds is far more satisfying.

Another major thrust of my interests was in learning how groups of people form and behave in organizations. After a stint in the Navy and a job in my father's lumber company, I had the opportunity to see how big business works when I was offered a position with the Raytheon Company. Several years later, I joined another large organization when I was recruited to join Honeywell. I began to see organizations differently, in that I observed lots of smaller groups within the larger organization rather than one monolith. These smaller groups were less formal and often more collegial. I found my major interest through an academic discipline called "organizational behavior," which I studied in graduate school. Research was underway on the groups, called "informal organizations," that form through personal association and mutual protection, and on how communication travels swiftly through them. Information travels much more slowly through the official channels. This efficiency is just one of the aspects of informal organizational research that fascinated me.

The next 50 years have been filled with all sorts of professional, social, and academic challenges. All of these were wrapped in the same sense of fitting in and standing out that I experienced early on at the Shady Hill School. Somehow life during this time was less what I was seeking than what sought me out. It was my choice to pursue.

Throughout this time, one additional quality has been present— as part of standing out, the quality to be remembered. I am often surprised when someone I meet says that he remembers me from years earlier. Even now, after I have retired from my profession, I seem to be remembered.

Being remembered is a wonderful part of anyone's life. Upon reflection, I believe two of my qualities contribute to this for me: first, my presence, and second, the easy curiosity bred in me. I was interviewed 30 years ago for an article in the *Boston Business Journal* about the "New Black Bourgeoisie." The author called me "a handsome man in his early 50s whose presence is felt when he walks into a room." I have used that to my advantage, in addition to my acquired skills and my curiosity. Over the years, I have conducted many interviews of candidates for positions as executives, engineers, organizational specialists, and even candidates for ordination in the Episcopal Church. My reputation is that of someone who asks the most penetrating questions with warmth and kindness. My natural curiosity allows me to step outside of myself and focus all my attention on the other person.

My latest triumph is that I have found a place where I can revisit some of my interests during my retirement. The Harvard Institute for Learning in Retirement (HILR) has given me the opportunity to continue to learn, lead, meet interesting people, and continue to act onstage in the theater. Even in retirement, I am managing to fit in and stand out. It has been a good life.

So, let me turn now to the wisdom I've accumulated about organizations. Over the last hundred years, organizations and the environments in which they operate have changed. Companies are more mobile, firms are more widely spread, and even religious organizations are becoming more malleable. Companies merge and sell off parts as a matter of course; this organizational churning has a major impact on working individuals and groups of workers.

Individuals can no longer count on permanent employment. Most employees are employed "at will" now. Thus, the old concept of "lifetime employment" has evaporated. A job is a short-term work situation. A career is a series of jobs in the same organization or, more likely, several different organizations. Human resource professionals used to reject job applicants with many different employers, calling them "job-hoppers." Résumé readers now have altered their view, so that an applicant who has been with only one employer over a long time may be seen as less flexible than others. This marks a sea change in organizational recruiting and admissions.

Given the mobility of organizations these days, individuals are constantly moving into new operations or organizations and must use fitting-in skills to position themselves to succeed. Fitting-in skills are a quiver of talents to influence others to accept a person into a group. These talents, which I learned early in my life, include presenting a good introduction, finding a good mentor or sponsor, and showing up.

A good introduction is a clear instructive statement of who you are and why you are there. This should be accompanied by intensive listening to how the respondent reacts to what was presented.

A mentor is an individual who seems interested in you and informed about the group or organization and its formal and informal practices. This person may be your hiring manager or another member of the group. A word of caution: Do not confuse a mentor with a sponsor. A sponsor will guide and inform you, but only up to a point, not risking his or her own organizational position. A mentor will guide you even to the point of risking replacement.

Woody Allen's quip "90% of success is showing up" is, in fact, an important part of fitting in. Making oneself available, being prepared, and being dependable are all important aspects of showing up.

My family and I are a family of firsts. My father was the first in his family to go to college; I was the first African American to attend Shady Hill; I was the first black in the Ceremonial Guard in Washington, D.C.; and I was the first black to be elected to the vestry, the governing body, at Trinity Church in Boston. When I delivered the eulogy at my Dad's funeral, I spoke of him as one who, throughout his life, plowed unfurrowed ground. I am proud that my son has continued this tradition by naming his not-for-profit "Unfurrowed Ground Foundation," a Community Tennis Association partner dedicated to "creating uncommon opportunities in common places."

I will end with one of my favorite Marshall Dodge stories. A Maine state judge was questioning an older Maine resident before receiving his testimony. The judge asked, "Where is your residence?" The man answered by giving his address. The judge then asked, "Have you lived there all your life?" The man answered, "Not yet!"

I'm not done yet either!

Reflections for Readers

1. What strengths might someone develop from having to overcome prejudices and acts of discrimination?
2. What distinguishes the person who meets the challenge of prejudice by rising above it from the person who succumbs to prejudice by getting angry or giving up?
3. What might someone want to "stand out" for, and when and how might someone want to "fit in"?
4. What qualities might lead to someone being remembered? How might a person enhance these qualities in himself or herself?

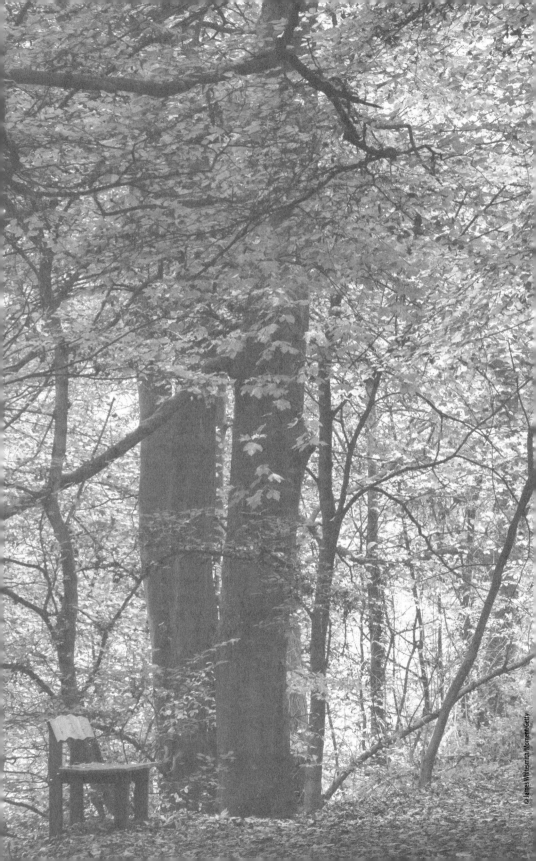

PART **VII**

Aging and Interpersonal Relationships

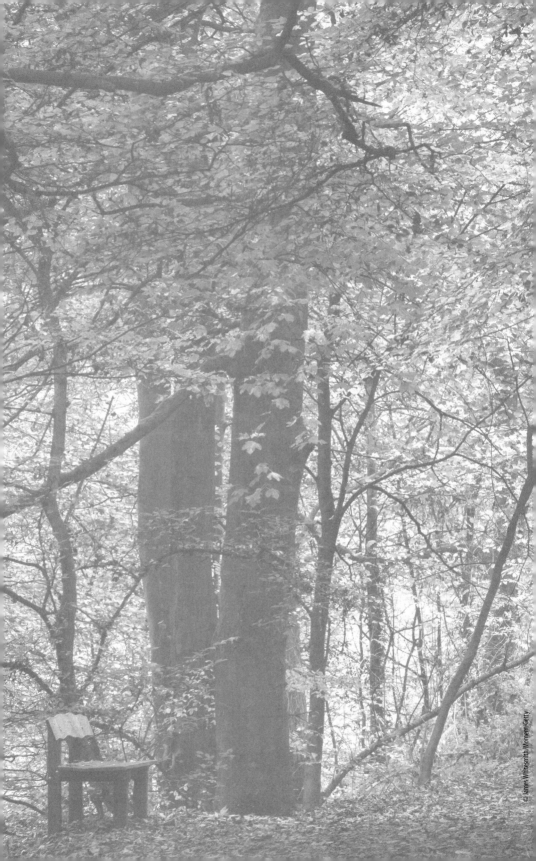

CHAPTER 38

Intergenerational Dialogue

Jenny Yen, PsyD
Post-Doctoral Fellow in Geropsychology,
Department of Veterans Affairs
Palo Alto Health Care System
Palo Alto, CA

As a little girl, I watched Lifetime movies and television shows that revolved around family values in order to feel a sense of togetherness. My family and I immigrated to the United States when I was three years old. We had no sense of community; survivorship and togetherness were all we had. While my family and I worked hard to take care of each other, we lost our own sense of community because my parents were working constantly.

Like many adolescents and young adults, I experienced immense academic and social pressures to be exceptional when I had little self-worth and only limited support. I battled against low self-esteem and loneliness, sought approval, and was perfection-seeking. My Eastern cultural background made no room for explicit encouragement, affection, or praise. Although my parents used their adversities, stories, and life experiences to teach and motivate me to work hard, I longed for the unequivocal validation that I had seen on American television.

Dorothy became an incredible grandmother figure for me. She is a petite, compassionate, hopeful, and independent woman. She had lived through the Great Depression, buried a child, and lost her husband and siblings. Despite her hardships, she always celebrated life by thoroughly engaging in it! She swam laps, held a part-time job working with computers and young adults after retirement, traveled, and preserved meaningful relationships.

Dorothy had a positive influence on me at a time when my identity was still fragile and taking shape. She generously offered me a luxury that my parents couldn't afford due to economic hardships. She had the *time* to listen and get to know me. She helped me with a school project and taught me how to knit. Dorothy also had this unwavering belief that I could achieve anything I wanted. In her eyes, I was easily that amazing! Her unconditional love and support for me was undeniable, and it fostered in me courage, confidence, and self-worth to reach for goals that my self-doubting mind would have otherwise hindered. I am blessed to have her as my life cheerleader!

Once I moved away for college, we began exchanging emails dating back nearly a decade ago. My emails to her almost resembled a diary because I was so open with her about daily occurrences, exciting new adventures, worries, and challenges along the way, and because I shared with her my dreams and accomplishments. We would write just to say we were thinking about each other and sent photos of beautiful flowers and plants so they would always remain lovely in our minds. Our emails became very special, as they demonstrated the support and unconditional love of our deep intergenerational relationship.

Personal email from Dorothy to me:

Dearest Jenny,

I've been thinking of you a lot lately. You, my dear, will always be special to me. I have every email you ever sent me. I really think that you are an unusual young woman and admire your efforts to become a successful person. I'm kinda at a loss for words. You have so much to offer! You will be successful! No matter what you decide. I am so proud of you!! I know how hard you have worked to get this far in your young life. WOW!!! I'm just delighted to watch your career develop.

Good for you for practicing your speech in front of the mirror. I have a feeling that you will do just fine. Take a couple of deep breaths and don't let your voice go too high. I know you will be fine and I'd be shocked if you weren't successful! I'll keep my fingers crossed.

Keep writing, Jenny; I wish I lived closer so that I could be of more help to you. I do know that your life is there and you should be there to fulfill your responsibilities, but I do want you to know if this gets so bad that you need to get out of it, I will be happy to have you here.

Be good, and if that doesn't work, then be smart!

Love you sweetie,

Keep in touch, I like hearing from you,

Dorothy

I hope that my relationship with Dorothy clearly and passionately communicates its significant impact on my development as I was a young girl emerging into adulthood.

Dorothy was essential and inspiring to me for three reasons:

1. She had the time to spend with me.
2. She consistently offered assurance and emotional support for me.
3. She demonstrated that aging was timeless and unrestricted.

Let's Talk—An Intergenerational Dialogue!

You can make a positive impact too!

An intergenerational bond and its positive influences on a young person's confidence, emotional well-being, and outlook on aging are meaningful and life-changing. Older generations represent to developing adults immense courage, survivorship, acceptance, compassion, and wisdom. It naturally comes with living a long time! You can offer the stability, limitless love, optimism, time, and guidance supporting values and morals from which young people such as myself (I am now 28) can greatly benefit.

In our youth-obsessed and perfection-seeking society, young people are increasingly isolated and pressured to excel with limited support. It is a shame that an intergenerational bond is often an unappreciated and untapped resource. We need to reintegrate to form an intergenerational community. This begins with awareness and an open dialogue, sharing wisdom across the ages.

Closing Thoughts

My final message illustrates the significance of older adults in a young person's life. From a younger generation to an older generation, I hope this message reaches your heart from mine:

I admire your courage to have lived a long life. Despite everything life has thrown at you, you are still here today. You represent to me an entity that is full of life, history, and stories. I wish to let you know that I see you, each and every one of you. You are not invisible to me, and I hope to bridge this gap that our youth-focused society has seemingly placed between us.

Reflections for Readers

1. How might intergenerational dialogue positively affect older and younger people? What do the parties on both sides of an intergenerational relationship derive from it?
2. How can someone develop intergenerational relationships? What must come from the elder? What must come from the younger person?
3. What makes intergenerational dialogue challenging?
4. How might these challenges be overcome?

CHAPTER 39

Reversal of Roles . . . Listening to My Children

Irving I. Silverman
Business Manager, Publication Division,
National Knitwear Association and
Proprietor of the Kosher Food and Jewish Life Expo (retired)
Dedham, MA
Age 97

As I have aged, assuredly I have learned and have continued to grow.

For all the years when my children lived with me, I tended to dictate to them, believing that "I know best!" I insisted that they listen to me and my suggestions for their behavior and my solutions to their problems. My children didn't always agree that "I was right!" They may even have voiced their criticism. I didn't always listen.

Now that my children are grown and living outside of my household, a new set of circumstances arises. Am I always right now? It has taken me a long time to recognize and accept that I am not.

This was demonstrably made clear to me when I was advised after a fall that I needed to accept new mobility devices. First, it was a cane. One of my children bought me a super-deluxe cane made by a crafts-man in Ecuador. That did it. I liked it, and it gave me the feeling that I was protecting myself when I used it. And I did use it for several years until I fell again, having lost my balance and becoming less stable in my walking gait.

Then came the intervention of the physical therapy professionals. They determined that I should graduate to the use of a walker. I objected strenuously, voicing the thought that that made me look frail and like an invalid. So I refused to listen!

My four children raised objections to my unwillingness to use a walker. What finally evolved was the expression of one of my children, "Dad, you need it and we want you to be safe."

A miraculous development occurred. I realized that my children were more interested in my safety and welfare than in forcing me to do something I didn't want to do. I looked around and saw many of my resident friends with walkers. They even looked cheerful! So I bit my tongue and ordered a walker for a trial period. I also felt pleased with the fact that I was listening to my children. "Yes, they could be right, and I could be wrong!"

When the walker arrived, I lost my sense of denial and agreed to use it, at first only when I was outside my apartment and walking around the campus of my retirement community. I was very surprised that no one looked at me with unpleasantness. On the contrary, several of my friends agreed that it was good for me to use the walker, even inside my apartment; and I was able to move around with confidence that I was safe and protected.

As I listened to others, I heard that they were not dictating to me, they were expressing their wishes for my welfare and enhanced mobility. Realizing this produced a major change in my attitude. I realized that I could and should listen to others, including my children. It was a total change, and, believe it or not, I liked the change.

This experience has had a tremendous impact on my relationship with my children. In reversing the roles from the time I dictated to them to the time when I now really listen to them, a new wave of appreciation of parenting evolved. I'm a better parent now, and a wiser and a better listener. It will translate into a better pattern of communication between my children and me.

A lot has to do with tone and communication. It wasn't so much a reversal of roles; it was an awakening to the realization that I had made a mistake in not listening to my children a long time ago. They had learned a lot from me and their mother, and they were worth listening to—*listening*, because it was a two-way conversation, with no one dictating to anyone else.

I'm a better parent now than I ever was, primarily because I am willing to listen. "Listen" does not mean "obey"; it means considering what someone else is saying. When my children were growing up, that didn't happen. I'm glad it can happen now.

Reflections for Readers

1. What are the benefits of listening to others?
2. Are there particular benefits to listening to one's children? Are there deficits? What are they?

3. What might make it hard for a parent to listen to his or her children? Does this depend on redefining "listen" to something other than "obey"?
4. What other lessons can someone learn about parenting from his or her relationships with adult children?
5. If you were advising someone who, like this author, always thought he or she knew best, what would you say about listening to others?

CHAPTER 40

Moving to Be Closer to Family: Pluses and Minuses

Irving I. Silverman

Business Manager, Publication Division,
National Knitwear Association and
Proprietor of Kosher Food and Jewish Life Expo (retired)
Dedham, MA
Age 97

I have lived in a variety of places, including New York City and West Hempstead, New York, with my first wife, Henrietta. And Roslyn, New York; Bernard, Maine; and Tucson, Arizona, with my second wife, Nancy. Nancy died in 2002, and I began living alone.

In 2010, I underwent brain tumor surgery and decided that I should no longer live alone. But that raised the question of *where* I would live. Although initially I had resisted the idea of moving into a retirement community, I eventually decided that doing so would offer me some important advantages. But *where?* Of my four children, one lives in Milwaukee, two in greater Boston, and one in Dallas. There were desirable retirement communities in all these areas, and all four of my children wanted me to be near them.

It was a hard choice for me because I love all of my children and wanted to be near all of them, which obviously was not possible. I chose Boston partly because two of my four children were there and partly because I still had a home in Maine where I wanted to spend my summers, and Boston is closer to Maine than any of the other choices.

The major reason for moving, however, was to live closer to at least part of my family, so I could benefit from their watchful eyes and care. Thus, I would say that the biggest plus of moving was that new closeness to family. Where I had been living before, in Tucson and in Maine, was nowhere near any family members.

Earlier, I alluded to the words *pluses* and *minuses* in relation to family. I recall one particularly pleasurable incident: my eldest grand-daughter, who joined me for brunch one Sunday morning, said to me, "Before you moved to your retirement home, I saw you once or twice a year. Now, I am able to be with you 10 times in the last three months." What a joy it has been to be with her so often.

Enjoying the holidays and birthdays with my family became treats for all of us. They often joined me for evening entertainment programs in the auditorium in my community. And when I was able and the weather was accommodating, they would pick me up, and we enjoyed attending concerts and visiting museums and just being with each other for the day. It was never boring. It was always joyful.

I shouldn't sugarcoat the decision to relocate. Moving from my former homes meant leaving communities that were dear to me. There were many friends I had made in both Maine and Tucson, and I would have much less opportunity to see them if I moved away. Both of those communities were familiar to me—I knew where the post office was, where local landmarks were found—and I had never lived in the Boston area, so everything would be new to me.

I asked my daughter, Ellen, and her husband, Donald, to scout for a suitable retirement home in their vicinity. They found one in Dedham, Massachusetts, called NewBridge on the Charles, which was an upscale continuing-care facility, consisting of independent living, assisted living, and long-term healthcare accommodations.

I wanted to have a major hand in selecting my new retirement home, which would be my permanent home for the balance of my years. I was 90 years of age at the time. My grandchildren participated in all the re-location decisions.

NewBridge was the right choice for many reasons. First was location: I could be close to two of my four children and two of my six grandchil-dren so that they could visit me and benefit from the proximity to their father and grandfather. Second, I was able to obtain a two-bedroom unit, with ample space for comfortable living. Third, the facility pro-vided restaurant-quality dining, health care, staffing, a fitness area, and a full program of social, cultural, and entertainment activities. The fact that NewBridge was populated by 800 residents with ages from 70 to 100 was an important consideration, as it meant I would have many possible new friends.

Now that I am 97 years of age, I find being in the "afternoon" of my life a rich experience because I have family and many friends nearby and always have something pleasant to look forward to.

I am now acknowledged as "the giraffe man," "the man who loves lighthouses," and "the man who optimistically expects to live to the age of 120"!

Will I make it? I hope so. Living a long and accomplished life is a joy! Authoring this book is a lasting legacy, hopefully to be appreciated by you and many others reading this book.

Reflections for Readers

1. What problems might seniors encounter if they live far from any family members? What about problems faced by their families?
2. How can a senior living far from family find substitutes in terms of care? In terms of companionship?
3. What suggestions would you offer to a senior who does not have any family?
4. In some families, there is friction between generations. How would you advise an elder with such a family about where to live?
5. Some elders resolve family difficulties by informally "adopting" others as additional or substitute children and grandchildren. What do you think about this solution? Do you think that it offers advantages to seniors in general?

CHAPTER 41

We Were Never Afraid to Try Something New

Murray Staub, JD

Business Executive and Attorney, Municipal Law (retired)
Dedham, MA
Age 91

When we are young, love comes on like a thunderbolt! Of course, it is primarily a physical attraction (with hoped-for passion), but most relationships flame out. The good ones get deeper as we get to know each other better. We spend most of our time together. We get to know each other's "hot buttons"; i.e., what to say or not to get a reaction from our partner. Hopefully, we get married!

The passion that comes with love is sensitive and sweet. We constantly tell each other how much we love each other.

My wife Rhoda and I have been married for 67 years! It excites me to remember all these years and how we expressed our love and passion for each other. We lived in the environment we grew up in. Family around us, good friends, some even from grammar school. We had three great kids, now all adults with children of their own. Several of the grandchildren now have babies, so we are great-grandparents. How wonderful to see babies take their wobbly first steps! We had a comfortable home in a nice community, good friends whom we entertained and who entertained us. We could gossip about others and revel in our own good fortune to have that necessary spark of love.

Our early days were storybook times. We spent summers on an island off the coast of New Jersey. We played on the sand with our young children, and then with our grandchildren.

It was easy, lying on the beach watching the waves, the soaring sea gulls, the boats on the horizon. Watching the sun sink below the horizon and light up the clouds in the blue sky was incredibly beautiful.

Then real adventure came along. I was asked to assume the management of my company's Far East offices, headquartered in Hong Kong. One of the "perks" that I insisted on was that my wife, at company expense, could travel with me whenever she chose to. We had offices in Korea and Taiwan that I visited at least once a month. Of course, she tired of that. But, how about visiting China, Japan, India, Singapore, Indonesia, Sri Lanka, Bangladesh, and Thailand? When we first arrived in Hong Kong, we met some of the old "China hands," as they were called, at a cocktail party. They talked about Abu Dhabi and Kowloon. We had no idea where these exotic-sounding places were!

This was just the beginning of many adventures that we never dreamed of. Many times, we were homesick, and we clung together to assure ourselves that as long as were together, that was enough. One example was a dinner party given by a very sophisticated Chinese couple.

We were picked up at our hotel (we were still looking for an apartment) by their Rolls Royce and taken to a beautiful apartment that overlooked Hong Kong Bay. I'm sure most of my readers have eaten at a favorite Chinese restaurant where the food was "family style," with platters in the center of the table. Well, not in this fancy place! The first course, served individually, was a plate with six rice birds that all stood erect, with their long necks and tiny heads. Rhoda and I grasped each other's hands under the table. What do you do with these things we had never seen or heard of! We watched the other guests carefully. They confidently picked up a whole bird with their chopsticks, put the body in their mouths, bit off the neck and head and chewed with gusto! With great trepidation, I followed suit, nearly choking. But I got it down. My poor New Jersey wife did the same. There were still five birds left, but we managed to move them around so they looked somewhat eaten. Several unknown courses followed, but the last course was overwhelming . . . it was a whole suckling pig!

Many food events followed. Without my dear wife by my side many times, I was forced to drink much too much. The Chinese service always included three glasses at each setting, one for wine (not French), one for beer, and one for a Chinese liquor that tasted like gasoline. Not knowing what to expect, I drank the three glasses quickly, trying to fortify myself before the food arrived. To my horror, the attentive waiter refilled the glasses quickly so I would have enough to return my host's toast! To add to my discomfort, my host's translator said, "The Chairman asks 'how do you like the food'?" I of course said, "Very good." So he called the waiter to refill my plate!

But to the good times. How satisfying to share an ancient site, a wonderful restaurant, a walk in a park surrounded by hurrying Chinese who look at you questioningly, a rickshaw ride on an unknown road in the dark, seeing little light in small houses, and hoping that the driver will really take us to the hotel! Believe me, our passion was in our clasped hands. Many of the places we visited had colonial backgrounds. In Shanghai, for example, there is the Bund, a waterfront promenade filled with large stone buildings with their previous ownership signs such as "Bank of England" or "East India Company." You can feel the past as you walk by.

We had many adventures together and loved them all. We were never afraid to try something new. We even saw the famous River Quai in Thailand, where the Japanese used their Western prisoners to build the famous bridge depicted in a film. Thousands died, and we visited the cemetery where they lie.

However, no matter how much you love your life, fate sometimes deals another hand. My wife, once an adventurous and passionate partner, has gone into a state of dementia. She no longer lives with me. Here is where your remembrances are all that you have. You remember walking together hand in hand in so many new places that we never could have imagined we would be in. She cannot remember anything. I tell her stories about events, such as when we were invited into a hall where retired geishas were rehearsing for a concert. The music was terrible to our ears, but we smiled and applauded and they bowed in return. In the same afternoon, we stopped and looked into an open shop that turned out to be a tofu (soybean) factory. The owner saw us looking and invited us in, sat us at a table, and served us several versions of her product. She was so proud of her tofu, and we exclaimed how good it was.

There is nothing to compare to adventures together. How much you want to share the moment with your partner . . . who is no longer there. As I write this little memo, old scenes come back to me, but they all include my love. The passion can only come from your love for each other. I remember, most of all, having our arms around each other, murmuring "I love you" and going to sleep.

Note: Between the time when Murray Staub wrote this chapter and the publication of this book, Murray's beloved wife Rhoda passed away.

Reflections for Readers

1. What is the value of occasionally trying something new in older adulthood?

2. What kinds of changes has this author seen in his 67 years of marriage? How has his perspective on relationships matured over this time?

3. How are relationships in younger adulthood similar to and different from relationships in older adulthood?

4. This author describes the sadness of having a partner who is still alive, but in a state of dementia. What resources can someone draw upon to ease the feeling of loss in such situations?

CHAPTER 42

Love and Loneliness in Older Age

Irving I. Silverman
Business Manager, Publication Division,
National Knitwear Association and
Proprietor of Kosher Food and Jewish Life Expo (retired)
Dedham, MA
Age 97

I have always been a very independent person, and from the time I was married, at age 23, I lived in my own home. After the death of my second wife and some health issues of my own, my children suggested that I move to a retirement community, preferably near at least one of them. At the time, I was moving seasonally between homes in Tucson, Arizona, and Mount Desert, Maine, neither of which was near any of my family. Initially I resisted their suggestions, but I eventually decided I would accept their suggestion. I therefore agreed to move to NewBridge, near two of my daughters.

When I arrived at NewBridge, I was greeted by many of the female residents with platters of cookies and other treats. I was not interested at that time in forming any new relationships, and I let that be known, gently, to the women who had welcomed me. However, as time went on and I became acclimated to living in a retirement community, I began to notice that several other unattached men had found companions among the female residents.

I was jealous! Why did they have the good fortune to find new companions in later life, while I was alone? I didn't like having dinners with no one to talk to. I missed the closeness of someone to go to the opera with, someone to share projects with. I learned, only too well, that loneliness was painful.

But, the other side of things was, forming a new relationship would be taking a risk. Could I, a person who had been widowed twice, bear it if I let myself love another person and she were to become ill? Could I manage the pain and strain of taking care of her? Could I handle yet another bereavement?

No matter what our stage of life, being open to a relationship means being open to loss. That's the trade-off for having love and closeness. I wanted the love and closeness but was afraid of the possible pain.

I tried to understand my feelings better. If I were to become attached to someone else, who would I want that person to be; what would be important to me? Both of my wives had been attractive women; I would want a new love to be attractive too. Both my wives were educated, and that was important to me also; it deepened the kinds of conversations we could have. Given my fears, it made sense to me that I wouldn't want to start a relationship with someone already ill; and it also made sense that I would want someone willing and able to help and take care of me.

I looked again at the men I knew who had found new companions. I thought my upset was that they started these new relationships soon after their wives had died. Were they being disrespectful to their wives' memories? That was something that might have deterred me in my early years of widowhood, but it didn't apply to me at NewBridge; my wife had died in 2002, and I didn't move to NewBridge until 2010. But as I thought about it, I realized that my upset was more about jealousy than it was about feeling that they were being disrespectful. They had achieved something I wanted but did not have.

I next had to look at how those other men felt about the possibility of loss. By and large, they seemed not as concerned about this as I was, therefore more willing to take the risk . . . and maybe happier in their couple-state than I was in being alone. Maybe the fact that I had lost *two* wives made me more fearful than someone who had had one long marriage. Maybe having traveled through life with a visual handicap made me more concerned that a partner would have to take care of *me*, and being vulnerable to the loss of a helpmate, as well as the loss of a partner, just seemed like too much to me.

I still am alone, and I still suffer pangs of loneliness. Not all the time, and I am grateful for that, and also for the strategies I have found to minimize the pain. Keeping busy helps. Helping others helps. Those are not merely distractions, but also ways to feel that I have accomplished something, ways to be recognized by others as a worthwhile person.

My recommendation to others who find themselves alone and lonely in their later years is to look deep inside themselves, to determine how best to balance possible love and possible loss. This is a very personal and individual decision. If you decide that you are willing and able to risk love again, look for a new partner, and remember, there are a lot of lonely people out there who are possible mates or companions for you. If you decide that there is too much risk of pain in giving your heart to another person, find comfort for yourself in being busy and in doing as much good for others as possible.

Reflections for Readers

1. Many seniors find themselves alone after long years of marriage. What are the benefits and risks of entering a new relationship in one's older years?
2. Is it disrespectful of a spouse's memory to enter a new relationship after that spouse's death? Why or why not? Is there a proper amount of time that one should wait?
3. What might someone do to relieve his or her feelings of loneliness in later life?
4. Like loneliness, jealousy is a difficult feeling. How might a senior feeling jealous of his peers process that feeling?
5. Should couples talk to each other about whether they would want the surviving spouse to marry again? What considerations should enter such a conversation?

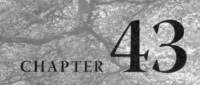
Love and Life

Ben Slomoff
Business Executive, Mediator, and Arbitrator (retired)
Walnut Creek, CA
Age 103

My life without love

Was bleak and bare.

I much preferred a warm hug

To a lonesome shrug.

What can replace

The ineffable joy of

My love's embrace

With that adorable smile

On her face?

You are gone but your

Picture is in its usual place.

When one phase of life ends

An innocent and meaningful glance

Can provide another chance

For Romance.

Love is nature's way of certifying life.

Don't count the ways of yesterday's sorrow.

Love can bring an eternal spring,

And with tender thoughts and smiling eyes,

A precious tomorrow.

First published in *A Stalwart Bends: Poems and Reflections* by Ben Slomoff

Reflections for Readers

1. How do you understand the line "Love is nature's way of certifying life"?
2. Does it require courage to seek a new relationship after the death of a spouse? Why?
3. This author writes, "You are gone but your/Picture is in its usual place." What remains of a loving relationship after the death of a spouse?

CHAPTER 44

Finding New Relationships in Later Life

Irving I. Silverman

Business Manager, Publication Division,
National Knitwear Association and
Proprietor of Kosher Food and Jewish Life Expo (retired)
Dedham, MA
Age 97

It is a sad truth that many elderly people find themselves single again after long years of marriage. This most often occurs because of the death of a spouse. It could also arise when a spouse suffers a prolonged and debilitating illness and the other spouse finds himself or herself effectively single even while the ill spouse is still alive. Especially for those whose marriages were happy ones, there is the desire to re-create the same kind of companionship previously enjoyed with one's spouse. Thus, more than in the past, elders are making decisions about remarriage or about creating new, serious nonmarital relationships, which may or may not involve living together.

Whether or not to enter into a new relationship in one's later years is a very personal decision, and different people will come to different decisions. There are some people who still feel married after the death of a spouse and are not willing to consider a new relationship. Others miss the companionship of a spouse so urgently that a substitute relationship seems necessary, as a way once again to experience the joy of togetherness. For some, what is missed is someone to care for or someone to care for you. Sometimes the lack of a sexual partner is what inspires a search for someone new. And sometimes financial considerations come into play, when the remaining person can't afford to live alone. Finances may also enter the picture when two seniors want to be in a relationship, but Social Security entitlements complicate remarriage. In these situations, both remarriage and living with a new partner become considerations, possibilities, or desirabilities.

For someone who has been widowed, it is a big step to say, "I'm ready to think about a new relationship." This will happen (if it does happen at all) on its own timetable, and no one else should tell you it's "too soon" if it feels right to you. You are not disrespecting your lost spouse if you choose to enter a new relationship; on the contrary, often the reason for wanting a new relationship soon after losing a spouse is that you found being in a loving relationship so good.

Someone whose husband or wife is still alive but suffering from dementia or for some other health reason is not able to be the same kind of partner as in the past, is in an even more difficult situation, and may receive a lot of criticism from others about forming a new attachment, even though he or she feels the need for companionship. Still, what is most important is to acknowledge your own feelings and needs.

For many seniors, sex remains an important consideration. There is great pleasure associated with being able to engage intimately with a partner, and some new relationships focus on this pleasure.

Seeing others forming couples might be what inspires two people to form a new relationship—maybe seeing such a thing for the first time as something both possible and desirable.

Whatever the reasons, we see more and more couples joining together. In the retirement community in which I now live, there have been numerous instances of living together, sometimes soon after a spouse passes, and not necessarily involving remarriage. Living together no longer has the stigma of "not proper" or "a disservice to the previous spouse."

It is important to recognize that the other person in a new relationship is not, and cannot be, a clone of one's lost spouse. The new person will bring strengths, talents, interests—and fears and weaknesses—all his or her own. For a new relationship to work, it needs to allow each partner his or her own individuality.

One should take into consideration all of the parties who will be affected by any new relationship. A new relationship in later life is likely to involve not just the couple, but possibly new (adult) children and grandchildren being "acquired" by one or both partners. How do you, as an elder, want to integrate these new family additions, and what effect might a new relationship have on the children and grandchildren? Family members may have issues about finances, including inheritances; they may also have feelings about whether a soon-to-be-remarried parent or grandparent will be buried with the deceased spouse or with the new partner. Talking to family members is important, as it will uncover their concerns and allow you to address them. Being sure that you have considered the feelings of all the adults and all the children involved will improve the probability of creating a happy and enduring relationship for everyone!

Being alone may no longer be an acceptable choice, for reasons of safety or avoidance of stress; however, entering into a new relationship just to have someone else take care of you is not the best possible motivation, as it does not allow much space for the other person's wishes or needs. Persons whose prime motivation is that they cannot live alone safely should find caregivers rather than looking to a new partner to keep them safe.

One thing I have noticed is that, even as we age, the idea of finding a possible new partner spurs people to become more sensitive to their appearance and outlook. This is not unlike regressing to your teen years, when you were so concerned about how you looked and what others thought of you. And finding new relationships becomes more possible in the age of the Internet, where dating services abound, including some aimed at seniors. "Why not?" has become the byword of many older people as they see relatives and friends who have developed new relationships in their advanced years. Indeed, "why not" find what will make you happy?

Reflections for Readers

1. What should an elder couple considering remarriage or living together talk about in advance with each other? What should they talk about with their respective children and grandchildren, and with each other's children and grandchildren? Which decisions do you see as the most important?

2. Can you think of characteristics that might distinguish the people who want to enter a new relationship after losing a spouse from the people who continue to feel married to the departed spouse?

3. Does sex still matter in one's later years? How should a prospective couple address this with each other?

4. Like young love, love in one's later years can be a heady feeling that pushes sober reflection to the side. Given an understanding of that fact, how and when should children and grandchildren express their questions or concerns about an elder's new relationship?

5. Is the age of a senior's prospective new partner a fair issue for children or grandchildren to be concerned about? What if the prospective partner is younger than the children? The same age as a grandchild?

CHAPTER 45

Grandparenting Is a Perk

Sherri L. Meade

Technology Executive, IBM (retired), and Real Estate Agent
Hatfield, MA

Having grandchildren is one of the primary rewards for having children in the first place. All those years when you thought you would never get through their infancies, childhood, adolescence, teens, and finally college, and all the mistakes you made and times you wished you could have a do-over; grandparenting is your chance for putting it right. The primary perk of aging, if you are lucky, is having a chance to enhance the lives of your grandchildren.

It is particularly amusing that sometimes, your grown children have revised history memories. They really can't (or won't) remember that you raised them to have the very values that they want to instill in their children. Somehow, they need to assert their authority as parents, to be sure that their children are looked after with appropriate care. When any of my children first became parents, before they would "let me babysit," they read me the ground rules and in one case, had me sign that I understood! Yes, a written manual on how to care for the child and lines for agreement with signature. But, you know, I happily signed and felt this small sense of pride that my children, now parents, were looking out for their babies.

The first time I held any of my grandchildren, the joy flooded me so much that I almost couldn't breathe. How could it be possible to have time reverse? Here you are holding "your baby" again. How wonderful is life and all its precious cycles. I am so happy to have this life-affirming opportunity again.

My love for my grandchildren has led to some crazy experiences. I remember once having to keep my overly tired 11-month-old granddaughter from falling asleep on a long car ride to a sleep doctor appointment.

I had to keep singing to her or telling her stories or getting her to laugh and not to fall asleep. It worked, but it was brutal.

I remember staying overnight at my daughter's house to help watch her newborn twin sons so that she could get some rest. The boys tag-teamed me, so that the minute I fed one of them and put him down, the other would wake up and need his turn. No sleep that night. But the look on each of those precious faces as I held them melted me. I am still melted even after 17 years.

In order to spend time with two of my granddaughters, I agreed to drive 200 miles each week to babysit, so that their mom could go to nursing school. Whether my son and daughter-in-law truly appreciated what I was doing hardly mattered. It was a sacrifice that I would make any day. After all, the relationship I built with those grandchildren can never be denied. There were many times that I did not pay enough attention to my own children (when I was younger and working); this needed redemption! It is quite remarkable that most of the things I would do for my grandchildren, I would never have thought to do for my children when they were younger. Is it that I now have more patience or appreciation? Probably! Otherwise, why is it that now I am willing to sit on the floor for hours and play games with my grandchildren? I think the wisdom of aging is acknowledging that time matters, attentiveness matters, and listening matters. I am determined to give my full self to my grandchildren so that each will feel undivided support and love. Errands and chores can wait this time!

One of the nuttiest things I have done for my grandchildren is to fly across the country (in the winter) in order to pick up their new puppy at a breeder. Yes, I flew from Boston to the Midwest, drove to a breeder's house, picked up an eight-week-old puppy, and flew with him to San Francisco. Crazy, yes, but the look on those kids' faces when they saw their new dog was priceless, and I knew that I was forever part of that story. Why wouldn't I do anything for my grandchildren?

My husband and I are blessed with nine grandchildren. Each child is so special, and each one has a unique relationship with me. I have tried very hard to establish different techniques and communications when spending time with each child. I want them all to feel like I know who they are and that each one is loved individually and unconditionally. I believe that the job of grandparents is to embrace each grandchild with unquestioning support. It is not our job to discipline or correct our grandchildren; their parents will surely do that. We can enjoy them for who they are and use every opportunity to "spoil them." I don't mean materially (although sometimes I do that too), but rather be there for them when they need unquestioning love and assurance that they are good people. What a fabulous thing it is to be able to make them smile and laugh, especially if they had been previously crying over some minor hurt. Yes, grandparents have that power!

We need to be role models for our children and grandchildren. We need to show them that aging does not mean giving up on love or time spent doing loving deeds. Family time is so special and gets more so as time passes. This understanding, this acceptance that after careers and hobbies, after other life goals, what is most important at the end is family and the love we share. My grandchildren are everything to me. I have worked hard (although *work* is really the wrong word) to be sure that each of my grandchildren feels that he or she can depend on me. I want them all to truly know that they deserve and are entitled to be loved because they are beautiful human beings. If I can instill this self-confidence in my grandchildren, I will surely have fulfilled my legacy.

Reflections for Readers

1. What is the "do-over" that grandparents get when they have grandchildren? Why might that be important to them?
2. When children grow up and have children of their own, how might *their* parents—now grandparents—renegotiate the relationship with their now-adult children?
3. What is the difference between being a parent and being a grandparent? What are the different responsibilities? What are the different rewards?

CHAPTER **46**

Water Play: Being Alec's Grama

Catherine Cobb Morocco, EdD
Educator (retired) and writer
Newton, MA
Age 76

"I found you!" Three-year-old Alec is beside my chair, beaming up at me with his wide, Howdy Doody mouth and cheeks, his red hair. His mother and father (my grown son) have just arrived at our extended family Thanksgiving. I have fallen in love again in my 70s, and it is reciprocated.

Some grandmothers live close enough to their grown sons and daughters to be a constant presence in their offspring's lives, even providing child care a day a week. My son lives in Brooklyn, my daughter in Denver, and my husband and I just outside Boston. When my first grandchild, Emma, was born in Manhattan, I clung to a fantasy that I would babysit a day a week—taking a train to Penn Station, a cab to their apartment, sleeping on the couch. Seeing how such a plan would wreck my writing life and complicate her nanny program, my daughter broke the news (gently), and I wept. They moved to Colorado, where I would be a visitor.

In Brooklyn, I puff after Alec as he races his scooter past smiling neighbors, crouching on one leg, holding the other in the air. We watch the tops of subway cars—"The choo!"—from a bridge over the tracks. In the Connecticut countryside, where my son and his wife have a cottage for weekends, we toboggan down their hillside in winter and roam adjacent meadows in summer. I learn to immerse myself in "special time"—devoted to activities that Alec loves—during the precious hours with him. "Water Play" is about one of those enchanted times.

Water Play

My son's three year old trots by me toward the meadow,

passing by swings. *Want to see the water—*

I follow, hearing sounds of water brush and tumble over stones

   rushing to join the Housatonic—

                        Go in the water—

He pulls my hand toward rock steps jutting down the bank,

without a railing. If I balance him in front of me,

holding his small arms high, water curling at our feet—

   Light flashes half-blind us.

I divert him to a path through grasses, tall, hiding a bog

with planks floating in muck, sucking as we teeter. I grasp

his jacket from behind.

The path opens to a pond ten feet across, water trickling

from crevices in a boulder, spilling drops of sunlight.

We touch pocked lichen.

                        Touch the water—

We bend over tree shadows rippling. If I dazzle

and he plunges, I will dive deep, then rocket from the water

with him in my arms, his sunflower face,

   both laughing that we are not . . .

   we are safe,

I listening for my son's whistle insisting

                        we return.

The sound-and-light show of water running over rocks in a stream is my "totem animal," my spiritual guide. I learned this during a writing retreat in Oaxaca, Mexico, in a sweat lodge that our host arranged. The presence of moving water that day with Alec, combined with the joy of being with this innocent boy, fearless and fascinated, drew me into a kind of trance.

In moments like this, I'm aware of a tension in my grandmothering between rapture and responsibility. I am attentive to Alec's safety and well-being as we explore. At the same time, I may become more child than adult, more seeker than caretaker, in the thrall of the child's pleasure, longing to feel the touch of water on my hands and body. My son is aware of this rapture side. His card for my 75th birthday is a child-like collage of a little girl in a swing, high in clouds, red hair (mine was strawberry blonde and now is white) streaming back in the wind, wide red mouth open.

In "Water Play," the grandmother is drawn to the stream, and is also careful to hold the child's shirt as they teeter over a bog. As they bend over the side of the pond, she is aware of the play of light and shadow that might "dazzle" her, and she indulges in a mythic fantasy of rising out of the water with him should he fall in. She is poised in a delicious reverie between being safe and not safe, expecting the son's signal, knowing that he will support her in being cautious.

I am well aware that this is a moment of "earned ecstasy." Opportunities to spend time with a grandchild are planned and coveted and most likely to occur if the older person is sensitive to the autonomy needs of the young family. Having special time with a grandchild brings the need to balance the grandmother's desire for this extraordinary relationship with the child with her desire for a strong bond with the grown son or daughter and his or her spouse. My daughter says, "Get your needs met, Mom," when I am reticent about suggesting a visit, because we have worked on our communications for a long time. My daughter-in-law, Alec's mother, lets me know Alec's boundaries in the city and country, and—in agreement over them—we all kick a soccer ball or build a snow igloo together.

My five grandchildren and I have much to help us connect from a distance—books that I send and we read together on Skype, photos that our grown kids text us or that we take and send, photo books that we make for each other. FaceTime links us suddenly in the midst of a busy day. When I'm physically with my grandchildren, I observe and listen to fathom where they have come and who they are now. I help each child say goodbye, with honest promises of when we'll be together again. Sometimes the child helps me leave by giving me a drawing for my refrigerator.

We grandmothers wonder how much of our grandchildren's future we will experience and are hungry for as much time as we can get. Should our grown sons and daughters move with their children to, say, California or Australia, we'll find them. As long as we are able.

Reflections for Readers

1. Grandparents can become young again playing with their grandchildren, but they also have a responsibility to keep their grandchildren safe and secure. How might grandparents negotiate the tension between those two aspects of their relationship with their grandchildren?

2. The author describes time with a grandchild as moments of "earned ecstasy." What is "earned" about such moments, and how? What creates the "ecstasy"?

3. In what ways do grandchildren represent a legacy to their grandparents, and how might grandparents work to provide a legacy to their grandchildren?

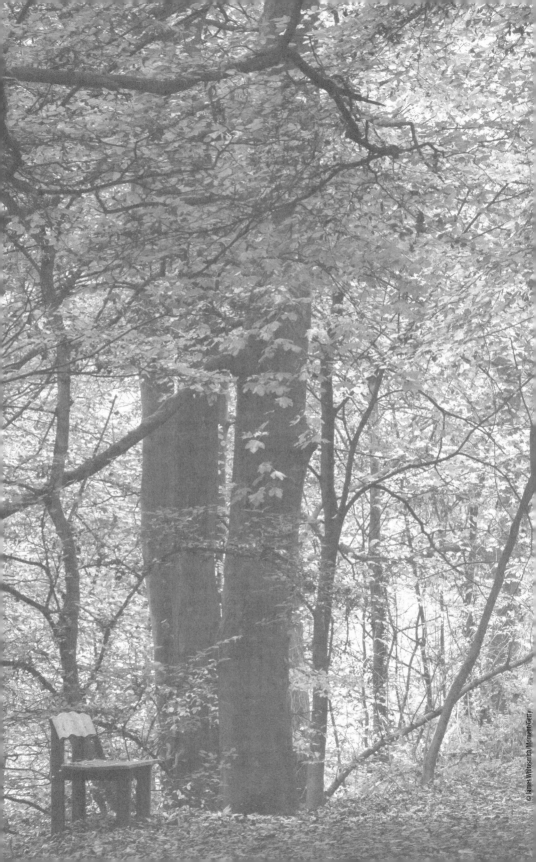

PART VIII

Overcoming Obstacles, Living Life to the Fullest

©James Whitesmith/Moment/Getty

CHAPTER 47

Caring and Being Cared For: A Reciprocal Relationship

(A tribute to Elsa Pollack, a beloved, wise elder)

Rabbi Judi Ehrlich
Chaplain, NewBridge on the Charles
Dedham, MA

As a Rabbi and Chaplain to the elderly and their families, I am in the privileged position of having many role models for how to age well and wisely. I have come to see how, despite illness, adversity, and losses, many elders manage to find joy and purpose in their lives. When I encounter seniors who, despite advanced age and declining health, display remarkable resilience and continue to live purposeful lives, I feel compelled to learn what it is that energizes and inspires them, so that I, too, can strive to cultivate this magical trait.

One of my many mentors in the art of wise aging was Elsa Pollack, who lived the last three years of her life in the Assisted Living wing at Orchard Cove, a retirement community in Canton, Massachusetts. Perhaps I admired Elsa so much because we shared many of the same values, the most significant of which is a love of people.

When I met Elsa, she was learning to cope with her diminishing independence and to accept her need for greater assistance with daily life activities. Having lived a full, productive, and independent life, this could not have been an easy adjustment. The most valuable lesson I learned from Elsa is that accepting care from others can be a mutually rewarding and reciprocal experience. Even when we are frail and dependent on others for assistance, we have much to offer because everybody needs to be cared for in one way or another.

Elsa had relished the social interactions she shared with other residents. She loved to engage in good conversation over dinner, sharing ideas and learning about the life experiences of her friends and neighbors. But now, as her strength waned, the effort of being in the dining room became too strenuous. Elsa found herself needing to eat in her room and had to limit her involvement in community activities. But although Elsa was no longer able to get out much, she created a meaningful social life within the confines of her own room. She took an interest in everyone who came to see her. Whether it was the housekeeper who straightened up her room, a waitress delivering her meal, the nursing aide who checked her vitals and helped her with her pressure stockings, or a dear friend who had driven 20 miles from Newton to visit with her, everybody who graced Elsa's doorway received a warm welcome and her full attention.

You know that feeling when you meet someone; they grasp your hand, look you in the eye, and make you feel like for that moment you are the most important person in their lives? That was Elsa. Initially, I thought it was just me, because we had such a special connection. But in conversations with my colleagues and with other residents, I was told repeatedly that whenever they went to see Elsa, she greeted them so warmly . . . because they had such a special connection! While I admit that it was a bit of a blow to my ego to discover that Elsa made *everyone* feel so special, I was intrigued by the ability of this unique woman, in her 90s, to have such a positive effect on so many people.

One of Elsa's housekeepers, who had taken a week off work when her mother died, made a point of visiting Elsa upon her return to check if there was anything she needed. The housekeeper later shared with me that she had gone to see Elsa to make sure that her room was in order and that her hearing aids, hairbrush, and telephone were next to her bed, where she could easily find them.

Elsa remembered why the housekeeper had been away. She invited her to sit down and tell her a little about her late mother. So she sat and they talked. And the housekeeper told me that for those few minutes, she felt her mother's loving presence surrounding her. She had gone to Elsa's room to provide care, and she left feeling comforted and nurtured.

I once praised Elsa for taking such a warm, genuine interest in her team of supporters, myself included. She explained that she could no longer get out into the world and mingle with interesting people in many settings, the way she had once done. But when people share their experiences with her, when they tell her about their concerns and their hopes and their joys, she feels connected to the world. So, although she seldom leaves her room, she feels enriched and her life expands.

Elsa told me that the less she has in common with someone, the more interesting it makes them. By taking an interest in this person's life, she learns about new ideas and comes to understand why people value something that had not previously been of interest to her.

Elsa also wanted to make it quite clear to me that she is no saint and that, like everyone else, she has her bad days. She told me that when she is in pain or feeling very weak, she doesn't always have the energy to reach out and connect with others. There are times when she feels sorry for herself and is frustrated that she can't participate in family events. There are times when she is grumpy and confused and feels that her needs are a burden on others.

However, she explained, she realized long ago that what makes her feel better most of the time is human interaction. And so even when she feels least able to be sociable, she knows that the best antidote to her woes is reaching out to others and returning the kindnesses that she receives from them. Through example and wise words, Elsa taught me that taking a genuine interest in other people expands our own horizons and takes our minds off our problems. She taught me that when we take a sincere interest in others, we feel engaged with and connected to the greater family of humanity.

Although Elsa was hard of hearing and had a weak heart and poor vision, she was a good listener and her heart was open to all. We all felt like she could really see us. And we knew that she genuinely cared for us. And so, we were fortunate to be nurtured and inspired by her deep insight and generous, loving spirit. Elsa modeled for us that physical disability does not have to limit our ability to continue to engage with the world and nurture others. She demonstrated the magic that happens when we care for those who take care of us. May her wise teaching be a blessing for all who seek lessons in living well.

Reflections for Readers

1. How might one's perspective on caring and being cared for change as one ages?
2. How did Elsa offer care to the people around her?
3. Do you agree that the people you have the least in common with are the ones you find the most interesting? Why or why not?
4. How might we best channel our "inner Elsa" and care for others with our full attention?

48

Living in the Real World, Not an Imaginary One

Helene Oppenheimer

Director, Tax Library, BDO Seidman (1983–1993),
New York, NY (retired)
Dedham, MA
Age 82

I ask the question "What is the real world?" Everyone will answer that question differently for themselves from the way others would answer it. Even people growing up in the same family would answer that question differently, according to their place in the family and how they see themselves in that place in the family.

What was the real world to you? What did you think a real grownup was? Look at your place in the family. Look at yourself as a child and as a grownup. Think of your family as you saw them when you were a child; think of your family as you saw them when you were a teen and as a young adult. Then think of your family when you became an independent adult, perhaps working and living at home. Then review your family if you married and had children, had responsibility for other people, and *you* had to become a real grownup.

What was the real world to you then? Was it difficult to accept the real world? We view our lives differently at different times of our lives. Think about spending your time as a child: daydreaming, playing pretend, playing house, dressing up your dolls, playing with your cars and trucks, pretending to be a fireman or policeman, and building sand castles at the beach. What did you feel when you were called to dinner and had to stop playing? The spell was broken. I know that I resented having to go to dinner and stop my world of make-believe.

Perhaps we were not aware that as children, we were living two lives: the real world of eating, sleeping, schooling—and play, lots of play. That was the imaginative world. This world involved telling stories to ourselves, to our playmates, even to our siblings and parents. We lost ourselves in that pretend world. There was a Saturday morning radio program when I was growing up called *Let's Pretend.* I remember sitting at the kitchen table being transported to the world of make-believe from that morning's story, probably a fairy tale. I cannot remember any of those stories now. Perhaps as a grown-up, I've lost the ability to pretend. Is that what happens to most healthy adults? Our attention is turned to other activities: we become absorbed in work, marriage, possibly more education; then care of our family, and perhaps care of our parents. No time for fantasy!

There are some professions that do allow a certain amount of pretend. The acting professions, both stage and screen, the fiction-writing profession, the screenwriting and stage-writing professions all allow the world of pretend to exist in their practitioners' lives. Movie stars and stage actors have refined their pretending into a real talent. But what happens to them after the performance is finished or when the show closes? What happens to the actor who has years of pretend? Some are able to see their pretend as a real job, a real stopping-point at the end of a day's work. Some are involved in other businesses, not just their acting jobs. So some do have a real life, but there are others who seem to have a life of despair: they cannot separate the two worlds in which they live. The pretend worlds of the stage and movies are so much fun, offer so much glamor, and all that applause to keep their egos intact. The real world becomes so hard for some actors to deal with.

And what about the fiction writers, whether novels or screen or stage writers? Is there another *Gone with the Wind* or *The Wizard of Oz,* or another *Alice in Wonderland,* around the corner waiting to be discovered? Most of the fiction written today seems to be based on actual historical happenings, not on imagination and fantasy.

I like to think that our childhood can carry us into the future by allowing us to enjoy imaginative acting and writing while living in the real world of work and family at the same time. Today's young adults seem to live in a different world, a world where they feel that only their peers understand them, that we as adults do not understand their needs and desires, and that we are perhaps too different, so that it is too difficult to let us in. But we adults were young once and had dreams, and we became responsible adults, ready to accept the world's challenges. Many of today's youths will do the same thing as they mature and realize that they have to live in the real world, as difficult as it may seem.

I can remember a semi-real-world incident when, as a young child, I went to the movies with my mother. I was age 7 or 8, resenting being indoors in late winter on an exceptionally springlike day. My mother loved the movies and often took me with her when we were going to her parents' house afterward. This particular movie took place in a city, in winter in a snowstorm, with high winds sweeping through the city. I can remember being frightened by the movie storm. My mother quieted me by saying, "This is only in the movie; there is no storm outside." But when we left the movie theater, we found ourselves in the middle of a snowstorm with high winds. We made our way through the snow to the streetcar, and by the time we arrived at my grandparents' house, the snow and wind had lessened; 45 minutes later, they had completely stopped. That incident left such an impression on me that I found myself believing that happenings in the movies were real. I have always avoided going to see violent movies, and if there is unexpected violence, I hold my head down, shut my eyes, and cover my ears; I do so to this day.

What do most people feel when watching movies? Is it an escape from their real world; does it make them feel better about their real world? Most people, I believe, would say that it takes them out of themselves; it gives them some time to avoid dealing with their lives; or it makes them feel that their lives are better than the movies.

Now let's look at the world of television: what it was and what it has become. Is it an escape or entertainment, a teaching tool, or a way to release inner emotions? Doesn't that depend not only on the program content, but on the person viewing the program content?

In Baltimore where I grew up, TV in its infancy consisted of three channels with limited on-air time. Watching TV became a family entertainment after dinner. There were few or no daytime programs until the "soaps" started. Even into the 1950s and 1960s, it was not a 24-hour occurrence. My children's TV time was limited to sports and historic events, and, I must admit, they were allowed to watch *Star Trek* and the Saturday-morning programs, even those awful cartoons. But limited they were, as my husband and I believed in outdoor activity, and we were lucky to own a house with a large, fenced-in back area where the children could run free with our dog. TV did enter our lives and stayed there, but not to the exclusion of play, which allowed the children to be imaginative and provided a release from the anxiety of their days of school, both secular and religious.

Eventually, the number of TV stations multiplied, along with the number of hours that the stations were on the air, and the size of the TV screens grew larger. More and more families bought more and more

TV sets. TV was often used as a baby-sitter, which tended to isolate the children from the rest of the family and limited their playtime, as they spent more and more time in front of their TV sets. After many years, 24-hour TV programming became the norm, and the channels became not only a source of entertainment, but a source for instruction and education, as well as a source for shopping. A grand resource for the housebound.

I do not know if any studies have been done to explain how people watching TV think of that time spent in front of those sets, but to my way of thinking, it is unreal to spend so much time just sitting watching, watching, and watching.

Many of the programs today are of the day's events, real news in the real world, but so many programs are just done for excitement. Crime shows have proliferated and some parents have opted for a "parental lock" so they could determine some of their children's TV watching. So depending on how TV is used in various homes, TV watching can be entertainment, instructive, or make one feel less fearful and alone. This TV watching can make a person feel that they are in the real world, but can also make a person feel they are in the land of make-believe.

We live in a much more complicated world today, and we might need our imaginations to maneuver in it. Is it a more imaginative or a more realistic world than the one we lived in when we were growing up? Today's world of information technology is certainly more complex. Reading Dick Tracy, could we really have imagined the smart watches and smart phones of today? No wonder it is difficult for some people to live in today's real world, because the real world of today is a complex, almost unreal one; and we need all of our imagination to survive.

About Older People

Having written about childhood and young adults, I will look at the elderly and what they have to deal with, day by day. I know there are elderly who live alone, and that this can cause sadness. My mother experienced this when my dad died at age 71 and my mom was age 69. My mom died at age 104 1/2, so there were many years for her to feel alone and to be sad.

However, I only remember her sadness until shiva[1] was finished, and she knew it was time to pick up her life again. She did this after every loss, especially those of her parents, whom we all were quite close

---

[1] In Jewish tradition, shiva is the seven-day period of mourning following burial, when the mourners all stay together and friends bring food and comfort.

to—we spent some time almost every weekend at my grandparents' house. (I was lucky to have had two sets of grandparents living while I was growing up, but we spent more time with my mother's parents.) My grandmother died at age 71 when I was 11 years old, and my grandfather died at age 75 when I was 15 years old.

My parents generally included my brother and me in their family talks because they wanted us to be prepared for illness and death of those whom we were close to and loved. However, my dad never spoke to us about his parents' illnesses (his mother died in her early 70s, but his dad lived to be 97), nor did he talk with us about his own illness as he aged. Perhaps this was his nonreal world, trying to protect us from sadness, and he may have thought of this as a gift to us.

After my father died, I spent a good deal of time with my mother: visiting family, traveling together, and having her visit with me, Martin, and our children three months every winter, and in the summers before the children went off to camp. We lived in New Jersey, and my mother lived in Maryland, where my brother and his family lived, as did my mother's brothers and sisters, and many good friends. I often traveled down to spend time with her, especially as she aged. But her day-to-day life was filled with activity, such as attending services at her synagogue and events at the Sisterhood there, attending classes and Hadassah meetings, meeting friends and family out for luncheons. These activities made her live in the real world.

We had many conversations about her health, especially when she was in her 90s and had a hip replacement due to a very bad fall. Luckily, she had moved into a retirement/medical community near her family. She was in relatively good health, and though she would not talk about a "Do not resuscitate" order, she did talk to me about funeral arrangements and the funeral service. She had made notes for my brother and me to read so that we would know her wishes. So it seems to me that my mother was living in the real world, being pragmatic.

Many elderly will shy away from such conversations because they are uncomfortable discussing these matters with their children; perhaps older people feel sad talking about their problems (health and others), or they feel that they are imposing on their children, or they are trying to protect their children. Their real world is not truly a real world; they live in a world of loneliness and pain until they are ready to face their aging head on. This is hard for them to do because they may not recognize their pain and sadness; they may not want to talk about their aloneness for fear of driving away friends and being even more alone.

As my mother aged past 100 years, she hesitated to talk about her feelings. I suggested that she might talk with her doctor or rabbi, but she told me that she would talk with me when she was ready. She seemed quite content with her life and never sad, except when we spoke about my dad. I do know that my mother was a strong and a strong-willed woman, but I often wondered how she managed to stay grounded in the real world after the love of her life had died. Of course, she immersed herself in everyday life, living it as it came, never complaining about her life as she lived into her 100s.

There was one thing that made our entire family sad: a very young baby grandchild died in 1963 of sudden infant death syndrome (SIDS). Of course, sadness was to be expected in this case. We all dealt with Suzanne's death by talking about it during shiva, and what could be done to prevent this from happening to other babies. My brother and sister-in-law, after talking with the medical examiner in Baltimore where they lived, formed a charity to raise money for SIDS research. My mom and dad joined in all the activities of this fundraising that took place over many years. So through their sadness, my family faced the reality of the future, being interested in the protection of many more families for years to come. Our talking with each other made this acceptance possible. Many families do cope with sadness by doing positive, but some families are not able to cope, and so they separate and live in their own worlds, not always a real one.

One thing that I am certain about is that sadness has to be dealt with, that loss of life has to dealt with, in order to live a real life in the real world. The elderly who cannot face the realities of aging, illness, and loss will remain alone in their sadness and miss out on the many wonderful opportunities in the real world today.

Reflections for Readers

1. This author contrasts the "real world" with the world of imagination and play. As children, most of us move easily between those two worlds; but what is the role of the imaginary or "play" world for adults?

2. Sometimes living in an imaginary world is not playful, but rather an exercise in denial of reality. Some people, for example, act as if things that are objectively not true are real because that is how they would prefer their world to be. As a professional, a family member, or a friend, how might you deal with a person

with this "perception" of reality? Would you behave the same in all these roles or would the roles dictate different attitudes?

3. The author writes, "We view our lives differently at different times in our lives." How does our aging process affect or change our view of our lives?

4. Do seniors ever have the same experience that children often have, of believing that something from the world of imagination is in fact real? If so, is this a good or bad thing? Why?

5. How important is it for adults to exercise their imaginations? For adults not in professions like acting or fiction writing, how might adults accomplish this?

6. This author contrasted her parents' different philosophies regarding talking about end-of-life issues with their children, one believing it was important for the children to "be prepared for illness and death of those [they] were close to and loved," and the other perhaps trying to protect the children from sadness. Which of these philosophies makes more sense to you when dealing with young children? With teens or young adults? With more mature adult children?

CHAPTER 49

Finding Meaning in the Face of Life Difficulties

Jason M. Holland, PhD
Assistant Professor, William James College
Core Faculty, Geropsychology Concentration
Newton, MA

The nineteenth-century existential philosopher Friedrich Nietzsche once wrote, "He [*sic*] who has a why to live can bear almost any how." Throughout my clinical and research career as a geropsychologist, as well as in my own personal life, I have found those words to be true. In our Stressful Transitions and Aging Research (STAR) lab, we have seen, time and time again, that those who are able to maintain some sense of meaning and purpose in life, even in the face of intensely stressful life events, are at a distinct advantage.

Research on Meaning Reconstruction

In particular, we have found that veterans returning from war, as well as other populations exposed to extreme violence, often struggle to reconcile their experiences with prior beliefs about the safety, predictability, and fairness of the world (Currier, Holland, & Malott, 2015; Holland, 2016). When left unresolved, these struggles can fester for years and possibly even follow veterans all the way to the end of their lives (Holland, Currier, Kirkendall, Keene, & Luna, 2014).

This search for meaning also seems to be much more than just an intellectual or existential exercise. Indeed, the outcome can mean the difference between life and death. For example, among veterans returning from Afghanistan and Iraq, those who were able to integrate traumatic experiences into some overarching worldview that subjectively made sense to them showed fewer risk factors for suicide and were less likely to engage in life-threatening behaviors, such as driving under the influence of alcohol or engaging in self-injurious behaviors like cutting or burning themselves (Holland, Malott, & Currier, 2014). In studies with older adults, we have also discovered that seniors who feel that they have made sense of their most troubling recent experiences, ranging from interpersonal loss to health problems, are significantly more likely not only to report being hopeful about their lives but also to show healthier salivary cortisol profiles, suggesting an improved response to stress even at a physiological level (Holland, 2016; Holland et al., 2014).

Fortunately, it seems that this process of integrating difficult life events into some broader frame of intelligibility occurs fairly automatically most of the time. Even after some of the most devastating events, like losing a spouse or a child, resiliency seems to be the rule rather than the exception (Bonanno, Westphal, & Mancini, 2011). People find ways to pick themselves up, dust themselves off, and keep moving, even if the path forward is not entirely clear. For a subset of individuals, however, professional consultation may be needed to facilitate the process.

Case Example: Gretta

Gretta was one such person. She was referred to me because of difficulties that she was having after a recent fall. About a year before, at the age of 85, Gretta had been knocked to the ground during a large and crowded outdoor concert. Ever since, her family and friends reported that she was somehow not quite the same. She had received a thorough cognitive evaluation, involving numerous batteries and follow-up assessments. However, the resulting pattern was quite inconsistent. On some tests and on some days, she seemed to show up and tested well within the normal range. On others, she didn't seem to be entirely there. Though a head injury or degenerative disorder could not be ruled out, Gretta's neurologist surmised that fluctuations in mood and motivation might help to explain her erratic testing, prompting his referral for psychological counseling.

At her first appointment with me, Gretta appeared quite anxious and was overwhelmed by so many concerns that it was difficult for her to maintain focus and articulate a clear narrative about what had happened to her. It was apparent that until quite recently, she had been fiercely independent and wore it like a badge of honor. Gretta rebelled against aging itself, in the way she dressed and talked, and felt intensely energized by being around young people. She prided herself on still keeping up with all of the local happenings of her community, even in her advanced age.

Thus, her fall during an outdoor concert represented much more than just an accident that required physical recovery. It was an assault on her most cherished values of independence, energy, and youth of spirit. On that day, she suddenly found herself helpless, laid out on the ground, not even entirely aware of what had just happened. "The rest was a blur," as Gretta put it, as ambulances and emergency personnel rushed in and assessed the damage. The physical repercussions initially seemed to be limited to a few facial fractures. However, after several months, the damage to her self-image and confidence was apparent. By the time Gretta came to see me, she was psychologically paralyzed, completely frustrated with her limitations, some self-imposed and others not, yet unable or unwilling to consider ways in which she might reconstruct a meaningful life for herself in the wake of her fall.

Given her restricted routine, in the early stages of treatment, I recommended that Gretta try to supplement each day with at least four pleasant or meaningful activities. Although social activities were encouraged, anything that she regarded as promoting a more positive mood was fair game, from knitting a scarf to going to a charity event. Although this increase in activity seemed to help stabilize her situation to some degree, Gretta still did not seem entirely engaged in the process, and her mood was only moderately improved.

After our fourth session, Gretta took a week off for a Caribbean cruise with one of her closest friends. Though planned for a long time, the timing of the trip was fortuitous, and Gretta returned for session five with a somewhat different presentation. She beamed as she reminisced about her trip, noting that it was the first time since the fall that she felt like herself again.

Exploring that theme further, Gretta and I engaged in a dialogue about what she made of that. How was it that she had only been able to feel like herself again on a trip far away from home? What was it about the new environment of a vacation that allowed her to try on new roles and explore new ways of being herself? As Gretta reflected on these questions, she became tearful, acknowledging that one of her biggest fears had been to resume her normal routine. What if she tried to go to a concert, just as she had done before? Would her worst nightmares be confirmed? Would she compare notes before and after the fall and find that her experience of life had somehow diminished? Beyond that, Gretta worried that her friends in the community would perhaps come to see her as an "invalid," if for some reason she appeared in public and seemed confused or showed an unsteady gait. She was far too proud to "accept charity" and resisted any displays that might prompt such gestures.

Hearing these two discrepant depictions of herself, I reflected back what I heard to Gretta, noting how she used words like *vibrant, youthful,* and *energetic* to describe herself before the fall. Now afterward, there seemed to be a totally different kind of vocabulary. Words like *invalid* and *helpless* started to come up. Holding these two depictions up to her, side by side, I asked Gretta to help me make sense of it. How exactly did her life story take such a sharp detour? Which strands of this painful narrative felt most difficult and discrepant from her core values? And alternately, which narrative strands remained intact? Did any personal characteristics or life themes survive the fall?

This exploration came to define our remaining work together, as Gretta started putting the pieces of this puzzle together and taking small risks in her life. On one occasion, for example, she accompanied a friend to the symphony at a venue she had not returned to since her fall. It didn't come as a tremendous surprise that she did in fact notice some differences in her experience. She felt somewhat unsure of herself now and worried that people were directing sympathetic glances her way.

At the same time, it was a tremendous relief to be out of the house, and although it didn't feel exactly the same, she began to notice remnants of her prior self bubbling to the surface. The music lingered in her head even after the concert was over, and despite feeling a little tired, Gretta got her second wind and joined a group that was going out for coffee and tea afterward. Once the awkwardness of the first few minutes passed, she found that most people treated her just as they had before, and she was still able to enjoy conversations, laugh, and bask in the glow of good company, as she always had. After a series of "small wins," like her successful trip to the symphony, Gretta gradually came to develop a new way of looking at herself. Though perhaps more vulnerable in some ways because of the fall, this event also came to represent one of her greatest protests against the physical and psychological forces that, from time to time, can pull us all down.

Conclusion

As so poignantly illustrated in Gretta's struggle for significance and meaning, difficult life events can hold tremendous psychological weight. They often defy rational integration and challenge even our most cherished notions about ourselves and the world around us. However, Gretta's story is one of hope. Despite the very real forces of aging, which likely played a role in her fall, Gretta still found ways to connect to the values that defined her through much of her life and flexibly reconstructed an image of herself as a woman who was now perhaps limited in some ways, but still had much left to offer the world. I find Gretta's story to be quite inspiring, particularly in those moments when I too must struggle with the forces in life that inevitably knock me down.

Reflections for Readers

1. How does having "a why to life" improve a person's quality of life?
2. What is the relationship between finding meaning in one's life and being resilient in the face of life challenges and even traumatic events?
3. What meaning can someone attribute when bad things happen in his or her life?
4. Do you agree that difficult physical life events can hold great psychological weight? How and when might you encourage a person who has suffered a fall or other physical injury to seek psychological help? How would you explain to that person why such help might be beneficial?
5. How would you go about helping a senior who has suffered a physical setback, restore a sense of himself or herself as an active, vibrant person? In other words, how would you restore the meaning that he or she had formerly seen in life?

References

Bonanno, G. A., Westphal, M., & Mancini, A. D. (2011). Resilience to loss and potential trauma. *Annual Review of Clinical Psychology, 7*, 511–535.

Currier, J. M., Holland, J. M., & Malott, J. (2015). Moral injury, meaning making, and mental health in returning veterans. *Journal of Clinical Psychology, 71*, 229–240.

Holland, J. M. (2016). Integration of Stressful Life Experiences Scale (ISLES). In R. A. Neimeyer (Ed.), *Techniques of grief therapy, Vol. 2* (pp. 46–50). New York, NY: Routledge.

Holland, J. M., Currier, J. M., Kirkendall, A. M., Keene, J. R., & Luna, N. (2014). Sadness, anxiety, and experiences with emotional support among veteran and non-veteran patients and their families at the end of life. *Journal of Palliative Medicine, 17*, 708–711.

Holland, J. M., Malott, J., & Currier, J. M. (2014). Meaning made of stress among veterans transitioning to college: Examining unique associations with suicide risk and life threatening behavior. *Suicide and Life Threatening Behavior, 44*, 218–231.

Holland, J. M., Rengifo, J., Currier, J. M., O'Hara, R., Sudheimer, K., & Gallagher-Thompson, D. (2014). Psychosocial predictors of salivary cortisol among older adults with depression. *International Psychogeriatrics, 26*, 1531–1539.

CHAPTER **50**

Accepting Help

Irving I. Silverman
Business Manager, Publication Division,
National Knitwear Association and
Proprietor of the Kosher Food and Jewish Life Expo (retired)
Dedham, MA
Age 97

The cardinal rule of aging is to ask for help when needed. All of us need help throughout our lifetimes—from parents, from siblings, from friends, from teachers, and from a range of other helpers.

Babies are unable to ask for help, even though they are dependent on help from parents and other caregivers, which hopefully is given generously. Receiving such help is essential for developmental growth.

As babies grow into children and eventually into adults, they become increasingly responsible for themselves. For some, illness, handicaps, and other obstacles make this especially difficult. With growth, we all have to assume responsibility for adjusting to or overcoming whatever hurdles we face.

For many of us, the need for help becomes pronounced when we reach old age. More things go wrong—health issues, losses, increasing weaknesses, and fears. All of this is sometimes exacerbated by choices that we made earlier in life. It's necessary to enlist the cooperation of others and to choose appropriate people to ask for help. Finding people who know your personality, interests, and choices and have faced similar challenges before can make this process easier.

Problems arise when someone becomes unwilling or unable to ask for help, believing that he or she is able to make all the right decisions alone. The opposite is also possible and equally problematic, that a person decides that he or she cannot function independently but needs to solicit ideas and suggestions from others on all things.

The path that one follows to achieve older age is not always easy, and learning to accept help is sometimes one of the difficulties. But: the bottom line is that life is worth living and pursuing. And one can achieve a successful life with a variety of steps along the way, never looking backward, but always looking forward with the expectation that tomorrow may be a brighter and happier day. It can and should be!

I'm a prime example of an aged individual who has lived through continued experiences of needing and accepting help. As I remember it, it was all done without embarrassment and without any serious objections. I knew I needed help and was receptive to the assistance that others provided. In early childhood, the assistance came from the teachers in the sight conservation classes that were provided for students with severe visual impairments. Help included access to large print books and other materials that were individually composed and enabled me to keep up with the learning process of my fellow students. I remember receiving additional psychological support so that I could accept the special materials without resistance. The special sight conservation teachers were trained to provide that assistance. The sight conservation classes in the school I attended were an accommodation that removed us from the mainstream into a special classroom, a sort of "one room schoolhouse" with 17 students of different ages. This was the era prior to the current use of special education classes for students with attention or behavioral issues. So much for the educational assistance I benefited from.

I had to devise ways to keep up with other children on the playground and in sports and had to learn how to ask for help in mastering the skills of playing sports. This was a strain for me, as it was hard for me to accept assistance from my peers. I suffered from always being the last to be picked for any team. That became a test of my psychological adjustment.

Accepting help became even more straining in college, where I was dependent on teachers' abilities to segment me out of the regular class structure without causing me to feel inconsequential. The mental adjustment was immense. One technique that I developed to deal with this was to foster close friendships with fellow students who could then assist me without making me feel incompetent or undeserving of respect. The skill of building friendships has continued through all my subsequent years and has been a source of not just help, but also comfort and mutual giving—a very important accomplishment that has carried me through my adult years as the need for assistance has become more pronounced. As I have aged, I have needed my friends to be more watchful to keep me from falling or otherwise endangering myself.

In the midyears of my life, I encountered other difficulties that caused me to look for help from others. For example, I have difficulty seeing and recognizing other people and that became an ongoing emotional challenge. It wasn't easy to accept the scorn that sometimes was directed at me for failing to recognize someone. It's not easy to feel different or incapable of managing the challenges of daily living. As I have grown older, I have found it easier to ask for help from other "olds," and from caregivers and aides who are accustomed to providing assistance to handicapped people. I've been privileged to find "guardian angels" who have miraculously appeared at the appropriate times to help me; all I had to do was to ask, and their response was immediate and affirming. It gave me the incentive, as I matured and grew older, to provide for the training of new "guardian angels" for other needy adults via providing philanthropic support to schools and training institutions.

What has made it possible for me to accept help—the *most* important thing—is the tone with which someone offers help. A recipient of help may be embarrassed, with feelings of inadequacy, and the tone that a helper uses can overcome those feelings. It seems so simple! Less simple is when the person needing assistance is unable to ask for help or articulate what is needed, but even then, a well-trained or well-meaning helper can usually figure it out in a way that preserves dignity and shows respect.

The need for asking for help is ongoing, and can apply to simple things like tying one's shoelaces, buttoning one's shirts, combing one's hair, and finding the way to a restroom, all of which become increasing challenges with age. It's important to develop the skill, and the willingness, to ask others for help in such instances. An example of this happened to me just the other day, when after attending an outdoor event, I became confused, unable to find my way back to my apartment. I asked a friend for help, which he immediately and graciously provided.

The problem of asking for help becomes more acute when one loses a partner, meaning that it becomes more necessary to ask for help from strangers. That represents a new learning experience. But it's all accomplishable!

At the age of 97, I have lived through scores of occasions when I needed help and found myself unable to communicate that need. How wonderful, when a helper can anticipate what is needed! Even to this day, I am continuously aided by such assistance. For instance, I was recently in a restaurant and the lighting was very poor. When the main course was served, I found myself unable to see well enough to cut the food on my plate. My friend noticed my hesitation and without my even asking for help, he came to my aid so I could finish my meal with pleasure and comfort. There's an art to this, which includes preparation by the person needing help and anticipation by the provider. When it was accomplished, it seemed so effortless but it did require forethought—and was very much appreciated!

Reflections for Readers

1. What can make it difficult for seniors to ask for help?
2. In what areas is it most difficult to ask for or accept help? What can helpers do to make asking for help easier?
3. What strategies can someone use to ask others for help? Would the strategies in asking for help from peers be different from the strategies in asking for help from professionals?
4. For people who have needed help all through their lives, is it harder or easier to ask for help? Why?
5. For many, helping others is a source of pleasure and pride. What can a recipient of help do to add to that feeling for the person providing help?
6. The author mentions that a "fringe benefit" of his needing help was that he developed the skill of building friendships. Are there other such fringe benefits from asking for help?
7. Is needing help incompatible with being independent? With feeling independent?

©James Whitesmith/Moment/Getty

51

Occupational Therapy and Productive Aging

Laura Lee, MS, OTR/L, CHT
Occupational Therapist, NewBridge on the Charles
Dedham, MA

As we age, many factors may limit our abilities to engage in the activities that are meaningful to us. These factors may be physical and anatomical limitations, or they may be cognitive or a visual limitation that is often associated with dementia or vascular disease. Activities like getting dressed, walking the dog, driving to the grocery store, and playing bridge may become difficult, may require more effort, or may become too challenging to perform at all. This is when a referral from a physician to an occupational therapist (OT) may help. OT practitioners are educated to address all aspects of aging, from recovery from an injury like a wrist fracture secondary to a fall or from a major medical event like a stroke. OTs have a special role in preventing injury and falls to fostering safety and independence with all aspects of daily living, from getting washed up and dressed to the occupational performance of driving and community mobility.

Specifically, OTs are skilled in evaluating age-related conditions and their associated impairments, like arthritis and hand weakness, stroke and arm pain, visual-perceptual changes and driving impairments, fractures, and limited active range of motion. Dealing with these and many other medical conditions that affect the older population, OTs strive to engage elders to perform the best they can at whatever activities are most meaningful to them. Older persons, like younger people, want to be productive, engaged and independent.

Case Example: Mr. R, a 77-Year-Old Male

Mr. R was referred to OT by his primary care physician following an embolic stroke with noted right dominant hand weakness and lack of coordination and with questionable impairment of cognition and visual-perception skills. His past medical history was remarkable for arthritis, total knee replacements, high blood pressure, and cataract removal. He is a widower and lives alone in a single-dwelling home, next door to his daughter and her family. Prior to the stroke, Mr. R was living independently, provided car transportation and child care for his grandchildren, and enjoyed weekly poker games with "the guys." As Mr. R entered the rehab gym area, he was observed to walk without assistance but with decreased right arm swing and slow gait. During the initial assessment, Mr. R reported generalized hand weakness, causing him to have difficulty cutting foods, opening containers, and tying his shoes, and increased effort carrying heavier items. He also noted that his right leg seemed weak and a bit off-balance, and a subsequent referral to physical therapy (PT) was initiated. But the biggest concern for Mr. R was: When would he be able to return to driving?

The evaluation tests and activities revealed a 75% loss of right dominant grip and pinch strength, a mild deficit with coordination and dexterity and minimal impairment of hand and wrist active range of motion. Upon assessment of his cognitive and visual perception skills, he was noted to have mild to moderate impairment of visual attention, attention switching, and upper visual field deficit. These findings concerned Mr. R most of all, as he was eager to return to driving as soon as possible as he frequently drove his grandchildren to and from school, as well as driving himself to his customary activities.

A treatment plan was established for Mr. R with his primary goals of returning to driving, to be able to complete all heavy household chores, as well as to return to all previous activities with ease. The first few OT sessions focused on regaining his strength and range of motion of his dominant arm. He quickly progressed from simple pinching and motion activities to tasks that required sustained grip, strength, and coordination in sitting and standing. Dynamic functional movement tasks were introduced in conjunction with visual-perceptual retraining activities to facilitate return to driving. Within four weeks, Mr. R's strength doubled and he had only mild to trace deficits in active motion, coordination and dexterity, as he was now tying his shoes, cooking his own meals, and maintaining his home again. His visual-perceptual skills and attention and awareness also improved so that he was able to return to driving during daytime hours and to familiar places. Mr. R was quite pleased with his progress toward his goals and continues with his home exercises for his vision-perception, cognition, and physical recovery.

Case Example: Mrs. M, a 95-Year-Old Female

Mrs. M was referred to OT from her neurologist secondary to painful and limited motion of her left shoulder. Her past medical history is notable for left shoulder arthritis and left-sided weakness, hearing loss, macular degeneration, and altered gait. She lives within a continuous care retirement community (CCRC), with 24 hours of assistance per week for housekeeping, dressing, meal prep, food shopping, and transportation to appointments. Mrs. M exercises three to four times per week and is active in community affairs. Mrs. M complains of painful and limited shoulder motion and increased hand weakness and numbness, which are currently impeding her ability to manipulate and hold common objects and causing increased effort and difficulty with dressing, as well as with walking with her rollator.

The evaluation tests and activities revealed that Mrs. M noted severely limited shoulder motion combined with moderate pain and weakness during functional activities of reaching, cutting food, and dressing, and with weight-bearing during functional mobility. Also notable during assessment of her hand, she presented with impaired sensation and decreased ability to identify common objects within her hand when her vision was occluded. Mrs. M asks, "What can OT do for me? Can I get any strength back? Can you make me better? Can you help me?"

After the evaluation results were reviewed, Mrs. M and the therapist identified Mrs. M's functional goals and determined a plan of care that would include OT two times per week for eight weeks, with the goals of increasing her arm and hand strength, improving functional shoulder range of motion to allow decreased effort and pain with all aspects of her instrumental activities of daily living (IADLs) and basic activities of daily living (ADLs), specifically cutting food, dressing, and moving things and herself in the environment. Considering the advanced arthritis in her left shoulder and noted weakness and lack of sensation in her left hand, Mrs. M was agreeable and motivated to try any therapeutic intervention that might help. Together, we set goals and determined an appropriate plan of care that included the use of progressive resistive activities like theraband, fine motor and sensory reeducation activities, as well as the use of pain-relieving modalities such as diathermy.[1] The therapist also explained

---

[1] A medical and surgical technique involving the production of heat in a part of the body by high-frequency electric currents, in order to stimulate the circulation, relieve pain, destroy unhealthy tissue, or cause bleeding vessels to clot.

the benefits and evidence of ongoing cardiovascular activity and how this could positively affect her overall muscle function and provide pain relief. Within the first two weeks of therapy sessions, an improvement in pain was already noted. Mrs. M reported decreased shoulder pain during a.m. routine activities like getting dressed, and only intermittent pain with walking with her rollator. It was with delight to Mrs. M that she had already gained two pounds of functional pinch strength and five pounds of grip strength. It was rewarding to see the doubtful Mrs. M encouraged and eager to make more gains toward a more confident and independent self. Her commitment to better her health and activity engagement is admirable, and she serves as a mentor to other nonagenarians.

These were just two case examples of how occupational therapy can facilitate the return to one's meaningful activities, despite significant medical conditions that may have affected these individuals' lives. It is without doubt that the older client faces numerous conditions that can affect health and the pursuits of daily living. Understanding how older people's medical conditions and/or impairments affect their well-being requires identifying how they interact within their environments and developing the right treatment path to wellness. An OT is an important type of health care professional who is prepared to meet the challenge of the aging population.

Reflections for Readers

1. How can an OT help reconcile an elder's functional disabilities with the elder's definition of meaningful activities?
2. What issues can occupational therapy address? How might occupational therapy play a helpful role with people that you encounter in life or at work?
3. How might an OT motivate a patient for the often hard work of improving functioning?
4. How might an OT help an elder with physical difficulties deal with the psychological issues around those difficulties?
5. OTs need to balance challenging patients to improve their capacities and modifying patients' environments so as to make it easier for them to function well. How might an OT working with a given patient find an optimal balance between challenging the patient and modifying the environment to empower the patient in what she or he can already do?

CHAPTER 52

How I Learned to Cope with Depression

Arthur Wood, MS
Biochemist (retired)
Newton, MA
Age 75

For many people as they age, depression becomes a companion. We lose loved ones and we lose capacities we used to have; that can be depressing! We also sometimes fall prey to our own biology: our bodies and brains just start operating in a different—depressed—way. What I'm talking about here is more than occasional sadness, but the kind of deep clinical depression that can cripple one's life. Having said all that, there are treatments available that can make a BIG difference.

I have been depressed for my whole life—at times, suicidal. But here I am, at age 75, still alive and kicking!

Let me be clear. I am not a psychologist, and depression is such a complex and varied disease that I would not claim that my experience has taught me all there is to know about it! But please read on, and if you find my words resonating with you, I hope you will try those things that appeal to you.

Did you know that you have many subpersonalities? I am not referring to "multiple personality disorders," where a person literally lives two very different lives and ne'er the twain shall meet! I am referring to ideas that are basic to therapeutic techniques popularized in the last 30 years, which have found it useful to entertain the idea that one has many "selves" or "parts" that coexist in your psyche. The selves can support each other or compete with each other in trying to influence your life.

What does this have to do with depression? As a young man, I often could not get out of bed in the morning. I would lie there going over every negative thought about my life and would sink into deep despair. This went on for a long time, and no therapist or drug enabled me to alter this behavior.

Then I was exposed to a technique called Voice Dialogue, where I was asked to imagine that I had many different internal voices and that I could learn about these voices and how they influenced my behavior. Pretty far out, aye! Please stick with me and realize that you don't have to swallow this hook, line, and sinker. Just entertain the possibility that this is so and think about how you might use these ideas to influence your depression.

What occurred to me one morning, as I was starting my plunge into the depths, was the following: Hey, wait a minute! It's not "me" who is depressed. It is just a subpersonality of mine that is depressed and I can make a choice here. I can let this part take over my behavior and lie here crying, or I can acknowledge the existence of this part and talk to it, reason with it. I would engage the part with respect and have a short but effective conversation with it, such as:

"I understand that you feel very negative about life and I empathize with you. But I need to get up and go to work. I would appreciate it if you would stop dominating my behavior right now."

Whether or not such a depressed part really exists, thinking about it in this way enabled me to get up and get going each morning. It did not make my depression disappear forever. But it did allow me to change my behavior. What a gift!

I delved deeper into the theory of Voice Dialogue and, having a very critical subpersonality, I naturally began to find things in the theory that I could not agree with. At that time, I learned about a similar theory and technique called "Internal Family Systems Therapy." This is not the place to go into the fine details of the therapy. Suffice it to say that both Voice Dialogue and Internal Family Systems Therapy are built on the basic idea of subpersonalities. Since most people have some familiarity with family therapy and the different members of the family interacting and having an effect on each other, it is not that much of a stretch to think of each individual as having an "Internal Family," composed of parts that have to learn how to get along with each other!

Unfortunately, while these ideas helped me tremendously, they did not "cure" my depression. Thus began my ongoing relationship with psychopharmacologists and an endless array of antidepressants. I am a biochemist by training and believe that depression is linked to abnormal metabolism in the brain. Therefore, I found it reasonable that drugs might be developed to modify this abnormal metabolism and nudge it toward normal.

There are many such drugs on the market now, and just trying one of them will not necessarily tell you whether drugs will help you. Your psychiatrist will prescribe a drug that your medical history indicates might be useful. From there, you and the psychiatrist may follow a trial-and-error approach to find the drug or combination of drugs that enables you to rise above your depression most of the time.

In my case, I have found such a combination of drugs. I'm positive that they work because if I forget to take my meds in the morning, I start feeling depressed, and that reminds me to take the meds, which brings my mood back up.

Having talked about therapy and drugs, but finding that both, while helpful, were not a cure, I now want to relate some of my experience with "Mindful Meditation." Most of you have probably come across such a term in the popular press. I became acquainted with it by going on short meditation retreats at Buddhist retreat centers. This is not Buddhism as a religion, but Buddhism as a science. Nothing to believe in—just techniques to try and see what happens. If they help you, then it is reasonable that you might modify your daily routine to incorporate time for meditation. I have found it incredibly helpful in dealing with my anger and my guilt, both of which are intimately connected with my depression and with my grief over the death of loved family members.

There are no magic bullets in dealing with depression, but there are plenty of approaches that can help. Reread them, evaluate them, and then make a plan to help yourself. I trust that if you try any or all of these things, you will experience enough positive feedback to keep you on track. Good luck!

For more detailed information and instructions in each of these areas, please see the suggested readings.

Also, for those of you who use Google, there is much information on the Internet, including individuals and organizations that can help you with your depression.

Reflections for Readers

1. What signs or symptoms should tell a person to seek professional help for depression?
2. What is the difference between depression and "the blues"?
3. There are many forms of therapy for depression, some of which are discussed by this author. How can someone with depression

find the right treatment for his or her particular depression? Are there other variants of "talk therapy" that a depressed person should also consider?

4. Some people deny their need for treatment, as they see depression as a (stigmatizing) "mental illness." How would you help a depressed person see that depression is not something to be ashamed of and that appropriate treatment would improve his or her life?

Suggested Reading

Salzberg, S. (1995). *Loving kindness—The revolutionary art of happiness.* Boston, MA: Shambhala Press.

Salzberg, S. (2011). *Real happiness—The power of meditation.* New York, NY: Workman Publishing.

Schwartz, R. C. (2001). *Introduction to the Internal Family Systems Model.* Oak Park, IL: Trailhead Publications.

Segal, Z. V., Williams, J. M. G., & Teasdale, J. D. (2013). *Mindfulness-based cognitive therapy for depression.* New York, NY: The Guilford Press.

Stone, H., & Stone, S. (1989). *Embracing our selves—The Voice Dialogue manual.* Novato, CA: Naturaj Publications. A Division of New World Library.

CHAPTER 53

How Not to Make Mistakes

Irving I. Silverman
Business Manager, Publication Division,
National Knitwear Association and
Proprietor of the Kosher Food and Jewish Life Expo (retired)
Dedham, MA
Age 97

We all make mistakes, but the repetition significantly increases as we age. That doesn't mean that we are born to make mistakes. They happen because of changes in our cognitive capacities. That shouldn't scare us because with training and resolute commitment, we can do something to prevent making mistakes. It does take an effort and a serious commitment . . . but there are tools that we can use to help us.

The first step is to anticipate the possibility of mistakes by writing down what you want to remember. A short note on a pad that you remember to carry with you might suffice. It's wise to cross off the note when you're sure that the incident has passed. Avoid making notes on scraps of paper that are easily misplaced or discarded. If there is the possibility of continuous recurrence of the mistake, don't delete or discard the reminder.

If the possibility of making the mistake again involves someone else, enlist that person's assistance in helping you. They'll be delighted to be your ally.

If repetition of the mistake might involve the loss of money, time, or another serious condition or matter, it might be best to enlist the help of the affected person or locale. What is important here is anticipating and finding tools to help you avoid repeating the mistake.

Most important: Don't blame yourself if you do make a mistake, especially if no one was hurt or inconvenienced. A brief apology will make the mistake a thing of the past, without any lasting consequences. Forgive yourself and move forward. One way to accomplish that might be by giving yourself a reward so you will have turned the mistake into a lasting benefit. Don't keep your accomplishment a secret; share it as a teaching experience for others—who may be mistake-makers too!

Remember that correcting mistakes is a learning experience. As an example, I have never been a writer of "clean copy"—that is, text material that reads perfectly the first time through. Give yourself a span of time to write and then edit a text; you'll be amazed with the improvement in what you have written. Gertrude Stein, the famous author, was notably a practitioner of editing and reediting. The "tool" here is time, which allows you to look at something freshly. In other realms, too, mistakes can be avoided or prevented by slowing down the process of decision-making. The old adage is true: patience is a virtue.

Human experience is rife with evidence of the need for better ways to do things. Sometimes several steps or stages are needed to reach a final and improved solution. It takes willingness to welcome change and not labor the thought that the original effort was either deficient or incorrect.

As a business executive, I had to make hundreds of decisions, and I wrestled with the possibility that I might make a mistake. I learned that not making decisions, out of fear of mistakes, was not an effective strategy: inactivity can be an even more horrendous mistake. We all know people and businesses that can't or won't make a decision because of that fear; and at the same time, we have all witnessed colossal mistakes being made by poor training and advice.

Despite the best of judgment or advice, mistakes will occur. We can maximize our capacities and minimize our mistakes by looking for tools to help us—and then using them!

Reflections for Readers

1. Elders are particularly susceptible to fears that if they forget something or make a mistake, it's a sign of dementia. How can elders differentiate between normal forgetfulness or mistake-making and the beginnings of dementia?
2. How can families of elders and the professionals working with elders deal with an elder's fear that making a mistake indicates a downward spiral into dementia?
3. In addition to the strategies mentioned by this author, can you suggest other strategies for preventing mistakes?

PART **IX**

Work and Retirement

CHAPTER 54

The Golden Years: Retirement and the Years That Follow … A Personal Reflection

R. Peter Shapiro, Esq.
Attorney, Civil Litigation, Tardiff, Shapiro, & Cassidy (retired)
Dedham, MA
Age 79

Let me use as a framework the teachings of Rabbi Gunther Plaut, as set forth in his book *The Price and Privilege of Growing Old.* I will begin with my journey into retirement and the years that followed, and then relate them to Rabbi Plaut's teachings.

I will preface my remarks by stating I always enjoyed the practice of law. As a colleague once said, "You need to have fire in the belly to properly represent your clients." I prided myself in giving each client my maximum effort. It was when I began to realize that "the fire" in my belly was not as hot and my work was beginning to be more perfunctory, that I felt I was not being fair to my clients or to myself. My initial reaction was that if I worked part time, I could practice at a level that would allow me to provide each client with the maximum effort which I considered to be my responsibility.

That was 15 years ago, and early one November morning, I sat down in my partner's office and said, "I intend to work half time starting July 1." He responded, "If that's what you want, it's OK with me." Later that day, he came to my office and said, "Stop by my house on the way home. We need to talk."

When we had that talk, the advice he gave me was that after 30 years, he knew that I could not work part time. He said something would come up that interested me, and I would not say no. He reminded me that I could not tell other lawyers or the judge that they would have to adhere to my schedule as I only worked part time. His advice was, "For your peace of mind, stay full time or retire." I took his advice, trusted my instincts, and the next morning, I told him I would be retiring on June 30.

How did I feel on June 30? I had taken the artwork home a few days earlier. I looked at the bare walls, clean desk, and worktable with some sadness as I closed my office door. After saying goodbye, I carried an empty briefcase and a cardboard box with some memorabilia out to the car. My first thought was, "Is this cardboard box all I have after almost 50 years as a lawyer?" Realization set in at breakfast on Monday, when I could relax and not have to rush out to court or the office.

I have never regretted my decision. As time has gone by, seeing a former client, or reading about events or cases similar to those in which I had been involved, brought me back to the profession I enjoyed. I have no regrets; the memories of the positive as well as negative experiences are the valuable material I took with me when I left the office, not the items in the cardboard box.

My wife has been supportive of my decision. I don't think I've been underfoot or that I have impeded her activities. I can recall one time when what I call "my boyish charm" may have worn thin. I reminded her that her mother said to her father, "I took you for better or worse, not for lunch." Betty responded "Lunch is OK—it's the rest of the time."

So, what did I learn from Rabbi Plaut? His first observation was that we need to adjust to the loss of our name. We thought of ourselves, more than others, in relation to our vocations. Peter the lawyer, Joe the dentist, Sue the artist, Todd the rabbi, etc. Rabbi Plaut observed that this change in status, real or imagined, was not an easy adjustment for many retirees. However, it was not a problem for me. Being a lawyer, while important, was not the center of my universe. My family was my number one priority, and thus in retrospect, I considered my primary name *husband/father*. That did not change when I retired except to add *grandfather*.

Rabbi Plaut's next observation was that those who said upon retirement, "I will do *x*," and listed what they would be doing seldom followed through on their statements unless they had previously engaged in those endeavors. If you had no interests aside from your vocation and family, it's difficult to engage in new interests unless you have supportive friends and family.

I was fully engaged in organizations and was supportive of those that involved my family. For me, it was a seamless transition from the practice of law to retirement. I remember saying on more than one occasion, "I ought to go back to the practice of law to get more free time."

Rabbi Plaut reminded us that as we age, our bodies shut down, and we need to care for our physical and mental health and learn to adjust to such changes. I might add that when I met Rabbi Plaut, he was in his late 80s. His congregants confirmed that he played golf and tennis three or four times a week. So far, caring for my body has not been an issue for me. My observation is that without proper advice, retirees may not appreciate those body changes. When they do, they often exacerbate the problem by overcompensation or by withdrawing from some or all activities.

I doubt the planners at Hebrew SeniorLife (the organization that owns and operates NewBridge, where I live) read Rabbi Plaut's book; however, their approach to integrating residents into the NewBridge culture of meaningful retirement addresses his observations. When moving to NewBridge, you feel like you are a member of an extended family. To the extent that the loss of name caused discomfort, at New-Bridge, one is given a fresh start. We are interested in who you are and how you interact with our community more than who you were prior to joining our family.

NewBridge offers a wide variety of programs. Many of them are designed to stimulate the mind and engender conversation. Opportunities for enrichment programs off and on campus are available, as well as participation in town government and the Intergenerational Program at the nearby Rashi School. Those who previously were involved in activities unrelated to their vocations have no problems continuing an active life. Those that did not but indicated on retiring that they would engage in such activities are encouraged and supported to do so by their immersion in the NewBridge culture.

Plaut's observation that our bodies and minds slowly shut down is addressed by NewBridge, where a special effort is made to ensure that we remain mentally alert and do not succumb to depression. Residents are encouraged to participate in physical fitness programs adapted to accommodate one's abilities. There is little chance that one might exacerbate a change in physical or mental status by overcompensation or withdrawal.

Moving to NewBridge was the second-best decision of my life. (The first occurred 54 years ago, when Betty and I were married. In case you ask, I have not determined if she agrees with my assessment. The lawyer in me recalls the old admonition, "Never ask a question to which you do not know the answer." The evidence suggests that she agrees with me, however, as she is still here.) I have no regrets, and the move to New-Bridge far exceeded my expectations. We were immediately welcomed as members of the family, and I seamlessly continued participating in cultural and physical programs on and off campus.

My father was fond of saying, "The golden years aren't that golden." I could understand his feelings. His friends had moved away or passed away. He and my mother could not drive, and there were few activities that they could engage in. Betty and I moved to NewBridge, where we made new friends; we continue to participate in those activities that were important to us and to explore new ones. These *are* truly our golden years.

Reflections for Readers

1. Of the things one keeps after a long career, which are the most important ones?
2. What factors should a person consider in deciding whether to continue working full time, work on a reduced schedule, or retire?
3. How does life, individually and as a family, change after a retirement? What might someone do to maximize the positive changes and minimize the negative ones?
4. What defines one's identity? How much of identity is determined by profession? How much by family roles? How much by other factors?
5. Does one's self-definition have to change upon retiring?

CHAPTER 55

Planning Ahead

Maurice Lesses, Esq.
Attorney, General Practice
Cambridge, MA
Age 84

I never consciously planned for the future except for two things: to save money when I could afford to, and (thanks to my late wife) to try spacing our children's births about two years apart.

When I was in college during the Korean War, I had no clear idea of what I would do next. I had an unfounded sense that a graduate degree was necessary in order to make a living, but no real knowledge of any profession other than medicine (my father was a doctor who worked seven days a week). Business as an occupation was an absolute mystery. My immediate necessity was to extend my student deferment for a few more years in order to postpone being drafted.

After eliminating the alternatives, but for no positive reason, I went to law school. The law was so unexciting that after a year or so, I thought about dropping out to go to architecture school. Upon graduating from law school, I became a commercial real estate broker.

Two years later, I had the opportunity either to join a bigger real estate firm or to start practicing law by working for a successful solo practitioner. By staying in real estate, I would immediately make more money. Becoming a practicing lawyer would mean a lower salary than I had been earning, and we now had two children. However, I felt guilty enough for not using the legal education that I had spent so much time (and parental money) on that I went to work for the lawyer. I believed that I could return to real estate if I did not like the law.

Practicing law soon became far more interesting, with an infinite number of problems to deal with. Ours was a general practice, so I had to learn new things regularly and quickly. Our practice included wills,

241

trusts, real estate transactions, leases, small business law, labor law, contracts, accident cases, divorces, probating estates, and going to court for some of these matters. A few years after I started, a new commercial real estate brokerage firm in Boston offered me a partnership, but the law had become too enticing to give up. It still is.

About a dozen years after I started practicing law, a Boston trust and investment management company recruited me to run its trust department and serve as general counsel. I worked there for the next 24 years until 1993, when a huge out-of-town bank acquired it and I retired formally. Since our finances would be okay for a couple of years, at least at that point, my wife-to-be (whom I had met before I retired) and I quickly adopted a plan for my retirement future. The major part of our plan was to spend a lot of the next year or two traveling to music festivals, mostly in Appalachia, to play old-time (Appalachian) music. Old-time music is largely square dance music, with fiddles and banjos as the lead instruments. I had become (and still am) very involved with the music, and my wife loves to dance. The rest of the time, I would work on building both a law practice and a small investment advisory business. That was my plan for the future, looking ahead a full two years.

However, a week after my retirement, the chairman of a Delaware trust company asked me to become its President. I agreed to do so on a temporary basis (I did not want to leave Cambridge permanently), so our travel plans mostly vanished. I left the trust company somewhat more than a year later, but began handling a lot of the company's legal work. And 21 years later, that company is still a client.

My general law practice—but no courts, no torts—developed, as did a tiny investment advisory business. Even together, they never became full time.

Enough legal work showed up, however, to help support us. Then my wife went to graduate school and became a psychotherapist. After working for a couple of institutions, she started her own private practice about a dozen years ago. It has become more than full time. She, too, has passed the usual retirement age and enjoys her work too much either to cut back or retire.

In my practice, I have found that nearly every legal matter presents at least a small, different issue, and many matters require new learning. Dealing with them is too much fun to think about stopping.

Besides legal work, I help my wife with her information technology (IT) problems and the business side of her practice, which she conducts from both our houses. Maintaining a couple of houses (and yards), with tenants in one of the locations, is also part of my job description. Once in a while, it can be fun.

Working on my own, but less than full time, allows me flexibility in managing my days. As a result, my schedule rarely controls me, and I have chances to do other things when I want.

Many of my friends have retired in recent years or are planning to retire fairly soon. None of them has indicated any interest in continuing the work (mostly professional) that they have done for so many years, even part time. All of them want to pursue or are already pursuing their avocations. My impolite response (either verbal or unspoken) when I hear this is, "Slacker!" More seriously, I occasionally wonder for how long their avocational interests will be both strong and time-consuming enough to replace their old jobs. So far, it does seem to be working for them. My approach, which developed free of any forethought, is working for me, too.

Reflections for Readers

1. What are the advantages of planning ahead? What are the advantages of making more spontaneous decisions? What might one lose by following either of these paths?
2. What factors enter into choosing a career? How would you rate the relative importance, for yourself, of financial reward versus professional satisfaction?
3. How might enjoying one's work influence decisions on when and whether to retire? What other factors would be important to evaluate?
4. What factors influence decisions about working part time?
5. This author mentioned his interest in old-time music and also that he takes care of IT needs for his wife. In your opinion, how might such diversity of interests contribute to a decision about working full-time, part-time, or not at all?

CHAPTER 56

Aging and Retirement

Gregory Ruffa

President, GRA Advertising

Plainfield, NJ

Age 91

When we think of old age, do we get an image of gray hair, someone with a weathered face and a mouth missing teeth or full of clackers? The expectation goes on—a feeble body with all sorts of aches or pains, walking with the assistance of a walker or scooting around in a wheelchair. Is that what aging is doing to us?

Of course, planning ahead for your advanced years when you are young can make a difference. We can do nothing about that now; back when we were young, we might not have bothered, thinking that we were invincible. We excelled in sports, we ran in marathons! Spending hours in the gym or health club was for the other guy; we thought we were indestructible, and since we watched our diet and checked our weight and vitals regularly, we would last forever. Right? Wrong! I find that in addition to all that, you need a very positive attitude, a good sense of humor, liking people, and being approachable and friendly. We all know you can't change your inner personality, but keep at least one or two of these traits in mind. People do respond to friendliness. Try it, practice it—it's easy to smile.

Most of us are not prepared for retirement. It's a time with all sorts of choices and challenges, like joining a weekly food program or joining a small group to do your periodical exercise. Even walking around a golf course, playing a game or two of tennis, squash, or volleyball, or taking a swim would be a good thing. Anything done on a regular basis can be good as a bodybuilder.

I am not here to advise, but to talk of planning in your working days to take you into retirement. There may be something here to help you . . .

Think positive. If there is a family, keep them close and express your love for them—every time! Every time!

There is another critical area: Money! Never let anyone other than a spouse know. A creditable fiduciary advisor is worth looking into. There are so many methods to avoid unhappiness and family squabbles about how the money was distributed. Be smart and work with a professional fiduciary; they are obligated by legal mandate to work for your benefit, not theirs, and to find a method of sensible care for your beneficiaries. I love the comment made by Warren Buffett, the financial guru of Omaha, who said, "Leave them enough to do something, but not enough to do nothing!!!" Some people want to give their beneficiaries the money while they are still here so they can enjoy seeing them using the funds. I would place some limits. Remember, this is your hard-earned money; you sacrificed and denied yourself to save it for your future. There are many government, national, state, and local programs to help you, regardless of what your income may be. You or a family member could look into these facilities for estate planning.

These ideas leave out two large segments of our population: those hanging on at or below the poverty level, and those high above the middle-class folks.

When calculating financial matters, it is necessary to know where you stand in comparison to the rest of the country. I was surprised to learn that between 11% and 15% of the U.S. population is at or below the poverty level, amounting to 50 million people, some stuck there from 1980 and not improved much since then. On the other hand, there are 3.1 million people earning between $200,000 and $500,000 per year and another 1.3 million earning more than $500,000 annually.

Why give it all away? There was a story as I recall some time ago: a widowed woman in her 70s told her family that she had no intention of spending her later years in one of those "nursing homes." Investigating the alternatives, she read about the *Queen Mary*, dry-docked in Long Beach, California. Comparing the costs of the ship to a nursing home, she decided to take a room for a month aboard that ship, which does not leave port. The stateroom was incredibly large, with all the amenities and comforts imaginable: room service for her meals, her bed turned down and made up daily. The observation bar had spectacular views, and dinner was available in several rooms, including the elegant Sir Winston. All sorts of entertainment and exhibits were available, free or for a very reasonable cost. An onboard, 24-hour medical service; tours of the historical icon, the ship itself. Of course, taxis were available to shop or visit shows. All this sounded more like a vacation than a retirement home. She decided to make it her permanent home. What a great solution! The cost of all the ship had to offer was much lower than the nursing home. This is not a commercial—I thought it was a great solution to her problem.

Stories like that one abound, limited only by the financial position that a person may be in. There are so many wonderful venues to visit or live in. My golf partner of some 40+ years moved to Florida from New Jersey, a widower of six or so years. He is an avid golfer and he wanted the good weather advantages. Sold his home and virtually everything in it. He stayed a month or so investigating available properties. He committed to one, and it failed the building inspection. Nice, but no dice, fugeddaboudit already. Then he found a beautiful little house, but much bigger inside. An artist in his own right, he decorated the interior very tastefully, and the 60+-inch TV fit the room design perfectly, with a large glass wall overlooking the golf course and clubhouse. That is one happy man. Taxes, huh? About one-fifth of what he paid on his home in New Jersey. So many other states and countries have as good or even better answers for the best retirement location. Check it out before you make a permanent decision.

If retirement means staying in your current home, life can be very comfortable knowing that you still have your friends and maybe nearby family. Knowing your community—the shopping, a favorite barber, a frequented bar or restaurant, etc. That is where you can enjoy and continue your life. The church that you attend may need your help or contributions; it is also a good place to frequent. Continue and increase your place in a greater and blessed future home.

Reflections for Readers

1. Retirement planning includes financial planning. What role can a professional financial advisor play?
2. How might engaging in financial planning affect family dynamics?
3. What is the value of remaining in your home (or community)?
4. What do you think about the retirement "solution" this author cited, that of making a permanent home on a luxury ship? Some people enact a similar solution by making a home in a hotel or resort. What advantages and downsides do you see in such solutions?

CHAPTER 57

Prospering in Retirement Versus Coping with Retirement

Leonard J. Green
Vice President, The Analytic Sciences Corporation
(TASC) (retired), Consultant
Dedham, MA
Age 84

Planning for retirement should become a priority for anyone contemplating retirement within the next several years. I have witnessed several people in my family and near-friends who spend more time organizing their next vacation than they do planning for several years of anticipated retirement. In several instances, when I have cautioned on the necessity of having some solid plans for work and/or recreation during the retirement years, the answer that I have received is, "Oh, I have so many projects and plans that I will never run out of things to do." And, in reality, the list of projects, etc. is completed within a period of months and a great amount of unfulfilling idle time remains. Another common response is, "We will have plenty of time to travel and see places we have always wanted to see." In fact, what happens ordinarily is that the retirees have the resources and the energy to take either one or two trips a year, which then leaves many empty weeks and months to fill.

One acquaintance who was a manager for a wholesale cigar distributor was anticipating his retirement-years-to-come for several years in advance. When he was asked what he would do after retirement, he often mentioned that he would work part-time in a retail cigar store and, through his years in the cigar business, there were several retail stores that would love to employ him on a part-time basis. When his eligibility for retirement with a small pension finally arrived, the popularity of cigar-smoking was greatly diminished, and of all of his potential employers, not a single one was interested. Following his retirement, this man spent endless hours nearly every day WATCHING TELEVISION.

Another close friend, still working after I had retired but disliking his job, was anxious to reach his retirement years, but he needed to reach a financial objective before doing so. During that period of anticipation, I often had the opportunity to counsel him on the need to plan his activity during his idle days. Well, he never did any planning or preparing, and when the time finally arrived, within two weeks of actual retirement, he took a job at Costco. The job that he accepted was to hand out food samples, which he came to hate almost immediately because he was standing at his station, on a cement floor, for hours at a stretch, while people whom he came to despise were pushing and shoving to get a free sample of the fare that he was offering. (He lasted there for several months because there was no other job opportunity available for a man nearing 70 with limited skills.)

In my own situation, I was employed high up in the organization of an extremely professional company when they offered an early-retirement package. I had not been considering retirement until this package was offered; and then I started to consider it seriously. When I talked it over with my wife, she became very concerned about what I would do "with my free time." She was concerned for me, and I did my best to reassure her that I had a number of tangible things in mind that were fairly readily available (one of which was being a radio talk-show host, with which I had some experience). I also believe, although never confirmed, that my wife was concerned that every day I would ask what was for lunch, and that her routine would be seriously compromised by "taking care of me."

After my actual retirement, I assure you that that never became the case. I have been semiretired for over 15 years, working 20 or more hours each week as a consultant, and I am busier than I want to be and more satisfied than I might have contemplated. There has never been any time in which I have not been employed.

One of the dangers of inactivity is falling into a state that the professionals would call "depression." In the cases I cited previously, both the cigar salesman and the sample-food dispenser exhibited symptoms that could be classified as "depression" due to lack of fulfillment during those later years.

In planning for the "golden years," I believe that there are many opportunities for volunteering one's time at schools, museums, hospitals, and entertainment venues as receptionists, ushers, and guides, and these can be explored well in advance of the time for actual engagement. In the absence of a part-time or full-time employment opportunity, the unpaid volunteering route can be very satisfying and fulfilling. However, I know from personal experience that almost nothing is as satisfying as receiving monetary compensation, as well as benefits such as health insurance, while doing something constructive.

In any circumstance, it is urgent that planning be done in advance to prepare for those upcoming years of leisure. I would strongly recommend that discussion be had with potential "employers" well in advance, whether it be for a compensated position or a volunteer assignment.

Reflections for Readers

1. When you think about your own future retirement, what would be important to you?
2. Different people opt for different approaches to retirement. Considering your own personality and circumstances, which would be better for you, to plan ahead for your retirement years or to approach them more spontaneously when you get there? Why do you prefer the approach that you have chosen?
3. How is the relationship between spouses affected by a decision by one spouse to retire? Does this depend on which spouse is retiring? Is it different depending on whether one spouse is still working or both spouses will be retired? How might spouses deal with these issues?
4. Is retirement really a time to finally tackle long-thought-about projects? What might get in the way of completing such projects postretirement, when presumably there is time to do them?
5. What aids might someone use to assess retirement plans realistically?
6. Does retiring foster a belief that now one needs to be "taken care of"? What would help someone maintain an independent attitude postretirement?

58

Once a Writer, Always a Writer

Harriet Segal
Novelist
Dedham, MA
Age 85

I began writing my first novel when I was about to turn 50.

I had always been a writer. In the third grade, I wrote long narrative poems and plays. For high school publications, I wrote short stories, and what would now be called op-ed columns, for the teen club newspaper at the Jewish Community Center in Wilkes-Barre, PA, where I grew up. For my second job in New York after college, I was a copywriter. Shortly after we were married in 1961, my husband and I moved to India, where he was a visiting professor at the government medical school in New Delhi, while I wrote for the U.S. Information Agency and edited a newsletter for the U.S. embassy.

During the years when my children were young, I was a journalist and freelance editor. It was not until my oldest daughter was a freshman at Dartmouth and the younger two girls were in high school that I found the courage to pursue a lifelong dream: to write a novel. Like many first novels, *Susquehanna* was set in my hometown and was inspired by my family history. The manuscript was 1,000 pages long. I wrote seven drafts on an IBM Selectric typewriter. It took almost three years to complete . . . and two weeks to sell.

There's always an element of luck in the success of a book. A friend had resigned from her job as editor-in-chief at a large publishing house, to become a literary agent. I was one of her first clients. She knew everyone in publishing. She submitted the manuscript to the top editors at four publishers and informed them that she would be in her office receiving offers on a specific date in two weeks.

That September day in 1983 was tense and exhilarating. I sat at home next to the telephone, while my agent was conducting an auction. Three of the four houses made offers, and the fourth asked for a few more days, which my agent refused. Not many literary representatives could do that.

We finally decided to go with Doubleday, which was a major player at the time. *Susquehanna* was scheduled for release in June 1984.

Then began the editorial process. I was naïve, to say the least. I had no idea how to proceed. My editor was a dynamic young woman who was making waves in the publishing world. She marked up my precious manuscript, indicating over 200 pages that she thought should be cut. Some of them were my favorite passages. I negotiated with her, and she gave in on a few selections, but she was insistent that most of the material that she had blue-penciled slowed the story down or was tangential to the linear plot. I had never taken a writing course—in fact, I had majored in economics at Wellesley. Working with the editor was like a seminar in fiction writing.

Just as the book was ready to go into production, we were hit by a bombshell. My editor was quitting her job; in fact, she was leaving publishing and going into a completely different industry, where she would be paid many times her salary as a Doubleday editor.

This was bad news. Overnight, I had become the dreaded "orphan author." You see, within a large publishing house, your editor is your advocate. She lobbies for your book with the editorial board. She fights for advertising and promotion money. She butters up the marketing staff and the sales reps. She uses her influence with the book clubs. And she argues with the art director, pushing for a smashing cover design. Without a strong editor representing me in-house, my book could "fall between the cracks"—another fearful publishing expression.

This was nail-biting time. For the next week or so, I was sure that my book would languish in the various departments that were part of the production chain. Here's where a savvy agent played a key role. The happy outcome was that one of the legendary editors who had guided many best-selling authors during her 20 years at Doubleday agreed to take me on. That was the good news. The bad news was that her views of the manuscript did not coincide with my acquiring editor's vision. In other words, each editor has her own taste and point of view. So we were almost back to square one, restoring some of the cut passages and deleting others. This was my *graduate* course in writing. I learned a great deal about the craft of editing, and it has served me well throughout the ensuing more than 30 years of producing six novels and any number of articles.

Susquehanna came out the summer of 1984 to critical acclaim and was a success, as first novels go. It was chosen by *Pittsburgh Magazine* as one of "The Best Books of 1984," and made best-seller lists in a number of regional newspapers—but not in the iconic *New York Times*. I did have a long interview in the Westchester section of the Sunday *Times*, which pleased the heads of marketing and publicity. My novel was selected for the Washington Irving Book List by the Association of Westchester County Libraries. It was bought for publication in a number of foreign languages, appeared as a series in a Norwegian magazine, and was a book club selection in the United States and two foreign countries.

I was feted at a reception and dinner at the famed Doubleday Suite, above the eponymous bookstore on Fifth Avenue. They sent me on a book tour to major cities around the country, scheduling talks at meetings of such organizations as the American Association of University Women, Women's Clubs, Hadassah chapters, synagogues, churches, and many, many public libraries.

It was a heady time. I was fortunate enough to experience publishing the way it used to be. It was exciting and, yes, glamorous. I was much in demand for signings in bookstores. There were many good reviews, and enough bad ones to thicken my skin. In every town where I gave a book talk, there would be articles in the local newspapers with pictures. That was better than advertising, especially in the important towns of Pennsylvania. There was one headline I will never forget: **LATE IN LIFE, A FIRST NOVEL!**

I am still writing, 32 years later. There was a long hiatus after *The Skylark's Song* came out in 1994, because my husband was diagnosed with the illness that caused his death. After he died, I moved from Manhattan to NewBridge on the Charles, a senior community in Dedham, Massachusetts. As soon as I was settled, I dusted off a manuscript that I had put aside six years before and went to work. By the middle of 2011, it was ready for release.

In my absent years, publishing had drastically changed. The major publishers that once reigned supreme were now down to the "Big Five," the largest having swallowed up many fine publishing houses, including my old outfit, Doubleday, which had become an imprint of Random House. Amazon loomed as this gargantuan presence, selling print books at a deep discount, undercutting other vendors. But the major change in book publishing was the advent of the eBook and devices such as the Kindle and the iPad. There's some debate about which was the first practical eReader, but the Kindle dominates the field. With public acceptance of these electronic readers came the prevalence of the independent or "indie" author. Such well-known writers as Stephen King, John Grisham, Tom Clancy, and Warren Adler (author of *The War of the Roses*) were self-publishing some of their books, selling them through Amazon, Barnes & Noble, and other distributors. It was a whole new world.

My agent had retired; it was a daunting task to find a new one. What's more, *The Expatriate*, my new novel, was exceptionally long, a saga. The estimated length of the printed book was over 700 pages. Publishers assess the cost of production and distribution—the quantity of paper, shipping weight, shelf space in stores—when they consider buying a book. I had been away from publishing for almost a decade. I no longer had contacts in the industry. If I were to get a new agent, and go through the process of submissions, it could be as long as two years before my manuscript was accepted by a publisher, and even longer until I would see the printed book in stores.

I made a rash decision: I chose a copublisher to format *The Expatriate* for all the eReaders—the Kindle, the Nook, the Sony Reader, the Kobo, and a bunch of others that you've never heard of. In less than a month, my novel was offered for sale all over the world by Amazon, Barnes & Noble, Sony, and dozens of other outlets. It was amazing and quite empowering.

I have just celebrated my 85th birthday, and I have recently finished a new novel, which I'm calling *First Among Peers*. I haven't made up my mind yet which path to follow—traditional or "indie" publishing.

It's nice to have a choice.

Reflections for Readers

1. What benefits does someone reap when her creative passion is also her occupation? Are there also costs associated with having these two things coincide?

2. This author noted that she put her writing career aside for several years to tend to her husband in his final illness. What are your thoughts on managing such collisions of professional and family interests? How important is the need to continue earning income, in your thinking? What other factors need to be weighed?

3. Over the course of this author's career, the nature of publishing books changed dramatically. For some seniors, it is difficult to accept or embrace changes from "the way things used to be." What can you suggest to aid other seniors in adapting successfully to change, as this author has done?

CHAPTER 59

A Scientist Retires

Muriel Trask Davisson-Fahey, PhD
Biomedical Researcher (retired)
The Jackson Laboratory
Bar Harbor, ME
Age 75

It seems a little presumptuous to write about aging when I am only 75, and only recently retired at 71. Yet already I can see a path forward into the next quarter of my life from the patterns that I have set in the last four years. What I write is also rather elitist because there are so many in our society in the United States and in countries around the world who live in poverty and do not have the means to take some of the advice that I am offering here. Retirement is inevitable for most of us who had working careers outside the home. Either we choose or are forced by regulations to leave our jobs. This chapter is directed toward those of us who held rather sedentary jobs, may or may not have exercised and eaten healthily, and have the luxury of retiring because of adequate Social Security benefits, pensions, or retirement plans. Of course, people who are "house spouses" never retire. Parents retire from child care when their children leave home, but many now return to caregiving as *their* parents age.

Not everyone chooses to retire. This is especially true of research scientists like myself. Several of my colleagues still have active laboratories and research programs. They are so passionate about their research that they do not want to stop. Some of my colleagues have passed on while still going in to their laboratories every day. Some, like myself, want to do something different. During my busy career, I set aside projects to do in retirement, when I had more time. Retirement gives us an opportunity to do something entirely different with the rest of our lives—in essence, to start a new life.

My biggest passion in retirement is gardening. I love digging in the dirt. Nothing brings you closer to nature. And it's good exercise. My quarter-acre vegetable garden provides all my healthy produce in season. My flower gardens give me immense pleasure. My volunteer work to help people gives me even more gardening opportunities (see below).

Also, I am very interested in history (although I nearly flunked a formal world history course in college). I have traced my family genealogy to find some inspiring stories about some of my ancestors. I am active in our local historical society, through which I am learning more about the place in which I grew up, in which I still live and where some of my ancestors were among the original settlers. I almost never think about science anymore, although I occasionally volunteer at the institute where I did research. The important thing is that I don't feel guilty about leaving my interest in science behind because I have moved on to a new life.

The Art of Giving Back

Throughout my life, I have donated financially to organizations that help people and animals. Now that I am retired, I have the time to physically help people, not just send money. I tried several different volunteer efforts, but even though I want to help people in need, I am not really an up-close-and-personal, people-person. A little searching led me to two volunteer efforts that help feed people in need. I discovered friends who have large gardens and grow and donate fresh produce to senior citizens in local senior citizen housing facilities and to women at the YWCA. Now I spend at least two mornings a week from June through October, providing food while doing what I love most. I also volunteer one afternoon a week at a clothing resale shop that supports our local food pantry serving families in need in my community. In New Orleans, I contribute food to Saint Anna's episcopal church food bank. These volunteer efforts are much more satisfying than sending money to some faceless charity.

Exercise

You have only to turn on the TV or radio or participate in programs for the aging to hear how important exercise is. I cannot say strongly enough how important exercise has been in my retirement. It does not have to be working out at the gym every day to be valuable. About a half mile down the road on which I live in Maine is a beautiful, classic lighthouse. Every morning, with only a few exceptions, I walk to the lighthouse and back—a mile. Nature surrounds me. The air is scented by the evergreen trees alongside the road and the salt air from the ocean. The trees are full of birds singing and calling to each other. Crows are perched in the tree-tops talking to each other. Then I reach the ocean, sparkling in the sun or shrouded by fog. Sometimes waves beat against the rocks, and the sucking sound as they recede is yet another voice in the sounds of my morning walk. The red beacon of the lighthouse reminds me of fishermen whose boats I can often see or hear in the fog as they haul their lobster traps. My world is alive. Often I meet friends and neighbors, and we greet each other or stop for a short chat. The walk is not strenuous and only takes 20 to 30 minutes, but it keeps my body physically healthy and I start my day mentally centered.

Three years ago, I began wintering in New Orleans, but I don't give up walking in those few months. A mile walk takes me along the Mississippi River in Crescent Park. I watch the ship traffic on the river and listen to the river sounds. Butterflies swoop among the plants, birds are chittering in the trees, and the coffee roasting at PJ's roasting facility scents the breeze. Or I walk along the levee in front of the center of the city, where the river sights and sounds mix with the sounds of street musicians and, at certain times of day, the music of the steam calliope on the steamboat *Natchez* and the smell of good food cooking in the restaurants and bakeries of the French Quarter. Whenever I don't walk for a few days, my body says "get out there and walk!"

Genetics of Aging

Longevity, aging, and life span clearly have a genetic component. Model organisms—especially short-lived animals, such as mice, fruit flies, and worms—are good models for human aging because many of their genes and their physiology of aging are similar to those of human beings. Research by many biologists has shown clearly that there is a genetic component to longevity in these model organisms. Genes and chromosomal regions in model animals have been associated with life span. A summary and detailed information on the genetics of aging may be found on the website of the National Institute of Aging (NIA), at https://www.nia.nih.gov/health/publication/biology-aging/genetics-aging-our-genes.

Yet epidemiological studies clearly show that we can modify our longevity and aging process by taking good care of ourselves—physically, mentally, and with our diet (again, see the NIA website). Only two of my six immediate ancestors (i.e., two parents and four grandparents) lived into their mid-90s—my mother and my paternal grandmother. My dad died at 53, my maternal grandfather at 66, and my maternal grandmother and paternal grandfather in their 70s. So far, I seem to have gotten the "good" longevity genes. I feel as healthy and am as active as I was at 50. I still drive 1,850 miles twice a year between my Maine and New Orleans homes. Of course, I still have a long way to go to 100, but the way I feel, I fully expect and look forward to living at least that long. And I believe that exercise, healthy diet, and a positive mental state of mind are more than half the battle.

Fear of Death

I believe that people who have a spiritual or religious faith probably do not fear dying. I cannot say, because I have neither, in the usual sense of these words in Western culture. I did fear dying when I retired—not fear of what happens, but not wanting to leave my life and friends. Retirement made me more aware that my time will be coming. Then, at 75, I discovered the precepts of Buddhism. I still do not want to leave my life and friends, but I have learned to live in the present and not worry about or fear the future. This has brought me a peaceful state of mind. At odd times, and unexpectedly, I find myself feeling suddenly physically joyful. The feeling is impossible to describe. It blends warmth, happiness, and a physical sense of well-being.

How Will I Be Remembered?

Most of my career, I did research in a biomedical research institute. My research was discovering and defining mouse models for human-inherited disorders. All of the mouse models I studied were made available to other scientists and contributed to basic biomedical research around the world—basic research that often led to lifesaving clinical research. As a scientist, however, I probably will be most remembered for creating the first viable trisomic mouse model for Down syndrome. These mice have an extra chromosome, with many of the genes present in three copies that are triplicated in people with Down syndrome. Since 1990, when my research group first published this model, much of the research on Down syndrome has been done using these mice.

But I hope that I also will be remembered by friends for whom I have been there in times of crisis and by those I have helped with my volunteer efforts. I hope that I have left my small corner of the world a little better for having lived in it and participated in it.

Reflections for Readers

1. What are useful ways for people to keep their world alive after retirement? Does it make a difference whether the passions that someone chooses for his or her retirement years are the same as or different from that person's preretirement passions?

2. How might retirement be different for people who identify themselves primarily by their work or career, as compared to people who have other major sources of identity, such as family roles or volunteer activities?

3. What is the importance of legacy in later life?

PART **X**

Housing Options and Solutions

CHAPTER 60

Housing for Older Adults ... HSL's Communities

Louis J. Woolf, MBA
President and Chief Executive Officer, Hebrew SeniorLife
Roslindale, MA

Today, our nation is entering uncharted territory. With over 10,000 people turning 70 every day in the United States, our aging population is growing more rapidly than ever before in our history. And because of the way members of "our greatest generation" and "the baby boomers" have lived their lives, there will be an unprecedented number of seniors who will want more services than are available today. Seniors who want—and in fact need—a range of options for housing; particularly housing that is vibrant, affordable, attractive, and secure, where they can remain healthy, independent, and socially engaged. The goal of Hebrew Senior-Life (HSL) is to provide those services for our seniors. We are committed to the notion that growing older does not have to mean growing inactive and frail.

Today, HSL communities provide almost 1,500 units of independent living for seniors in the greater Boston area. The majority of these units are government-subsidized, and all of them promote extensive resident participation—from physical, cultural, and multigenerational activities to program planning, community philanthropy, and volunteerism.

With the opening of Orchard Cove in 1993 and of NewBridge on the Charles in 2009, HSL expanded its offerings to provide housing for seniors who have resources and are making a decision to use their own funds to be part of a vibrant, independent community. Serving these seniors became part of our mission, alongside meeting the long-term care needs of seniors receiving Medicaid funding and providing subsidized housing. And because HSL knows the value of multigenerational

261

programming and interaction—it's an opportunity to keep the old young and to expose the young to the wisdom of the old—we have made sure to integrate seniors and young people by colocating the Rashi School, a K–8 Jewish day school, right on the NewBridge campus.

We at HSL believe that seniors need more than places to live—they need communities in which to engage with each other, support each other, and grow together to the benefit of the community. We don't think of retirement as retiring from anything, but rather as a time of discovery and enrichment. Our communities reflect that orientation; they are active, lively, and engaging—because that's what seniors want and need. According to HSL's Chief Medical Officer Helen Chen, the keys to a longer life are staying socially active, physically healthy, and mentally engaged. Isolation, she says, can be a major problem as people get older and can often lead to depression and declining physical and cognitive function. I have recently heard a number of people use the expression "Loneliness is the new smoking," and I believe that this is very much the case.

HSL communities encourage people to engage. Engagement is the opposite of isolation, and it forms the basis of new, deep, and important friendships. We encourage residents to meet in informal groups to play cards, discuss politics, and enjoy culture together; to choose from a wide array of classes, programs, and activities ranging from watercolors to bird-watching to social networking to the latest yoga techniques; and to join in classes at local colleges and universities through our partnerships with those institutions. The goal here is to ensure that residents lead full and fulfilling lives.

Our landmark Vitalize 360 program is an example of how we see—and are redefining—aging, and how we are meeting the objective of helping seniors continue to grow. Vitalize 360 is an integral part of life in all of our communities, and it has been adopted in other communities across the country. It is about seniors taking control of their life goals and developing personal plans to achieve active, interesting, and meaningful lives, no matter what their age; it is shattering the image of seniors leading sedentary and complacent lives. It helps residents make lifestyle changes that lead not only to improved health, but also to a richer quality of life.

Vitalize 360 looks at the entire well-being of a person, the 360-degree view. It encourages residents to consider all aspects of their lives, including health, nutrition, physical and mental fitness, community connections, lifelong learning, and spirituality. A holistic program, Vitalize 360 coaches each senior to set and accomplish personal goals. It challenges residents to think about their legacies and create full, vibrant lifestyles.

The program provides support as well as programming opportunities to help residents achieve their personally defined life goals.

The creation and nurturing of "community" is especially important as people get older. A continuing care retirement community (CCRC) provides an opportunity for seniors to make new friends and learn from and support each other as they continue to grow, flourish, and develop new skills and interests. Having a community and making new friends are particularly important to seniors who may be enduring the losses of partners and close friends.

We also recognize that many, as they age, worry about how future health changes could affect their lives. Accordingly, HSL communities have been designed to provide a full range of healthcare and social services—and the peace of mind of knowing that, even if needs do change, the services and supports are already in place to ensure that our seniors continue to live their best possible lives. Our residents have a full spectrum of options, including independent living, assisted living, memory support, rehabilitative care, and long-term healthcare services.

At the foundation of everything in this chapter is that we at HSL understand that seniors continue to have much more capability than what many give them credit for, and we aim to help our residents build upon those capabilities. We recognize that someone in their 80s or 90s still has goals, aspirations, and a passion for life. Just as all of us are always looking for ways to make our children's lives and their futures better, we should all be looking to do the same for our parents and grandparents. Our goal is to redefine a "senior moment" as enjoying a new or previously enjoyed activity, striving for and reaching an ambitious new goal, or passing along the value of one's experience to a youngster. Our commitment is that our senior living communities not only look at aging differently, but also reimagine what's possible.

Reflections for Readers

1. In your opinion, what would be the ideal housing situation in older adulthood? Would this be the same for all seniors?
2. What aspects of senior living would be most important to you?
3. How might taking a holistic, 360-degree view of older residents' needs improve senior housing?
4. How should an individual decide whether independent living or assisted living is more appropriate for his or her needs? How should that determination be made with respect to someone with an active mind and a frail body?

CHAPTER **61**

Why Moving to a Retirement Community Was the Right Choice for Me

Irving I. Silverman
Business Manager, Publication Division,
National Knitwear Association and
Proprietor of the Kosher Food and Jewish Life Expo (retired)
Dedham, MA
Age 97

When I was 89 years old, I had surgery to remove a brain tumor, and my children suggested that I move into a retirement community. I wasn't ready at that point, but a year later, I decided that it would be beneficial for me to do so. For me, it has been the right choice, even though I knew no one when I first moved in and was apprehensive about meeting people and feeling comfortable.

I believe that living in a retirement home for elder persons is much more desirable than living alone in one's home or apartment, with little access to well-established—or new—friendships. You do not have the burden of shopping, preparing meals, or housekeeping, and you don't need to endure the difficulties of lonesomeness. I'm a great testimonial for communal living and benefiting from social and other enjoyable activities within a retirement community.

I have found most living experiences in NewBridge, the retirement community that I moved to, very satisfying. Everything is under one roof, including whatever healthcare situations needed to be addressed. Staffing is courteous and considerate and everything is well administered. There are many memorable activities, including musical programs, lectures, enjoyable dining times, fitness activities, and religious services.

Being part of a community has given me people to talk to. It is easy to develop close relationships with individuals and even couples. There has never been a shortage of things to talk about, from past experiences, politics, and visits to the opera and musical programs. Life alone was boring in cloistered surroundings. And even more upsetting was the possibility of needing some physical help because of an accident and finding no one available to help.

I have found that being part of a new community means that there are others interested in learning about my many experiences. I've been invited to deliver several talks to the community, which I very much enjoyed doing. The community has also provided opportunities for me to use my expertise. For example, as a lifelong organizer, I undertook organizing programs for the community, such as a Nonagenarian Day to celebrate residents who were at least 90 years of age. (We started with 29 people attending the first year, and it has grown to the point that we had 130 attending in 2015.)

For someone who is alone and aging, it can be a burden to take care of even small things on your own. It's a pleasure to be able to call housekeeping, engineering, or information technology (IT) for help. In addition, I found that moving into a retirement community meant that I was no longer burdened by having to care for a large living space. In all of my previous homes, I had between six and ten rooms and the burden of managing everything. In those large spaces, I was always looking for my glasses that I had left in one of those rooms, either reading, watching TV, or doing some craft work that I enjoyed. I have found it a relief to downsize and simplify my life by having less to care for and be concerned with. I have also found it beneficial to get rid of many of the items I had accumulated that no longer are necessary for comfortable living.

One other aspect of living in a retirement community deserves mention, and that is the availability of finding supportive care. For most of the first five years of my residence at NewBridge, I lived pretty independently. But that changed with the occurrence of several falls and health interruptions. So I decided to engage a caregiver several days a week, a few hours each day, to accompany me to doctors' appointments and shopping, to keep me company, and to do all the other simple chores that would enable me to live alone. As time went by, I increased the number of both days and hours that the caregiver would be with me. I tried several caregivers before I found one who pleased me, who didn't boss me around or spend endless hours on the telephone while working for me. Obviously, one could have a caregiver in one's home or apartment without entering a retirement home, but that would never have satisfied all my housing needs. Because I am a gregarious person, I needed the time and attention of someone I could be comfortable with and whose presence I would enjoy, and I wanted all that and being in a friend-filled environment too.

Moving into a retirement community, while the right decision for me, had a minus element too, because in a large community populated by aging people, there would be a continuous progression of life and death occurrences. I have found it difficult to accept the repetition of birthday celebrations and funerals, all of which serve as reminders of aging and as markers of loss. In a community where everyone is older, there are more of these events than would be the case in a community of mixed ages; and of course, some of the losses are difficult to endure, as I have developed social relationships with residents who became dear friends. But: having lost two wives, I am no stranger to losses, and maybe that helped me count my blessings for all of the friendships that I have developed, even if there are losses too.

Reflections for Readers

1. The author provides several reasons why moving to a retirement community made sense for him. Can you think of other advantages a senior might find in moving to a retirement community? What possible downsides do you see to seniors making such moves?
2. Are the advantages and disadvantages of moving to a retirement community the same for people in their 60s, 70s, 80s, and 90s? What about for men and women?
3. What should someone look for in choosing a retirement community? In choosing the "right" level of care for himself or herself in such a community?

CHAPTER 62

Living and Learning in a Retirement Community

R. Peter Shapiro, Esq.
Attorney, Civil Litigation, Tardiff, Shapiro, & Cassidy (retired)
Dedham, MA
Age 79

My uncle and aunt relocated from Albany to Syracuse, New York, some time ago and suggested to us that when and if we decided to relocate, it should be a joint decision, to be made when we were not under any pressure to decide and when we could still be active members of our new community. We followed that advice in moving to NewBridge, which has several advantages for us. Newbridge—in Dedham, Massachusetts—is near Boston, a cultural hub and a city with a vibrant Jewish community. It is close to our eldest son, who lives in Belmont, Massachusetts. Moving to NewBridge meant that we would not be as isolated as we were in our former home in Concord, New Hampshire, where many of our friends went away for four to six months every year.

NewBridge has exceeded our expectations. The people have been warm and friendly, welcoming us into what I like to call the NewBridge family. The staff here makes a conscious effort to see that we are physically fit and adhere to a healthy, wholesome diet. There is programming, on and off campus, designed to stimulate the mind and engender conversation; by no stretch of the mind is it merely "busy work" to relieve boredom. NewBridge has been a place to foster what I refer to as "lifetime learning."

All of us are learners from cradle to grave. We acquire knowledge in formal and informal settings, from parents, friends, teachers, and our most intimate associations, as well as from the broader community. Our first lesson is to suckle, then to eat, crawl, walk, and talk. Structured education begins in preschool and continues through high school; some people go on from there to college and graduate school. The skills acquired become our passport to the workforce. And our education does not end once we leave school.

Let me tell you a story. I had been practicing law for about six months when one day, I was called into a senior partner's office. He said that I seemed bored with my assignments and he knew that I wanted to spend more time in court. He told me that many years earlier, he had been in my position. When he realized that each assignment and each person he met was different and unique, he was able to learn from all of those experiences. Being inquisitive had helped him make work interesting and had also increased his store of knowledge, his understanding of people, and his appreciation of the nuances of the law. I said thank you, but I was skeptical of his advice—until the next morning, when I had an experience of my own that taught me that I had received sound advice.

What happened was this: A woman brought me an old deed that she had found in her mother's effects and asked me to see if her family had any interest in the property. The grantor of the deed was Daniel Webster. Listening to my mentor's advice allowed me to appreciate the uniqueness of the situation and has served me well in my personal relationships, as well as in the practice of law.

We learn exponentially. Each new experience adds to our store of knowledge and informs our interpersonal relationships and our vocational skills. This process affords us the ability to establish our place in society and enhances our economic opportunities. However, for the knowledge to have value, it requires interaction with others, personally, professionally, or commercially.

Retiring does not change our course as lifetime learners. Learning's primary purpose is to enrich one's life and provide personal enjoyment. That doesn't end when we get older. We continue to have new experiences and to benefit from sharing them with others. For example, we might commune with nature by watching a glorious sunset or sunrise, taking a fall foliage tour, sitting by the fire looking out at the fresh falling snow, watching the waves on a stormy day, or watching the birds at the feeders. We get enjoyment and enrich our lives by attending theater, museums, concerts, sporting events, and the movies. We gain knowledge by participating in seminars, chat rooms, and lectures, and by reading. We can add to our store of experiences—and knowledge— by volunteering, being active in politics, running for office, and serving on boards and committees. We can manage our assets and advise family and friends.

For me, the number one activity here at NewBridge is the Intergenerational Program. Working with the students at the Rashi School is like having 40 more grandchildren. They read to me, and I am inspired when I see their improvement over the course of a year. We celebrate holidays and I attend special programs at Rashi. I currently am reading Steinbeck's *Of Mice and Men* in preparation for a discussion with seventh graders. The older students help our residents navigate the complexities of using computers.

A close second, in terms of importance to me, is the weekly Torah study group.[1] During the past 25 years, I have been fortunate to be able to study with rabbis at my synagogues and as a member and officer of the Union for Reform Judaism. The group at NewBridge is led by Rabbi Judi, who is an exceptional teacher, always prepared, able to adjust the subject matter to accommodate to the interests of the class, willing to research questions to which she does not have an answer, and always respectful of the views of the participants. She is a superb facilitator, giving each person his or her due and preventing anyone from dominating the conversation. Torah study is special not only because of Rabbi Judi, but also because of the knowledge and enthusiasm of our class.

I don't believe that a lifelong commitment to learning will extend one's life. On the other hand, retirees who do not continue their educational pursuits risk shortening their lives. That is, the failure to use our minds leads to boredom, depression, and the deterioration of our mental well-being, which could result in a loss of the will to live and possible premature death.

I want to say that longevity is important, but only when paired with a good quality of life. Seeing oneself as a member of a community, not simply as an individual, is important. Being part of a family or community culture encourages one to see that the community does not become stagnant, does not deteriorate and metaphorically die. The primary vehicle to enrich our lives and maintain a vibrant community is education. For those of us who live at NewBridge, we can keep our community vibrant by keeping abreast of how NewBridge functions, voicing our opinions, and participating in its governance and committees. We can also support the wide variety of cultural programs, lectures, and musical presentations at NewBridge and at other venues. This has the greatest impact when what we experience individually is discussed and shared.

---

[1] The Torah is the Jewish scroll of scripture. It consists of the first five books of the Old Testament.

The most appropriate definition of what it takes to be a dedicated lifelong learner can be found in the Talmud.[2] When asked "Who is a wise man?" Ben Zoma[3] responded, "He who learns from everybody."

Reflections for Readers

1. To what extent do you agree with this author's view that "longevity is important, but only when paired with a good quality of life"?
2. What is most important to you in terms of having a good quality of life?
3. How might lifelong learning experiences enhance one's quality of life? Will it also extend one's life expectancy?
4. The author suggested several activities that provide opportunities for continued learning for him, such as interacting with young students, studying religious texts, and participating in community governance. Can you suggest other activities that could also provide opportunities for ongoing learning in later life?

---

[2] The Talmud is an extensive body of rabbinic texts on a variety of subjects, including Jewish law, ethics, philosophy, customs, history, lore, and many other topics. The Talmud is the basis for all codes of Jewish law and is widely quoted in rabbinic literature.

[3] Ben Zoma, meaning "son of Zoma," was a rabbinic scholar who lived in the second century AD.

CHAPTER 63

Maintaining Independence: Staying in My Home

Irene F. Smith, RN
Nurse, Rheumatic Research (retired)
Alexandria, VA
Age 92

I am 92 and maintaining my independence is extremely important to me. The longer I can live on my own, go where I want, do what I want, and continue to make my own decisions, the happier I will be. I do not want be a burden to my children or grandchildren, and I do not want to be overly dependent on anyone. So far, I have been very fortunate and am able to drive during the daylight hours and live in my own family home.

I was married to my husband, Ray, for 56 years before I lost him in 2002. We had bought this home in 1974, when my husband started working in the Washington, D.C. area. We loved our house and its location. It is in a small cul-de-sac, which has developed into a little community of close neighbors. I have had the same wonderful neighbors for over 42 years. To a large extent, our cul-de-sac is akin to an extended family, and there is great love and friendship between us. Actually, it is the closeness of my neighbors that gives me additional security and makes it possible for me to stay in my home. I know that they will continue to check on me and are there for me if I ever need any help. By coincidence, they have each lost their own mothers and maybe I serve in that role, but just a little. They are primarily close friends who emotionally support me by being there. They occasionally call and say, "Would you like some dessert?" They also have keys to my house (and there is a lockbox), so they can verify that I am all right if I haven't been seen for a while. To be extra safe, I wear an alert button that is connected to a medical alert system. So I know that in an emergency, I would be able to get help instantly.

I love being in my house. It is true that it is a large, four-bedroom house that stays pretty much unused most days, as I really only use two rooms: the eat-in kitchen and my bedroom. Yet, I still enjoy the extra space and the memories that surround me. I think of my husband in this space and sometimes even engage in a "conversation" with him. It is warm and comfortable for me and really not hard to maintain. I have outside help with cleaning and other chores that large homes require, so it is not as cumbersome as some might think. My neighbors even help me with recycling and garbage cans (but only if I need it). True, my bedroom is on the second floor, but I only go upstairs once a day, to go to sleep. I do still go downstairs to the basement to do the laundry, but this is actually OK and affords me some exercise. If I couldn't continue to do the laundry, I know I could get help with this, so I am not concerned. I also have a den on the first floor that has a sleeper couch, so worst-case scenario, I could stay on the first floor if I needed to.

Since one of my sons lives only about 20 minutes away, he and his wife often call to make sure that I am doing well. They also are very generous about including me in many of their social events and arranging transportation for me. I know that my family is watching out for me, and I am very confident that they are assessing my health (particularly mental). If they felt that I was failing in some ways that I did not notice, they would discuss this with me in a timely way. I think that is also true for some of my neighbors, who could tell if I were "off." I guess this is part of my security system.

Additionally, my three local grandsons like to come over and spend some time with me. (I like seeing them too!)

Having enough space to entertain my family is very important. I want to be able to house my daughter and her husband, who live in Arizona, and my son and daughter-in-law from Massachusetts, when they visit. I could not imagine *not* having them stay with me, as our visits truly center around the house, with lots of cooking, eating, and playing games.

I have to admit that I don't mind my own company and I enjoy my privacy. I love to read and spend time alone relaxing. I worked as a nurse for many years and took care of my family, which included my husband, my three children, and my mother-in-law. Of course, I loved caring for my family, but there were many years (17 that my mother-in-law lived with us) when I felt like I had little privacy and time to myself. I miss my husband very much, but I am not overly lonely. I spend my life now doing my own thing and knowing that I am independent and not burdening anyone.

Fortunately, I can still get around with a cane, even if not as fast as before. I can do my own errands, like shopping and going to appointments. If I get lonely, I can go visit friends or play bridge or see plays. I still can participate in my synagogue and do some volunteer work with a group that helps homeless people. I do not need lots of activities planned for me, which I know differentiates me from others who look for that in senior centers.

Thank goodness, I can still take care of myself and all my financial responsibilities. I pay all my bills by check and balance my checkbook monthly. Eating healthy meals, including lots of protein, is not a problem for me, as I am able to shop and cook. I track my weight and blood pressure and know that I am in good health. I should do more exercise (walking) and will see if I can improve that!

When the time comes and I can no longer get around by myself, I will probably bring help into my house. I think about going to live in "senior housing," but I don't believe that is the right place for me. I worry that it will be too expensive and that I will lose too much independence. Some of my friends are excited about moving to senior living facilities, but not me. In all, I am very content as I am and want to stay in my house as long as I can. I hope I never have to change this decision.

Reflections for Readers

1. Some elders want or need the activities and sense of community offered by a continuous care retirement center (CCRC), while others place more value on aloneness and privacy. How might you help someone see where she or he fits on the spectrum of social contact needs?

2. Fear of mutual interdependence can be crippling. When does an elder's fear of losing independence become more of a burden to children and grandchildren? When is an elder's independence more of an illusion than something real? If this is the case, how might the family address the situation? How might a professional do so?

3. How might staying in his or her home facilitate someone's maintaining a continued bond with a loved one who no longer is physically present? Would moving decrease access to memories of the loved one and shared times? For some, might the reverse be true, and if so, why?

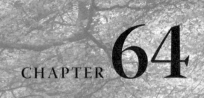

CHAPTER 64

Treasuring the Past, Enhancing the Future

Irving I. Silverman

Business Manager, Publications Division,
National Knitwear Association and
Proprietor of Kosher Food and Jewish Life Expo (retired)
Dedham, MA
Age 97

There is a big difference between treasuring the past and living in the past.

I want to tell a story about my sister, Beatrice, who lost her husband almost at the same time that my wife, Nancy, passed away. Beatrice's husband, Nat, had furnished their condominium in Florida, and after Nat's death, Beatrice refused to consider moving to a retirement community where she could meet new friends and create new life experiences. Even after I did this—and found the experience enlivening—Beatrice insisted on staying where she was because she thought that was the respectful thing to do. "My husband would have wanted me to stay in the same apartment we shared for 20 years." As a result, she was surrounded only by memories of the past and the caregivers who took care of her, a highly isolated life.

And here is what happened to her.

Unlike me, surrounded by new friends and opportunities to engage in social and cultural programming, Beatrice had no one to talk to except her aides, and nothing to keep her mind active and engaged. She became more and more isolated; and in her isolation, she became increasingly bitter about the course of her life. Whenever I spoke to her—and I tried to call her daily—her conversation was an endless rant about how unhappy she was. Now, it's true that Beatrice had a difficult life: she had lost her husband, and she had also lost their only child several years before Nat's death. Her mind kept looping back to how sad she was, how lonely . . . and yet she did nothing to change her situation.

Beatrice and I, the two youngest siblings in our family, were the only ones still alive. However, listening to her complain made me angry and uncomfortable, and eventually I too pulled away from her, calling her only once a week and not really listening to what she had to say. By living so consistently in the past, she estranged herself from the one person in the world who was most disposed to be close to her.

I too treasure the past, but I don't live in it. I keep photographs of people and places I have loved, and I share them with my new friends. I talk about my experiences, and I encourage others to do so too.

Instead of bemoaning my wife's death, I have taken great pleasure in remembering her gifts and finding ways to "embroider" them as I interact with my new friends. One example: I gave a lecture to the community I live in, NewBridge on the Charles, about the lighthouse that she had built as a gift for me.

Let me not conceal the fact that there are times of loneliness, but with my new friendships and acquaintances—the gift I gave myself by moving into a retirement community—I am able to live in an enhanced future.

The future is what we make of it. For us to close ourselves in a "closet" is a negative behavior—one that could destroy our zest for living and impair our joy and contentment. I believe in making constant efforts to extend my life into the future and to share it with others. Hopefully, doing so will extend my life; and in any event, it will add to my peace of mind.

Reflections for Readers

1. For elders especially, reminiscence is valuable—but at what point does reminiscing turn into living in the past?
2. How can someone use his or her treasuring of the past to enhance the future?
3. What is the value for seniors of a future orientation?
4. Faced with an ever-diminishing circle of family and friends, how might seniors manage rifts in long relationships?
5. How should someone deal with unpleasant—and therefore *not* treasured—memories?

PART **XI**

To Drive or Not to Drive

CHAPTER 65

Continuing to Drive Keeps Me Independent

Irene F. Smith, RN
Nurse, Rheumatic Research (retired)
Alexandria, VA
Age 92

Driving is the very definition of independence, at least for me. My ability to go where I want to go, when I want to go, is of utmost importance to my sense of well-being and self-worth. Driving enhances the quality of my life and enables me to continue to live in my home. When I can no longer drive, I think I will feel that I have truly lost my independence.

I have been fighting for self-reliance my whole life—92 years. When I was younger, I believe that my struggles for independence probably caused issues between my mother and myself. I think some of my siblings had similar problems with our parents. Yet, this drive to make my own decisions and to take care of myself has continued throughout my life. It is not that I don't appreciate cooperative teams; certainly, I enjoyed my time working with others during my long nursing career. I also had a wonderful and successful marriage partnership for 56 years with my husband, Ray. We always worked together on decisions, and I had my areas within our household that were mine to manage. I always was able to drive where I needed to be and take the children where they needed to go. But the years living in close quarters with my depressed mother-in-law were difficult, depriving me of privacy and frankly, it felt somewhat judgmental to me. So now, at this stage of my life, I want to be able to decide when, where, and how I live, and certainly how I go places. My driving provides me the tool to accomplish this and allows me the wherewithal to direct my activities.

Recently, I decided to give up nighttime driving. I felt uncomfortable with the oncoming headlights and the decrease of sight in the darkness. I became more convinced that driving at night might be potentially dangerous, both for me and for others. It was a very difficult and conflicted decision, as many of my social events occur at night. But safety comes first, and I have stopped driving once it gets dark. To facilitate some activities, I have begun taking taxis and accepting rides from my family and friends. Although the additional cost from cabfares is not terribly extravagant, I feel like it is discouraging me from going out at night. This could be the first notch out of my "independence belt." I hope it will not greatly affect me.

I have a friend who cannot drive at all anymore. She had become increasingly dependent on me to drive her around. In fact, she required so much time and effort from me that I started to feel her needs encroaching on my freedom. This has led to two results. First, it has affected our friendship and I no longer want to spend time with her or to be her chauffeur. Second, and much more subtle, I think it has reinforced the importance of my own driving requirements. If I can no longer drive, will I become as "needy" on others? Will I become a burden (as my friend did)? I really don't want to find out!

My family and my neighbors have agreed to let me know if my driving skills begin to deteriorate. I am smart enough to know that I cannot drive if my sight goes or my reflexes slow down too much. Of course, if I start to show signs of significant memory loss, I will not chance driving a car and getting lost or worse. For now, I enjoy driving to stores, doctor appointments, hairdresser appointments, and daytime social outings. I can manage all my daily activities and food/drug needs by using organizing techniques like putting my keys in the same place, making lists for shopping and to-do's, and using marked pillboxes for medications. All the places that I go are well known to me and are really not that far from my home. I get around with a cane, just not so quickly! My car is my good friend and takes me where I need to go and allows me to stay in my family home.

Unfortunately, if the day comes when I can no longer drive, I will need to make some serious decisions and/or adjustments. Do I move to a senior housing arrangement where a van is provided to take me to the places I need to go? Or, do I stay at home and bring in all the help and supplies that I need? If I don't leave the house, will that lead to a lack of socialization? Will the loss of driving change the contentment that I now enjoy? How will I avoid dependency on others? How will that change the quality of my life?

I do not spend time worrying about what will happen in the future. I continue to take each day one day at a time and enjoy my good life. To tell you the truth, I hope that when my time is up, it is quick and easy.

Reflections for Readers

1. For this author, being able to drive represents independence—but is this universally true? Does driving have the same meaning to someone living in Manhattan that it does to someone living in a rural or suburban area? What about someone who, for reasons of poor vision, has never been able to drive?

2. Some people become unable to drive because of cognitive problems. How is that situation different from the situation of a person who can't drive because of poor vision?

3. How and when should children or other family members intervene to take the car keys away from an elder? When should they enlist the help of a physician?

4. What other losses might have similar meaning for an elder as losing the ability to drive? How might elders be helped in dealing with all such losses?

5. How does the ability (or inability) to drive affect the decision about where to live?

CHAPTER 66

We Need to Talk—When Is It Time to Hang up the Keys?

Emily Grossman, MSW, CMC
Life Care Manager, LifeCare Advocates
Newton, MA

American iconography has represented the car as the vehicle that gives you the choice to pursue whatever path you want. From the very beginning, cars were advertised as giving you the freedom to go anywhere, to be mobile and completely unrestricted—to be able to "hit the open road." Nothing is quite as quintessentially freeing as getting behind the wheel—even if it's as simple as doing an errand or going to visit a friend. Driving represents the ultimate in independence. It is no surprise, then, when senior drivers are reluctant or downright adamant that they do not need to give up driving. No one wants to talk about it, think about it, or plan for it. It's as if ignoring the warning signs will stop the inevitable conversation—"Dad, we need to talk about the car."

Research shows that the normal process of aging affects one's driving ability, and yet there is no set age that makes you unsafe to be behind the wheel. But older people cling to their cars as the very lifeline that allows them to be "independent." Why is driving so important to our older population? What does independence actually mean?

For many, it means not having to reach out to family, friends, or neighbors just to get a gallon of milk or go to the pharmacy. Driving means not being dependent on anyone; it allows us to do what we want to do, whenever we want to do it. This is especially pertinent for seniors who live in suburban or rural areas, where daily needs and social outlets are spread across greater distances and not easily accessible by public transportation.

If you think about it, driving is actually a very complicated task. You have to aggregate a lot of information at once—sights and sounds—as well as be able to obey traffic signs and laws, be on the lookout for pedestrians and bikers, all while reacting quickly to the events unfolding around you in real time. For older drivers, this can be difficult due to a number of factors, including certain medications, medical conditions, deteriorating eye sight or hearing, and slower reaction time or reflexes. According to the National Highway Traffic and Safety Administration, of traffic fatalities involving older drivers in 2012, 75% occur during the daytime, 69% occur on weekdays, and 64% involved other vehicles. This certainly disproves the common wisdom that driving during uncrowded weekday hours is somehow less dangerous.

So how does one begin to broach this difficult conversation with an older driver? The most important thing to keep in mind is that this is a conversation, *not* a lecture. Recognizing the psychological importance that seniors place on driving is an important part of the process. Additionally, being proactive and starting the conversation early so that you can plan together is paramount to a good outcome. Allowing time for planning and exploration of options is better than waiting for a crisis or accident to occur. Moreover, your loved one needs to know that losing the ability to drive does not have to mean the end of independence. So long as she or he is presented with viable alternatives for transportation, such as private drivers, Ubers, or taxis, giving up the keys may seem like less of a big deal.

What do you do in the special circumstance of an older adult with memory problems? Relying on the ability of a senior to recognize the risks of continuing to drive can be tricky when the person has dementia or other cognitive impairment. People with memory issues are unlikely to be able to accurately assess their own driving skills. Dementia comes in many forms and is a progressive disease. In the early stages, individuals can have memory loss but still be high functioning and able to perform many daily tasks without issue. They might lack insight into their deficits and would be very unlikely to agree with you regarding the idea of stopping driving. In these cases, where a direct conversation might not work, enlisting the help of a professional, such as a life care manager, can be invaluable, as these professionals can help you plan and use new strategies to facilitate the situation.

What are some of the signs that an older driver may need to stop driving? According to AAA, receiving multiple violations can be one of the predictors of the greatest risk for a collision. Additionally, "fender benders," such as parking lot accidents, sideswiping cars and inanimate objects, and rear-end crashes are among the most common accidents for seniors with diminishing driving skills, depth perception, or reaction time. If a senior driver has been issued two or more traffic tickets or citations, or has been involved in two or more "near misses" or collisions in the last two years, he or she is at greater risk of having an accident. Additionally, ignoring traffic signals, having trouble staying in the correct lane, or driving well below the speed limit (and getting honked at frequently) are all indications that it may be time to give up the keys.

We are lucky to live in an age of new technology that offers up many alternatives for those who can no longer drive. Applications such as Lyft or Uber (for those with smartphones) or Go Go Grandparent (for those without a smartphone) offer a ride for substantially less than a traditional taxi. In many places, there is subsidized transport for seniors in both urban and suburban locations, often with door-to-door service. Additional options include hiring a car service or a companion or home health aide who can act both as a driver and a companion. While this may sound pricey, it is often less expensive than the cost of owning and maintaining a car, the insurance payments that may increase due to accidents, etc. We have to move past considering using someone else to drive as an "extravagance," particularly if this service avoids a potentially fatal crash.

In addition to the various driving replacement services available, it may be time to start talking about alternative housing options. Senior living communities expand the number of options that a senior has for social engagement; learning and cognitive enrichment; healthy meals; and general day-to-day interaction that elders might not get if they were still at home, even if they did continue to drive. Independent living and assisted living settings have built-in social networks and supports, as well as transportation options available to residents. Many have weekly scheduled bus trips to grocery stores, pharmacies, and other common destinations, in addition to providing personalized transportation options such as car services (often free or low-cost) for local travel. In this type of setting, not being able to drive becomes much less of a stressor, and often the person thrives due to the enhanced social setting and services offered.

There is no exact formula for figuring out when it is time for someone to stop driving. It's a process that begins with an assessment of driving skills and a series of conversations with family, friends, and the senior's physician. Be sensitive to the fact that to elders, you are talking about taking away what they see as their vital link to the world outside their home. Without the ability to drive, many worry they will become housebound and isolated—or worse, have to rely on others to get their basic needs met. By approaching the topic gently—and by being prepared with strategies for "life after driving"—the conversation will most likely have a better resolution. Let seniors know that you are concerned and that you want to help, not scold or threaten them. Make sure that they feel that they are part of the decision, not that it is being made for them. Most important, be prepared to have multiple conversations on this topic. Giving up driving isn't an end to a senior person's path of independence. It is a new fork in the road.

Resources

Professional help:

- Aging Life Care Manager: www.aginglifecare.org
- Your local Area Agency on Aging can help you find services in your area. Call 1-800-677-1116, or go to www.eldercare.gov to find your nearest Area Agency on Aging.

Warning signs and workbooks:

- *Driving Decisions Workbook*: https://deepblue.lib.umich.edu /bitstream/handle/2027.42/1321/94135.0001.001.pdf?sequence =2&isAllowed=y
- http://seniordriving.aaa.com/resources-family-friends/know-when -be-concerned/

Driver evaluation programs:

- AARP: http://www.aarp.org/home-family/getting-around/driving -resource-center/info-10-2013/driver-safety-refresher-course -2014.html
- Driver improvement courses: http://seniordriving.aaa.com /maintain-mobility-independence/driver-improvement-courses -seniors/
- Online driving evaluation: http://seniordriving.aaa.com/evaluate -your-driving-ability/interactive-driving-evaluation/

Conversation starters:

- http://www.aarp.org/home-garden/transportation/we_need_to_talk/

Reflections for Readers

1. When family members are concerned about an elder's driving, who should talk to her or him? Do you have suggestions for such a conversation?

2. Many elders feel threatened when someone suggests that they should stop driving. How would you handle such a situation, to put an elder person at greater ease while ensuring safety?

3. Elders sometimes use the fact that they are still driving to convince themselves that they are "independent," but in some cases, the "independence" is illusory, as they are unable to maintain their homes properly, to eat healthily, etc., without substantial help and support from others (which may impose a burden on family). While this is not true of all seniors, it is true for some. How would you deal with a senior who employs this logic?

PART XII
Money Matters

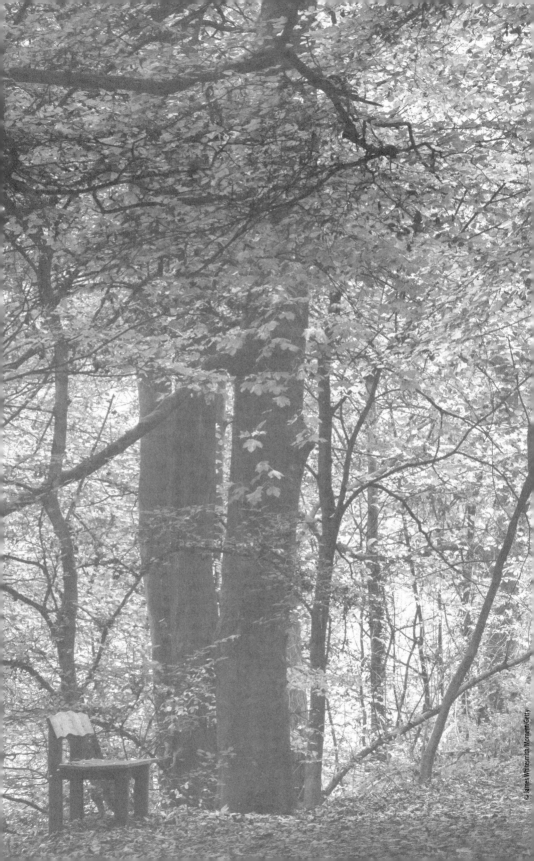

CHAPTER 67

When Social Security Is Not Enough

Ellen Beth Siegel, JD, PsyD
Clinical Psychologist
Cambridge, MA

For people with limited financial resources, the prospect of getting old is especially worrisome. Social Security offers a bare minimum of funding for elders. Someone who has worked—full time—at a minimum wage job throughout a 35-year career can expect Social Security payments of approximately $640 per month, and someone whose work career spanned half that many years—a situation disproportionately affecting women—can expect only about two-thirds of that. Needless to say, someone with a minimum wage history probably is not able to save toward retirement and probably does not have a 401(k), any other employer-funded retirement plan, or an Individual Retirement Account (IRA). Many elders feel that they have to continue working just to make ends meet, regardless of other desires or of the increase in medical issues that accompanies older age.

Worries about how one is going to live in one's later years plague many elders and soon-to-be elders, and this may lead to depression, anxiety, and other psychological disorders. These fears are realistic.

Case Example: Arish[1]

Arish, an immigrant from India who was born in 1952 and just turned 65, came to the United States about 20 years ago, when he was offered an

---

[1] To protect confidentiality, the patient's name and certain identifying details have been changed.

acting role in a movie. He has remained in the United States ever since on a visa that allows him to perform, but not to work in other capacities. He has appeared in a variety of commercials, regional theater, and TV shows over the years, but his income is spotty and he lives a rather marginal existence. Arish is aware that in his field, appearance matters a great deal, and he knows that he is not the strikingly handsome man he was when he was younger. He also has arthritis, which is beginning to interfere with his ability to perform. He has accordingly begun to think about a future in which he would no longer be earning any money. He came to therapy as he began considering his very limited options for retirement, stating that maybe it would be best if he just ended his life.

Arish has made a home for himself in the United States, and for that reason, as well as for reasons connected to his family of origin, he does not want to return to India. However, he sees no way to take control of his financial situation as he enters his later years other than the extreme measure of ending his life. He has minimal savings, would be ashamed to ask for governmental "hand-outs," can expect little from Social Security, and worries about what will happen to him when—not if—he is no longer able to work. As he says, "It's hard to be poor."

Lack of money interferes with Arish's ability to eat healthily, to engage in pleasant activities, and to interact socially with others. When he is not working, he spends most of his time alone in his apartment, leading to social isolation—and that, in turn, leads to further depression.

Although my usual role as a psychologist is not to offer advice or provide pragmatic solutions to someone's psychological difficulties, the situation with Arish is different. His depression and anxiety are caused by social circumstances, and it therefore seems appropriate to intervene on the social level. Accordingly, I've been working with him to think about getting a different kind of visa or becoming a permanent resident, as those steps would permit him to supplement his work as an actor with other kinds of work. I have explored what other kinds of work he might be able to do or want to do. We have talked about his moving back to India or to some other country, though up to this point, he has not wanted to do either of those things. We have looked at how his depression and anxiety are affecting his day-to-day functioning and have laid out plans for maintaining a healthy diet and finding activities with little or no cost involved to keep him active and socially involved. And we have looked at what his Social Security benefits are going to be and what government resources are available to him to supplement his Social Security. Unfortunately as a noncitizen, he has even more red tape to wade through than a citizen, and less assurance of finding safety net help.

This is hard work for Arish and for me. It's heart-wrenching to hear him talk about having to forgo fresh fruit and vegetables because they are too expensive, or not being able to further his career by attending workshops or other artists' performances. I see him come to our sessions, time after time, in old clothes. He talks about the difficult choices that he sometimes has to make: Will he pay for the medications he needs, or will he pay his electric bill? Unexpected expenses create chaos, as he has so little in the way of reserves.

Poverty is a real and pressing issue. Arish is struggling now, financially and psychologically, and has reason to worry about how he will manage in the future. He is worried—and I am worried for him.

Reflections for Readers

1. Seniors who live in poverty may find it more difficult to work than younger people, as both discrimination in the workplace and health issues may limit their opportunities. Where should seniors turn for help? What kinds of help are available, and what sorts of professionals can provide it?

2. Depression is a serious problem among the elderly. How can professionals dealing with seniors in various contexts—physical or occupational therapists, for example—recognize depression and help the seniors find appropriate treatment?

3. Many forms of economic assistance are available to people with little income, but for seniors especially, there is often a great reluctance to ask for or accept help; this is a matter of shame. How can a senior in this predicament be assisted to get past such feelings of shame?

68

Living Well on a Fixed Income

Roberta Horn, PsyD

Psychotherapist, Neponset Health Center (retired)

Quincy, MA

Living on a fixed income is often a major life disruption for senior citizens or younger people who have, for one reason or another, lost the ability to generate earned income. The fixed income is probably considerably less than the amount that previously came in on a regular basis. There may be a retirement fund in place, or there may be family members who can help out, but many do not have these additional sources of income. Social Security may provide some financial support, but it was never intended to be anyone's sole source of income and is generally insufficient even for daily living expenses (i.e., food, housing costs, heating, utilities, and clothing). Medical, dental, and medication costs are often financially out of reach. The newspapers are full of stories of impoverished people who have to choose between medication, food, or heat. The affected people often describe having previously had comfortable, middle-class lives, and many express bewilderment at their impoverished situations.

There are also many others in less dire circumstances who, despite having a limited income, can cover their basic expenses but would like to find ways to live more pleasurable lives.

Getting Help from Government and Social Service Agencies

There are multiple agencies and nonprofit organizations at the local, state, and federal levels that can and do offer various forms of help to low-income people. For example, some states provide heating assistance and other help. The help available may vary according to political policies (state and federal) and the financial concerns of the agencies or nonprofits in question. Each one also has its own set of guidelines to determine eligibility for aid. For instance, it may be possible to just show up at some food banks, but the food stamp program is run by the federal government and requires documents that verify income.

Income verification documents also may be required as proof of need when applying for other state, local, or federal assistance. Because state and federal agencies have stringent requirements, it is important that persons applying for aid keep careful records, including statements of heating costs, rent or other housing expenses, electricity, and other expenses. It will be equally important to retain all annual statements from Social Security, copies of income tax records for the past seven years, and all bank statements.

Fraternal and service organizations quietly help citizens in many ways. The Lions Club offers free eyeglasses, and Habitat for Humanity builds homes for people who are willing to put in their own sweat labor.

Making a file box or a computerized list of all the resources that are needed can be a big help. When I worked in hospice, my file box included categories for Wheelchairs and Walkers, Wigs, Churches, Drivers, and multiple others. Your file box might include State Social Services, Area Agencies on Aging, Senior Centers, Food Banks, Farm Programs, and others that you will think of as time goes by. By setting up your own resource file, you will avoid having to look things up continually. Professionals helping seniors can give such lists to clients to make things easier for them.

Finding Help with Food

Local areas have food banks, often located at churches or at town halls. As a general rule, churches and synagogues do not limit their donations to members. Other possible food sources are restaurants that offer senior discounts and farms, which offer crop-sharing in season.

Some techniques that my clients and their families have used include comparing prices in the weekly grocery flyers, looking for the reduced price table in the market (which might include day-old bread products and items no longer being stocked), using coupons, trying less-famous brands of canned goods (often stocked on the lower shelves), and, when they have sufficient cash, buying in bulk. It is also helpful to belong to a buyer's or discount club, but that does mean paying an annual membership fee.

Shopping

Shopping becomes a major issue when one has a fixed income, but there are many options that can help. Many stores, museums, movie theaters, and restaurants have senior hours or senior days when they offer discounts. (This might be a category for your filing system.)

Thrift shops and consignment shops are especially helpful for bargain shoppers. The Yellow Pages, local newspapers, and the Internet are all good places to start. Many thrift stores and consignment shops, including Salvation Army and Goodwill stores, have brand-new items along with others that are lightly used. Habitat for Humanity stores have incredible buys in furniture and lighting.

Salvage stores, which specialize in overstocked goods of all kinds and sell them at rock-bottom prices, are another useful resource for discounted clothing, sporting goods, flooring, small appliances, and food items. Yard sales, sidewalk sales, dollar stores, rummage/white elephant sales, and library book sales are excellent, but more random, sources for shopping.

Remember that stores want to sell. When someone needs or wants a large or more expensive item that he or she cannot pay for outright, it might be worthwhile to ask whether the store has a 0% payment plan. This is a plan that offers an interest-free period in which the buyer makes monthly payments. This method of buying requires careful and vigilant attention to the timing of payments because the onus lies entirely on the buyer. If the last penny of payment is made one day after the deadline, then an ultra-high interest rate is added to all the money due under the original agreement.

Health Insurance

Medicare and supplementary insurance, which covers the part of the medical bill that Medicare does not cover, are extremely important insurance policies and important budgeting items. Even one day in the hospital today can "break the bank" for most families, so both forms of health insurance are necessary.

People with limited resources especially need neutral but informed assistance in choosing the company and plan that is best for them. Impartial, informed help is available at or through the state agency of aging, which protects and supports the decisions of senior citizens.

Staying Active: Socializing and Volunteering

Having friends and being social have been proven to be major factors in elder health. Senior centers offer numerous opportunities for friendship, and membership is usually inexpensive. Activities might include art classes, games like bridge and Scrabble, local events, and even trips. Senior centers also have access to various senior discounts and might offer services such as foot care or gentle forms of exercise such as yoga.

Libraries and the local "Y" provide free or almost free activities like movies, art exhibitions, and "Meet the Author" events. Some have knitting groups, and others host concerts.

Colleges and universities are now offering low-cost "Senior College" courses in a wide range of subjects, like classic movies, writing your own memoir, learning a new language, and jewelry-making. High schools also offer classes.

People on limited incomes have become valued volunteers. Seniors are welcome. Volunteering costs nothing but gas money and time—and remember what a gift that time is. Volunteers are paid with the warm feeling they get inside from helping others. Many volunteers find that they receive far more than they give.

How Professionals Can Help

There is no shame in needing help. One way that professionals can help is by reinforcing that message. Many people have been raised to believe that they *must* be self-sufficient, yet they find that they do need help. The purpose of social service programs is to support self-esteem while giving people the boost they need. Practitioners, understanding the need for self-respect, can offer suggestions in a natural and neutral manner, conveying "The logical thing to do is . . ." rather than "poor you."

Living on limited incomes sometimes creates a focus on loss and difficulty in seeing what one *does* have. A good listener is helpful, and professionals of many types can fill that role.

An important note: Some seniors are not capable of gathering and maintaining records or of taking care of themselves in general. In such cases, professional help becomes essential. Professionals can evaluate the senior's needs and facilitate the appointment of a guardian to handle financial or other major decisions. This guardian might be an attorney, a trusted family member, or a friend; the senior will make this choice if she or he is of sound mind.

Finally, professionals need to encourage and celebrate the joy of what individuals *do* have, as opposed to what they have lost, and can cultivate the concept of making money stretch as a meetable adventure and challenge. When it is seen as a challenge, it is easier (and more fun) than concentrating on the negative side.

Reflections for Readers

1. Why might people on fixed or limited incomes feel ashamed of their financial situations? What can be done to reduce this feeling of shame?

2. How can someone on a fixed income best be helped to set and live within a budget? What are the "essentials," and what expenses are "optional"—and how might these differ from one person to the next?

3. What value might a senior accrue from volunteering?

CHAPTER 69

Challenges for Low-Income Seniors: The Not-So-Golden Years

Janet Gottler, LICSW
Social Worker, NewBridge on the Charles
Dedham, MA

The National Council on Aging estimates that over 25 million Americans aged 60+ are economically insecure, living at or below 250% of the poverty level ($29,425 for a single person). Richard Johnson of the Income and Benefits Policy Center at the Urban Institute reports that 14% of older adults, or 6.5 million people, do not have enough income to meet their needs. Most of their income comes from Social Security, and they spend much of it on housing.

To put things in some historical perspective, older adults have made some tremendous gains over the past generation. Johnson reports that between 1966 and 2013, the official poverty rate for older adults fell from 29% to 10% ($11,770 for a single elder). This was largely attributable to a set of increases in Social Security benefits. However, adjusting for out-of-pocket healthcare costs, the poverty rate for older adults is closer to 16%. These older adults struggle with rising housing and health care costs, inadequate nutrition, a lack of access to transportation, and diminished savings. One major life event can lead to a cascade of troubles.

The Center for American Progress reports that most elderly poor are women, and very elderly women have even higher poverty rates. A lifetime of lower earnings due to wage discrimination, absence from the labor market while raising children, and having jobs that are less likely to have employer-sponsored retirement plans takes its toll. Single, divorced, or widowed women do not have spouses, with the additional sources of income that they bring to a household.

Elderly people of color are more likely than Caucasian Americans to experience poverty. Rural elderly have higher rates of poverty than the urban elderly, and rural areas tend to have a higher percentage of elderly in their total population. Older adults with disabilities—defined as having difficulty living independently—are more likely to have inadequate incomes than those without disabilities.

Seniors living in poverty face many challenges. Many among the cohort reaching the age for Social Security have to delay retirement. Elderly Americans' limited budgets are strained by healthcare costs, including copays and prescription costs. The Center for American Progress reports that healthcare costs have contributed to the rise in bankruptcy filings among the elderly. They also face the challenges of rising utility costs, poor nutrition and hunger, lack of accessible transportation, and predatory lending.

Housing Needs as Low-Income Seniors Age

While healthcare costs dominate the debate about older adults' needs and preparedness for retirement, older adults spend more on housing than health care. Housing costs are significant for low-income seniors, who devoted 36% of their household expenditures to housing in 2013. Older renters spent 43% of their income on housing, substantially more than the 30% cutoff commonly used to identify burdensome housing costs. Strikingly, the lowest-income older households, with incomes below 125% of the federal poverty level (FPL), spent 74% of their income on housing in 2013.

The lack of affordable housing for older adults is a significant challenge across the United States. AARP estimates that 13 million Americans over the age of 50 can no longer afford their housing costs or live in inadequate housing. They found that there are only 44 affordable housing units for every 100 people in need.

As people age, they may face new issues of mobility and other physical limitations. Only 3.8% of all housing units in the country have design features to accommodate moderate mobility limitations, according to the Bipartisan Policy Center's Senior Health and Housing Task Force, and these are not necessarily affordable for lower-income people.

The housing crunch will likely worsen as more people live long enough to become seniors—and longer thereafter. The Harvard Joint Center on Housing Studies reports that by 2024, an additional 1.8 million senior households—a total of 6.5 million—will have less than $15,000 a year to live on. The Bipartisan Policy Center's task force recommends more affordable housing for seniors, including the model of Supportive Housing, which incorporates supports for in-home health care and supports for daily tasks.

House-Rich but Cash-Poor

The "American Dream" fostered in our culture is to achieve "middle-class status." For so many, this was the achievement of home ownership and the sense of dignity and security that home ownership provides. Many older adults want to be able to "age in place," yet our housing stock was not designed to accommodate an aging population, particularly in urban areas with multilevel homes and multiapartment buildings. Combine this with the challenge of living on a fixed income, deteriorating housing stock, and a reluctance to move, and we find seniors living in homes that are falling apart and badly in need of repairs.

When I worked at Kit Clark Senior Services in Dorchester, a working-class section of Boston, I collaborated with our Senior Home Improvement (SHIP) program. This program, and others like it across the country, provide free and low-cost repairs for low-income seniors, veterans, and people with disabilities. They found people with leaking pipes, broken windows, or failing furnaces. They found people in their 90s heating water on the stove to put in their bathtub as their only way to warm the water up. There were people who were heating their houses by turning on the stove and opening the oven door—a dangerous practice.

When people find themselves unable to cover unanticipated expenses such as home repairs or modifications necessary for their safety, programs such as SHIP and Rebuilding Together Boston can step in. When Mrs. C returned from a hospitalization and rehab stay with a wheelchair, her family found that she could not move safely around her home. During National Rebuilding Days in Boston, a team converged on her house to construct a wheelchair ramp, widen the bathroom doors, and install a more accessible toilet. For seniors struggling to maintain their family home and live out their remaining years in their familiar neighborhood, programs such as these are models for replication.

Supportive Housing and Affordable Assisted Living: Aging in Community

For many seniors, remaining in their homes becomes an isolating experience. They may lose old support systems as familiar neighbors die or move away, and family members may live scattered across the country.

Traditional affordable housing does not have the types of support that frail elderly need, and they may enter institutionalized settings prematurely.

Supportive housing and assisted-living communities are two successful models of support for older adults as they age. Supportive housing models provide affordable housing, along with supports in the building: Personal Emergency Response systems, access to health care on site, social workers/case managers, and availability of an on-site meal once a day. In some buildings, there is the availability of fitness equipment and some on-site programming that provides stimulation and socialization.

Assisted living is a growing option across the country, and many seniors are opting for this alternative: the ability to remain independent in one's own apartment, with gentle "wraparound supports" of care assistance on site, three meals a day, and enriched cultural and stimulating programming. Transportation for shopping and medical appointments can be available. Most importantly, the opportunity to "age in community" reduces social isolation, and that reduction can have a major positive impact on health, nutrition, and risk for depression.

Unfortunately, these options are vastly underfunded compared to the needs in our communities. There are long waiting lists for these affordable options, a source of frustration for seniors and their families and providers alike. I recall a fragile elder I was working with who resided in the Mission Hill neighborhood of Boston. She lived in an apartment in isolation, with no old friends remaining in her neighborhood. Mrs. D suffered frequent anxiety attacks and often ended up in our local emergency room late at night with shortness of breath and palpitations, to rule out cardiac involvement.

Mrs. D's daughter lived in Newton, a suburb of Boston, and placed her on the waiting list for one of the few affordable apartments that would become available in a new assisted-living facility opening in Newton Corner. Appropriate applicants would be chosen by a lottery system. I received an elated call one day from Mrs. D; she had "won the jackpot" and would be moving to Newton to live closer to her daughter. When I followed up several months after her move, I learned that she had not experienced any further episodes of palpitations and shortness of breath. Her nighttime trips to the emergency room miraculously ended, and she began to thrive in this social environment. Mrs. D was a poster child for the model of "aging in community."

These wonderful models represent both the hope and the tragedy. The hope is: We are developing models of caring in community that are proven successes in promoting health, dignity, and security for low-income elders in our communities. The tragedy is that our country's priorities ignore the seniors who are our national treasures, who have built our communities and nurtured younger generations, and these proven models of care are woefully underfunded to meet the growing needs of our senior population.

As Sandra Henriquez, CEO of Rebuilding Together, has said, "A lot of people who have spent good years helping their communities now need some help themselves. We take seriously that we are our brothers' and sisters' keepers."

At Hebrew SeniorLife (HSL), where I now work as a social worker, we take seriously the mission to "honor one's father and mother." HSL has several models of affordable supportive housing, in Revere, Brookline, and Randolph, Massachusetts, which integrate health services and social supports with housing. We also have a wonderful assisted-living residence in Dedham that includes a specialized assisted-living, memory-support community, but not yet an affordable assisted-living option. We continue to strategize on our mission to expand these options to all seniors in our community.

There is much work to do.

Reflections for Readers

1. From a policy perspective, how would you design an economic safety net that would meet the needs of seniors? What priority would you put on expenditures for housing, health care, and other needs?

2. Taking into consideration the increasing frailty that seniors often experience as they age, what features would you want to see in housing designed for seniors? How do you think these housing needs could be provided on an affordable basis?

3. Some seniors want to "age in place"; others prefer to "age in community." How would you evaluate these two models of care, and which is likely to be more affordable for the elderly poor?

CHAPTER 70

Living on the Edge: The New Economy for Aging Americans

Laura R. Reiter, MA
Writer, educator, and researcher
East Brewster, MA
Age 78

The question is asked of me—How, as an aging woman, do I manage on my limited financial resources? What can I do and what can I *not* do? Let's just say from the beginning that part of the aging process is that there are places and things that don't have the same importance that they would have had when I was younger. For example, I don't want to own a house. The thought of being in a relatively permanent place would stifle me. What would happen if I didn't like my neighbors, or worse, what would I do if I didn't have the money for repairs? Scratch that one out.

I never wanted to be married to a man who wanted a wife to stay at home. I still don't have any desire to pursue a relationship at this age, even though it might be financially rewarding. This I cannot do.

I think of myself as an atypical older woman. A woman who adamantly does not want to spend time with my age group. The thought of living in a "village" comprised of seniors in cookie-cutter apartments on a fixed income turns my stomach inside out. Perhaps I am unrealistic to think that I will find a better solution when I no longer have the money for first, last, and a month's security to get into any type of housing. In other words, I am living in the present, and since I have managed to find creative ways of living, I will continue to be positive about my outcome regarding housing.

In order to do what I want to do, there is always an element of risk involved. So long as I am physically and mentally healthy, I continue to take risks with my money. For example, I don't know how I paid off $3,000 worth of dental work or over $1,000 in eye care recently. I have little actual money in the bank, but I have excellent credit from paying off my credit card debts over many years. Hence, I use those handy monthly credit card checks to pay off my debts. Once my retirement money is gone—which will be within the next year—I will be faced with a serious financial problem. But then again, I might be dead. So, I want to work on my present situation and think of creative ways to keep myself positive. I remember a close friend, who was a university professor and who had a great deal of money, who repeatedly told me to file for bankruptcy during my university career. I never listened to her. She kept warning me that I would end up in the poorhouse. I hope not, but she is long dead, and her money did not go with her. So, what is the moral here? I continue to trust myself that I will somehow figure out what to do when I only have my Social Security to live on.

Even if I had an unlimited budget, I have no desire to go out to fancy restaurants. My happiness comes from going to an arty café and getting the latest book on Paris life or reading *The New York Times,* or reading about life in Africa, similar to the likes of the writer Alexandra Fuller, who currently lives in a yurt in Wyoming. Perhaps there is some hope in my creative writing, the fulfillment of the written word that will continue to nourish me, maybe not financially, but in ways that will keep me positive to make the right decisions in the future.

In addition to the above "what I can/cannot do with my limited resources," I will mention that I have had to make choices on the matters below. They seem minor decisions, but they do have an impact on my budget.

1. I am unable to visit my family on the West Coast on a regular basis. Until October of this year, I had not seen my daughter, grandchildren, and great-grandchildren for over two years. However, since we are all facing financial difficulties, there is a lot of stress between us. Perhaps it is better not to see each other several times a year as I wished.

2. Instead of going to Bloomingdale's or an upscale retail store for clothes, I am a thrift shop guru. I know my brands and I love multiple colorful layering, so I am happy with that, so long as the climate is cold and not hot throughout the year, as in Los Angeles where I used to live.

3. I tend to shop at discount stores like Ocean State Job Lot for my kitty litter and sundries instead of going to Whole Foods or

Trader Joe's. One Reynolds aluminum roll is the same in both stores, so I hide my pride behind my dark glasses. Job Lot does have its tacky stuff, but I am a good shopper, so I know what is a good deal or not.

4. I truly miss the fact that I don't foresee any European travel in the near future, but I can keep up with what is going on in the various countries that I would want to visit, simply by clicking away on the Web.

5. I would like to hire my own personal computer consultant for my many frustrating situations with my computer, printer, and phone. But instead, I have to depend on the trusty consultants at my local Staples store.

This is my life now . . . not quite invisible in society as yet. The reason: I refuse to conform to what society in the United States expects from a 78-year-old woman in 2017.

Reflections for Readers

1. This author is faced with very difficult circumstances but still maintains a positive outlook—that "somehow" she will manage. What do you take away from reading this story?

2. What kinds of tangible help do you think would be meaningful to someone in this author's position? What kinds of emotional help?

3. The author mentions that age has led her away from desiring certain things that she might have wanted when she was younger. What other things might someone no longer want as she or he gets older? Are there new things that elders want that they didn't think about when they were young?

PART **XIII**

The Meanings of Success

CHAPTER 71

How Does One Achieve a Successful Life?

Susan H. Green, MBA

Administrator, Massachusetts Association of
School Business Officials (retired)
Dedham, MA
Age 83

The meaning of success in life is certainly defined by the belief system of the individual contemplating the question. There is, therefore, no one correct answer for an individual or for members of an affinity group. By reading obituaries in the newspapers, one sees the highlights and sometimes the details of the deceased's life. The reader is then able to make his or her personal assessment of the degree of success achieved during that life. Some lives would obviously be evaluated by almost everyone as making very successful contributions to the world. Conducting research leading to lifesaving advances in medicine, discovering technical advances that improve daily existence, introducing and fighting to implement major changes in law or government, and even amassing significant wealth used for philanthropic causes or fulfilling family goals may be examples of what many consider success.

However, there are many other valid ways to measure success. For example, those individuals who have raised families, or those who have provided for a loved one in need of help, or those able to have overcome and live through their own physical problems, can also be deemed to have successful lives. I will also include those individuals who follow through to implement commitments that they have made to others regarding projects or activities.

My personal definition of success, and what I have made a priority in my own life, is to maintain positive and productive relations with family, friends, colleagues, and even acquaintances. I spend very much time reaching out to others by having long phone conversations, making and sending greeting cards, planning special family trips, arranging shared meals, and facilitating holiday, birthday, and anniversary celebrations. When extra support would be helpful, I try to provide it in whatever way seems appropriate.

A successful life can only be achieved once the individual determines his or her own personal idea of success, whatever that may be. By setting goals, establishing priorities, and taking the necessary actions to make the planned-for outcome a reality, the individual should be able to experience a feeling of success in life.

As I write this, I have become aware that there are things missing in my life that detract from my feeling successful. For example, my priorities do not include, nor does time permit, my taking other than minor actions to improve our country's government, to support Israel or Third World countries, or even to recognize all the residents and staff at NewBridge, where I live. But I have established my priorities, and I will continue to live with (and by) them!

After reading the above, you can see that the subject of successful living is extremely personal. Therefore, I have asked several additional NewBridge residents to join me by also writing for this book. In that way, we will be able to more easily sense the diversity of ideas, feelings, and opinions on the subject of success held by different people.

Reflections for Readers

1. How can thinking about your values help you fulfill your personal vision of a successful life?
2. What steps can one take to move from thinking about values to setting goals to changing behaviors?
3. What is your personal definition of success?
4. Does one need to achieve success outside of one's family in order to really be successful?

CHAPTER 72

Thoughts on Success and Failure

Brenda Keegan, PhD

Deputy Superintendant of Schools, Newton, MA (retired)

Dedham, MA

When I graduated from high school, I was voted the girl "most likely to succeed." I had earned top grades, played three varsity sports, acted in many plays, and captained the cheerleaders. I had also won a scholarship to Wellesley College, and I set off into my future with few doubts about whether I would succeed. However, some 50 years later, when I wrote my report for the reunion book at Wellesley, I questioned whether I had, in fact, succeeded.

Recently, I expressed this concern to a number of friends (especially after I was asked to write this piece), and they were aghast. I had, after all, taught for many years at the high school and college level; earned a PhD in English literature (in my 40s, while working full time and raising children); became assistant dean at SUNY/Empire State College; twice served as English department head at excellent high schools, including Newton North; became principal at Newton South; and retired as deputy superintendent for the Newton Public Schools. After retiring, I returned to teach in the MAT program at Brandeis University and eventually became principal and director of secular studies at a Jewish day school. At 75, I feel I am still able to do valuable work.

So, why do I still question whether I have "succeeded"? Some of this doubt stems from my decision to go to Wellesley College. I actually preferred Cornell (where I was also accepted), but I thought I had a better chance of marrying a Harvard man if I went to Wellesley. This reasoning would seem outlandish to a young woman today (the very people who preferred Bernie to Hillary), but one must remember that

I was making the decision in 1958. The key to success was making a good marriage (preferably soon after graduation). And I achieved that goal in 1962! Moreover, for about 30 years, it was a good marriage, as we raised two wonderful children, enjoyed the benefits of my husband's successful career in banking, and enjoyed spectator sports, theater trips, and gourmet food together.

Another of my goals was to live in a mansion. Although that seems somewhat bizarre to me now, as a middle-class girl in rural Pennsylvania who regularly read the society pages of the *Philadelphia Inquirer*, that dream of living in a great stone house on the Main Line represented concrete success. Eventually, we did buy just such a house—and loved it—though we had to do a lot of restoration work to make it livable. Later, in other cities, we restored other big, old houses, including one with a secret staircase in the library. My youthful fantasies had been realized.

What I had not imagined as I dreamed of success as an educator, a wife, a mother, and a homemaker was what a toll it would take. Like many other optimistic feminists of my era, I learned that "having it all" often meant "doing it all." I was exhausted most evenings and fell asleep every time my husband and I settled in to watch a movie. I preferred bringing home Boston Chicken to roasting a bird of my own à la Julia Child, that icon of my honeymoon years. In middle age, I never found time for the exercise I needed to stay in shape.

In 1998, my husband left me. And, in spite of all my best efforts, he has not come back. My friends tell me it is crazy for me to feel that I haven't been a success because my husband left. They point out the remarkable success of my children, the number of former students who find me on Facebook and testify to the positive effects of my teaching in their lives, the former novices who thank me for making them into excellent teachers, and the continuing success of my work at Brandeis and Torah Academy.

I have had flings with old and new beaux, including a beautiful seven-year romance with a wonderful poet I had dated in college. And I have maintained a pleasant relationship with my husband, where we go to family events and even Red Sox games together regularly. However, I still feel that I have failed.

Reflections for Readers

1. How is it that someone whom others would describe as having lived a successful life could still view himself or herself as not being successful?

2. Are there areas of your life that are so important to you that being unsuccessful in those areas would overshadow all the successes in other areas? If so, does this create a need to become more successful in the (so far) less successful areas, or a need to reevaluate your priorities?

3. This author notes that her feelings of unsuccess are grounded in the era in which she grew up, and that young people today might find some of the goals she aspired to "bizarre." What are the kinds of goals young people today aspire to? How do today's young seek to balance multiple roles in their professional and home lives?

CHAPTER 73

My Thoughts on Success, Developed in Childhood

Barbara Okun, PhD

Professor Emerita, Counseling Psychology, Northeastern University
and Clinical Instructor, Harvard Medical School (retired)
Dedham, MA
Age 80

I believe that the seeds of one's values and concepts develop in childhood and are influenced by immediate and extended family, as well as the community in which one is raised—neighborhood, school, religious institution, etc. Larger sociocultural variables, such as the era into which we were born, play a significant role. So consider that I was born in the 1930s, and raised in the 1940s and early 1950s. I was influenced by my family's experience with the Depression, World War II, and the postwar era.

In my family, the concept of success involved achievement—based on performance and others' approval. I was a good student, got into a "good" college, and was considered successful by my family and peers. My early adulthood focused on career and then graduate school performance, choosing a mate who was a true egalitarian partner in every sense of the word, and producing three children. We shared parenting, activities, interests, and friendships, as well as financial responsibilities. And we each assumed space for individualism. Our parents' values of material and status success faded as we gained experience in a rapidly changing world and broadened our understanding of diversity.

As I continued to develop, my notion of "success" no longer focused on performance and achievement. Success, for me, became based more on internal feelings of gratification with family and extrafamilial intergenerational relationships. As I have aged, my concept of success has focused increasingly on the development and maintenance of relationships. Since my profession focused on teaching and psychotherapy relationships, there was congruence among my different selves.

Another aspect of success for me in my later adulthood concerns taking responsibility for living a healthy lifestyle and maintaining my health to the best of my abilities. Success also involves adapting to changes, accepting limitations, and being open to reflection and new and differing perspectives. My notions may change with time and circumstances, and I wish for patience, tolerance, and self-compassion as I experience increasing losses, physically, mentally, and with relationships.

We develop our own personal concepts that are indeed shaped by the larger world, but our concepts need not be fixed and unchallenged. Changing notions of well-being and what we consider successful living are part of lifelong development.

Reflections for Readers

1. How are one's thoughts about success shaped by childhood experiences? By the values taught in childhood by one's elders? By the larger society? By one's peers?
2. Does "achievement" define "success"? Why or why not?
3. How does approval from others affect one's feelings about having lived a successful life?
4. How might one's assessment of what is successful change as one ages?

CHAPTER 74

Success Means Having a Positive Impact

William A. Gouveia, MS
Director of Pharmacy, Tufts Medical Center (retired)
Dedham, MA
Age 74

Success is a widely used term that can mean many different things to different people. Our society uses the term to indicate someone who has amassed great wealth. But wealth alone is not the only indicator of success. Success is not due to a single factor, but rather to a constellation of people, a supportive family, and business opportunities.

It is achieved by those who have had a positive and lasting impact on society or in their chosen profession. Investment in one's children and family can be the most important contribution to success as members in society.

Teachers, whose salaries are at the lower end of the scale, may be most successful, in having a lifetime full of students whom they have mentored and nurtured over the years. How many successful men and women attribute their success to a teacher who stimulated their interest in a topic they knew little about?

Social media (e.g., Facebook) can assure that an individual receives attention by placement of a posting on the person's website. The use of social media can be a powerful tool for giving attention to a given person's life or career. It is not real success, but the appearance of success that must be viewed through other sources.

In summary, success is determined by individuals who can assess for themselves, based on their own values and experience, whether they are indeed successful.

Reflections for Readers

1. What constellation of factors would you consider as you evaluate what makes a successful life?

2. In your opinion, does having or making a lot of money qualify as having a successful life? Would you differentiate between those who have themselves made a lot of money and those who simply *have* a lot of money, as through inheritance?

3. Do you agree that having a positive impact is an indication of a successful life? Does it matter whether the impact is on society at large or more narrowly focused, on one's profession or family, for example?

Passion, Authenticity, and Dedication: The Formula for Success

Clara Melendres Apodaca
Former First Lady of New Mexico
Albuquerque, NM
Age 82

I am an 82-year-old mother and grandmother . . . but if you scrutinize my résumé, you will see how I have succeeded in my life and how I have tried to set an example for women who are pursuing new careers or making changes in their lives. I have had a long and full career, but in the last 10 years especially, I have demonstrated that a person can open new horizons at any age.

I am a 14th-generation New Mexican, raised by a single mother after my father passed away when I was seven years old. My early years began in a small farming community in the southern part of the state, but by the time I was 10 years of age, we made the move to the city of Las Cruces, New Mexico, where I was raised and educated. My mother was an educator and instilled in my sister and me that we should be strong and independent, traits that have helped me throughout my life in social and professional situations.

From 1956, when I married at the age of 22, and for the next 20 years, my personal life was dedicated to my family and assisting my husband in business and in his political career. My professional aspirations took a back seat. At the time, that was my choice and it was a decision I never regretted.

In 1974, when I was 40, my husband was elected Governor of New Mexico and I became First Lady. Many observers agree that I was a major factor in my husband's political success. It was during my years as First Lady of New Mexico that I started to develop my own voice and knew I wanted to do something in the area of the arts, which my mother had exposed me to early on and which always excited me. I was not the one elected to an office, but I realized the power the First Lady could have on projects and community participation. I always believed—and still do—that you have to love what you are doing and stay with something that makes you happy. And I strongly believe that you must take advantage of all your opportunities and make them a success for you. That is what I have always tried to do.

During the four-year period of the Apodaca administration, New Mexicans began to notice and appreciate some of my talents and my involvement in many community organizations and the arts. I always felt strongly that our cultures and arts should be made available and accessible to all New Mexicans. I also believed that the arts were a strong economic engine for our state that our local citizens were not adequately enjoying. The arts became my primary interest, and four months after the inauguration in 1975, the "Governor's Art Gallery" was opened with a successful exhibition of works by Georgia O'Keeffe, with Miss O'Keeffe as the honored guest. To accomplish this, I designed a multi-element, achievable plan, and for the first time in the history of New Mexico, visitors to the state capitol could browse through a gallery exhibiting the arts and the crafts of regionally and nationally recognized New Mexico artists.

Besides the art gallery, I started "brown bag concerts" in the capitol rotunda, promoting several facets of New Mexico artwork and making the arts available to the people, from jazz to opera, chamber music to bluegrass, ballet to flamenco, and the musical theater.

Starting with some small ideas, I established important programs that will last a lifetime. Others can have such accomplishments too!

In 1984, at the age of 50 and with the responsibility of rearing my children behind me, I made a new start, believing that it is never too late to start a new career.

After working for the City of Santa Fe as a marketing director for a short time, I was asked by the Governor of New Mexico to head the New Mexico Department of Cultural Affairs. The department became a cabinet position under my leadership, in large part because of the energy

I brought; my ability to gain the confidence of all the department's employees, including the security guards, staff, curators, and heads of all the state museums; and my establishing strong working relationships with legislators. It took communication and administrative skills, which are always needed to be successful.

I believe that nothing happens for you if you sit back. In 1988, I moved to Washington, D.C., where I promoted myself vigorously, introducing myself to many people who helped me build a network in the competitive environment of D.C. Through one such contact, I was introduced to a well-known personality in the district: Elliot Richardson, former U.S. Attorney General under the Nixon administration, who was also chairman of the Hitachi Foundation Board. At a small reception, I visited with Richardson and mentioned to him that they had no minorities on the board—and of course I meant "Hispanic." Within a few weeks, he called to see if I would have lunch with him; and about two months later, I was invited to join the foundation board. I immediately responded that I was willing to serve and stayed on the board for 12 years—just one example of how one can get ahead at any age, but you have to make it happen.

I spent 18 years in Washington, D.C., and then was recruited to return to Albuquerque, New Mexico, to become executive director of the National Hispanic Cultural Center Foundation. Even though my roots ran deep in New Mexico, it took me two years to reestablish myself in the community. During my seven-year tenure in this position, I raised $5 million for the foundation to help the National Hispanic Cultural Center, a state agency, for all their projects. It took countless hours of dedication and reconnecting with my former contacts and political associations. In 2013, I retired from this position but have stayed active by taking positions on five boards and becoming very involved in the political arena.

My strongest advice to anyone is to always be yourself and never forget where you came from. Next, it is important to work hard at anything you want to accomplish. I believe that it is critical to have a positive attitude and be surrounded by positive people. If you have friends, relatives, or business associates who are negative and bringing you down, it is important to get them out of your life.

There should always be a sense of adventure in every task or position you take. No matter what you choose to do, do it with passion and determination. And know that if you are not successful at the beginning of a project, the next year will be better.

Reflections for Readers

1. How does setting an example for others contribute to a feeling of success? Would you say the same thing about mentoring others?
2. Is it possible for someone to open new arenas for personal success in later life? Why or why not?
3. How does loving what you do help you be successful?
4. Can one achieve success serendipitously, or must success come from following a plan?
5. This author mentions communication and administrative skills as characteristics that are needed to be successful. What other personal characteristics would you add to that list?

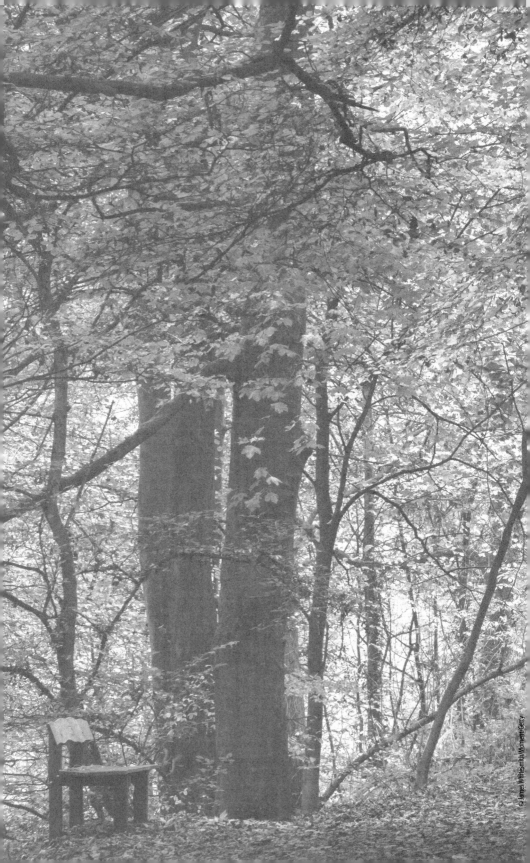

PART **XIV**

Finding Fulfillment in Older Age

CHAPTER 76

Life's Legacy

Stephen Colwell, MBA

Executive Director, NewBridge on the Charles
Dedham, MA

As Walt Whitman wrote in the poem *0 Me! 0 Life!*:

> That you are here—
>
> that life exists and identity,
>
> that the powerful play goes on,
>
> and you may contribute a verse.

Robin Williams quotes this poem in the movie *Dead Poets Society*, and then asks his students, "What will your verse be?"

The question is full of possibilities. It invites you to look into what legacy you wish to bring to the world. If life is indeed a play, we provide a verse regardless of our thinking. The question leads me to ask if one recognizes the *intentionality* of our legacy.

A legacy, by its inherent nature, is about the perceptions of others. Its calculus is stunningly simple: Have you made a difference in another's life? Note that it needn't be a positive influence. Parents can leave a legacy of emotional scars on their children. A teacher can humiliate a child into learning never to speak. A person can diminish others with an acerbic comment. Or in each case, one has the opportunity to be a presence that makes a positive difference. If one takes the time to think about their actions, one can make a meaningful—positive—contribution to another's life.

When I was a child, like many other children, I dreamed of fame. Maybe I would become the greatest second baseman in the history of baseball, or President of the United States, bringing it out of its darkest hours; or maybe I'd be part of a musical group more popular than the Beatles ever were. In my dream, I would be honored, respected, and special. People would seek me out for interviews, hoping to glean some nugget of my brilliance. In short, living a legacy was living large.

The fantasies never contained any family because I never could picture what they would look like or what their personalities would be. The stories would go exactly as I wanted—there was never any stress because I knew how the ending would come, and I was in the comfort of my warm, childhood home.

Life carries on, and I soon discovered I was not the best ballplayer on my team, much less the league, the town, or the state. Musically, I was pretty good, but again, I started to realize that I wouldn't be part of a cool rock band. My political passion was never strong enough to weather the difficulties and rejections that came with this lifestyle. I detested school politics; I would never have the patience to do it on a bigger scale and certainly would never attempt to become president.

Discussions of legacy often refer to big and permanent things in life, as if one must have a bridge, statue, or story dedicated to be a legacy for the world. One must become a governor, a chief executive officer, or an architect of great contributions to the world. Legacy is too often about largeness. The world builds monuments to great legacies. Yet as Shakespeare wrote, "Not marble, nor the gilded monuments of princes, shall outlive this powerful rhyme."

Perhaps my dreams are typical of one's youth, a time when anything (and everything) seems possible. Soon, though, as we grow into an adult life, we recognize some of our personal limitations and find that things don't flow the way we dreamed. The optimism of our youth shifts to the practicalities, and perhaps cynicism, of the realities of life unfolding around us.

Initially, I looked at my legacy as being something big—larger than life, something *historical*. I became sad that I wouldn't be all the things I thought I might become when I was a child. Life became routine. I became a father. My career became more typical than idyllic.

I noticed a shift as I began to realize how my family, friends, and mentors touched me.

As I aged and became wiser from experience, I started to see legacies all around me of a different kind. The soft kindnesses of people making differences—the volunteers in a soup kitchen, a scholarship created, or simply recycling our resources. I think now of my parents who taught me right from wrong, not from their words, but from their daily deeds in the world. As a small example, my mother taught me the value of fairness and honest communication. My father taught me to think of others before I took action. Through what I've learned from them, I am their legacy.

Yet one's legacy is not simply a culmination of a life. Everyone has the opportunity to begin their legacy at any time. This book, this collection of stories, is an example of a man in his mid-90s wishing to give back to the world. We all have the opportunity to look around us and choose to make a difference.

My personal legacy, as well as my parents' and their parents', will live on in my children, and perhaps their children. My legacy will continue with those I have mentored and with bosses for whom I made a difference. My legacy also comes from the frivolous: holding a door open for another, admiring someone for the difference that person made to me, etc. *AND* my legacy comes from all those times I wish I could take back: hitting my brother when we were kids, lying to a girlfriend, or ignoring my children when something other than them was on my mind.

So, we can live our lives in resentment and resignation, or we can choose to make a positive difference. If we choose to pursue a life of contribution, we get a sense of what our true legacy may become.

For some, this may be pursuing a career that matters, or dedicating our lives to children and family. Some may wish to change their community through outreach or politics. Others fulfill their passions through the choice of work. But the key ingredient for all of these is an action that fulfills your life's purpose and makes a difference for others.

We all have a chance to perform in this play. Our part has not been written, and yet *the powerful play goes on, and you may contribute a verse.* What will your verse be?

Reflections for Readers

1. Through the way we live our lives, all of us create legacies that we leave to the people around us. What kind of legacy do you wish to create, and what steps will you take to do so?

2. Some people have legacies that are "writ large," in the public sphere; and all of us have smaller, more personal legacies we leave to family and friends. Can you think of instances where someone's public and personal legacies are very different? How would you evaluate such a life?

3. Are you concerned with what others will think of your legacy? Should you be?

4. How have your own thoughts about creating a legacy changed as you have gotten older? What is most important to you now?

5. This author writes of both positive and negative legacies. Given that all of us have made mistakes and done things we later regret, what would you now like to change in the legacy you have thus far created?

CHAPTER 77

Still Finding Pleasure After 90

Eli Botkin, MS

Principal Engineer, Grumman Aircraft Co. (retired)

Dedham, MA

Age 91

I was lucky to be able to earn my livelihood doing what I enjoyed. My lifelong interests have been math and physics, so "playing around" with equations that mimicked the behavior of physical systems, at a company that produced the manned lunar lander, along with various defense systems such as fighter aircraft and reconnaissance satellites, was, for me, much like playing in a sandbox.

So, here I am, at age 91, still with those interests, but now retired from productive employment. How do I keep that sandbox feeling?

By fortunate chance, a nearby K–8 day school has provided an outlet for that continuing interest. I volunteer to spend time in seventh- and eighth-grade math classes where, along with their class teacher, I answer students' questions, helping them to understand their assigned algebra and geometry problems.

These youngsters, aged 12 through 14, are at a most knowledge-acquisitive stage, eager to understand the mathematical reasoning offered in their math books. I do more than offering problem help; the class teacher frequently grants me class time to present lectures on selected algebra and geometry topics that, as she says, stretch the students' thinking beyond the range of their elementary textbooks.

For example, math curricula at this level do not disclose that the number system that the students take for granted, the system of 10 digits, 0 and 1 through 9, referred to as the *base-10 system,* is actually an arbitrary selection for numerical calculation. What likely led us humans to using 10 numerical digits is the fact that we have 10 fingers!

In a slide presentation, I showed the class that other base systems, using fewer or more numerical digits, are also possible for doing the calculations that they so naturally do in base-10.

The student reactions to gaining this new understanding is very gratifying and keeps me interested in seeking other advanced math topics that I can present to a group of delightfully bright seventh and eighth graders.

The kids show interest and appreciation for my contributions and gain an intellectual understanding that matches my emotional satisfaction in sharing the fun of learning!

Reflections for Readers

1. Having work that one loves can be enormously fulfilling, and mentoring others in that work can be as well. How would you compare the pleasure and fulfillment that come from work with the pleasure and fulfillment of mentoring younger generations?
2. What benefits do seniors accrue by interacting with young people? What benefits do the young people get from the interactions?
3. This author writes that he was lucky in that a nearby school welcomed his contributions. In the absence of such "luck," how might someone interested in continuing to feel pleasure from lifelong interests find ways to do so?

CHAPTER 78

Being Passionate About the Things You Love

Irving I. Silverman
Business Manager, Publication Division,
National Knitwear Association and
Proprietor of the Kosher Food and Jewish Life Expo (retired)
Dedham, MA
Age 97

I became passionate about things I loved long before I knew what the word *passionate* meant. While many other kids collected baseball cards or stamps, I chose to collect other possessions. I became interested in fancy printing type, which appeared in a variety of places: newspaper advertisements, posters, and other printed matter. I literally devoured magazines that included fancy printing typography, which eventually led me to the idea of collecting antique printers' wood type.

At my first job, where I would go to the printing plant that printed the magazine at which I was employed, I had my first experience with collecting wood type. I noticed a workman carrying two trays of wood type out the door of the plant. "Where are you going with that type?" I asked. He responded quickly, "To the dump." Bluntly, I said, "No, you can't do that. I'm taking that type." I further explained the reason: "Because I collect wood type."

This wasn't true, actually, because I had not yet started collecting wood type. It came to my mind on the spur of the moment, and became a passion that lasted for 40 years. I was entranced by the variety of wood-type letters and numerals, all in different sizes and fonts. When I realized I could actually own some of this type, I became passionate about collecting it. This was in the early 1940s, when wood type was becoming extinct in printing usage as a result of advances in technology. Nevertheless, there was still a tremendous amount of wood type available in printing plants, newspaper plants, and other such locations. Fascinated by the endless variety of type styles, with the assistance of my wife, I undertook to find as much of this printing material as possible.

I began an ambitious search for type, pleasing many printing plant owners, who were desirous of getting rid of this "junk." Becoming passionate here led to the accumulation of a gigantic amount of stuff that—for me—became a prized possession.

Other collectibles that I was introduced to were political posters and buttons of election campaigns. When I was a voracious young adult, my brother Harry took me to visit the campaign headquarters of several politicians who were running for office. I began collecting posters from these campaigns, as well as buttons and other political items, especially those that had interesting slogans and typography. These items were abundantly available before present-day political campaigning became more of a television enterprise.

In my 80s, I became aware of the great variety of African masks, in all different sizes, shapes, and constructions. They taught me a lot about different lifestyles and the rich artistry of African tribal artists who captured the lifestyles of their people in these artifacts. My home is adorned with many of these masks.

Over the years of my adulthood, I developed many other passions. I became interested in—and then passionate about—lighthouses when my second wife, Nancy, introduced me to the state of Maine, which has the second-largest number of lighthouses in the United States. What appealed to me was the sheer beauty of these structures, which were designed over centuries of usage to provide safety for mariners. Lighthouses have been erected all over the world in different sizes, shapes, and constructions. But equally important, they became repositories of endless stories and histories, as told by the men and women who inhabited them.

I was captivated by these stories, especially because they included accounts of the many occasions when shipwrecks were prevented by the beacons. My interest in lighthouses only grew when I began conducting interviews with lighthouse keepers and their families; and that, in turn, led me to another passion—conducting oral histories of people whose lives needed to be recorded.

Over a period of 30 years, I was privileged to record the life stories of over 200 people, and gained an amazing insight into their families and life experiences.

Another passionate interest developed when, upon visiting the local zoo, I noticed the giraffes. Giraffes fascinated me not only because of their large size, but because of their unique status in the animal kingdom. In Africa, for instance, where they mostly are found, giraffes are easy prey for lions and other predators because of their inability to defend themselves vocally. Since their necks are so long, it is difficult for them to create vibrations in their vocal cords, and this limits them to making only barely audible sounds; thus, they are voiceless, and largely defenseless. I began a search for giraffe replicas in different sizes, styles, and materials. I have shared my passion for these majestic animals by distributing over 1,000 giraffe replicas to others as keepsakes. Sharing my love of giraffes has itself become a passion.

I have never understood why many people never seem passionate about a special interest or extension of their lives. For me, my passions have been such an enriching factor, and I would hope others could experience their own versions—not necessarily loving wood type, African masks, or giraffes, but finding their own passions and living deeply through them.

Reflections for Readers

1. How might turning an interest into a passion enrich someone's life? Is this something that one can do as a matter of will, or must it just evolve over time?
2. This author writes of his passions for a wide variety of objects. Do you see certain passions as more important, memorable, or worthy than others? Why or why not?
3. How would you compare passions for things to passions for the people who populate your life?
4. How does establishing a collection relate to establishing a sense of order in one's life? To establishing a sense of control?

CHAPTER 79

Making Violins, Learning Patience

James E. Van Lanen, Sr.
Real estate broker (retired) and hotel owner
Two Rivers, WI
Age 84

My life has always been very busy. Selling real estate, constructing buildings, developing and building a hotel with 100 employees. I could not have done this without the help of my wife and four children.

At age 75, I was visiting a priest friend in a building once used as a seminary. Walking through the large building, I noticed a retired priest sitting in his favorite cove outside the main building. I struck up a conversation with him, and we happened to get on the subject of woodworking. He told me that early in his career, he had constructed two violins, and he was still experimenting with a formula for homemade varnish.

I told him that I had started to make a violin at age 55, that I had purchased tools, wood, and hide glue, and that after cutting corner blocks, I had heated up the hide glue to glue the blocks into the mold. Leaving it to set for 24 hours, I had moved the mold, and one of the blocks fell out. I immediately felt that in heating the glue, it was either too hot or too cold, and I did not know who to turn to for accurate information; I ended up placing the violin on a shelf, and it had been there for 20 years.

The retired priest said, "Bring it to me and I will show you how to make a violin." His name was Father Bede, and he was a good Polish boy from Chicago. That conversation started a five-year stint of me traveling one hour to his residence each Wednesday. We met in his kitchen with a fresh cup of coffee, and from 12 until 1, we discussed the progress I was (or was not) making; then we went to his carpenter shop.

We would work from 1 until 2:30, at which time we'd stop for more coffee and more discussion; then we would go back to the shop until 4. Based on this schedule, we never felt that we were overworked, and we always looked forward to the next weekly session. This schedule continued for five years, and together we made eight violins.

Out back, there was an abandoned chicken coop. One bright afternoon, Father Bede invited me to tour his varnish-making lab. The building was about 10 × 15 feet. On the shelves were many small bottles, all labeled and partially filled with varnish. He made this varnish by taking sap (resin) off pine trees and then bringing it up to a boil. After each batch, he would brush some on wood to see how long it took to dry, and if it dried hard or soft. What did the color look like? By the looks of this lab, he had been at this endeavor for many years.

It was then that he told me that the two violins he'd made over 50 years before were still not varnished. Striving for a perfect varnish, he had kept trying to change the formula of boiling temperature, length of time, type of sap (resin), and ways of straining impurities off. Each time he would test the new varnish on different types of wood, but it never quite reached the perfection he was looking for.

His enthusiasm never varied. I offered to purchase a supply of varnish to complete the two violins he had made, but he immediately declined the offer; it was not in him to place cheap varnish on his masterpieces.

After five years, we completed eight violins but had only varnished the first two. His advice was "Always leave a little work for tomorrow," and "If you make a mistake, don't admit it—just say I designed this one a little different."

I cherished the time I spent with Father Bede as he discussed his lifetime of teaching—19 different subjects in high schools, none involving woodworking. He was never a pastor of a church but had helped out weekends at over 500 parishes in several states. His violin collection numbered over 50, many given to him by friends, none of them purchased. Some had found him in strange ways. For example, once he went shopping around 2 a.m. and while riding down a city street the day of garbage pickup, guess what he found: a violin.

A lady once brought him a bass fiddle that her husband had used for many years while playing with a polka band. He had died many years earlier, and now the grandkids wanted to play the instrument. It was in bad shape, and most repairmen would have discouraged her from spending any money on fixing it, but not Father Bede. He never worked by the hour but more by the job, and if he really enjoyed himself, the fee could be almost free. For him, this project, massive as it was, was done from love. The top had to be removed and the bass bar glued in place. After filling a hole in the side of the instrument, he took on the additional task of trying to make all the scratches disappear. Even the case had to be repaired. Finally, it did look good. He charged the lady $100.

Taking these old violins, repairing them back to playable condition, and then passing them on to an up-and-coming student, was his enjoyment in life.

Father Bede was always looking for a valuable Stradivarius instrument. There were more fake labels put in cheap instruments with the word *Stradivarius* than other makers by far. The design might have been similar, but it may be safe to say every genuine Stradivarius has been found and documented. After years of looking and acquiring many copies, Father Bede did find an instrument that had a great tone—and a fake Stradivarius label. He gave me this violin, promising to make his own authentic label for me to place in the violin.

It is amazing how he can do crossword puzzles and other word games daily. Keeping his mind sharp and witty, he can carry a conversation on almost any subject. Now confined to a nursing home, with his woodworking days behind him, he is nearing his 88th birthday. I thank him regularly for taking the time to pass on his techniques of violin making—and so much more.

Reflections for Readers

1. This author writes with fond appreciation of the long, laborious hours that he spent with someone else, perfecting a craft. What would you say was valuable in the interactions between these two men?
2. In your opinion, what did the writer learn?
3. What was fulfilling about the kind of work these two men were engaged in? How might the way they went about it, with a regular schedule, work breaks, and conversation, have contributed to that sense of fulfillment?

CHAPTER 80

Schubert at Harbor View

Geraldine Zetzel, MEd
Poet, teacher, and meditation practice leader
Lexington, MA
Age 89

Praise be to the two young women walking onto the stage,
    for they are lovely and slim as herons in their flowing
    blue skirts.

Praise be to the violinist's Slavic cheekbones and the ice-blue
    eyes of the pianist; they flash fire as she bends to the
    runs of the scherzo.

Praise be to the articulation of the fingers, the opposable
    thumbs, the joints of the wrists;
    their beauty is as the dance of the bees.

The violinist's whole body dances with each stroke of her bow;
    praise be that her body is unable to resist the music.

The pianist's feet caper over the pedals;
    praise be the fifteen bones in the foot.

Give thanks for the brightly lit hall, the comfortable seats,
    for the American flags with their gilt tassels.

Give thanks for the old, who sit in rows to hear the music,
    whose hands and bodies and feet remember, who drink in
    the music, who float in the music
    like seabirds on the swell.

Behold: their walkers and wheelchairs are ready, waiting to
   fly up in a cloud, like a host of swallows at evening.

Behold: the hearing aids and glasses, orthotics, braces, and
   canes—they lift up their heads like young colts let out
   to pasture.

Yea, out of nights in the belly of freezing caves,
   out of being born and dying and a need beyond language
   came the two-note flute carved from the bone of
   a mastodon—came music.

Yea, out of a young man on fire, tramping through the slush
   of Vienna to his cold room; from his pen,
   his ink, his lamp, his scraps of cheap used paper,
   this music.

O give thanks for a soul that could imagine such
   a beautiful noise.

First published in *Traveling Light* by Geraldine Zetzel (2016)

Reflections for Readers

1. This author has created an ode to all she found pleasurable in attending a concert. How do you think her attention to detail augmented her pleasure? How did it aid her communication to readers?
2. What is the connection, as you see it, between the music-makers and the elderly listeners? Is the pleasure inherent in the concert the same or different for the two groups?
3. What is the significance of the fact that the concert attendees were elderly? How do you think that fact affected their appreciation for the music, the musicians, and the concert experience?
4. After reading this poem, might you experience concerts in a fuller way? How would this poem make that happen for you?

CHAPTER 81

Art as an Aid to Senior Living

Natalie M. Wolf

Art Consultant (Volunteer), Hebrew SeniorLife

Roslindale, MA

Age 96

Several years ago, I was asked by Maurice May, then the head of Hebrew SeniorLife (HSL), to create a major art and decorative arts collection for the entire HSL family of eight senior living homes. He was familiar with me through my mother, who served for 40 years on the HSL Board of Trustees, and from my work as a National Master Flower Show judge. In 2009, the task expanded when Len Fishman, who succeeded May, asked me to concentrate on NewBridge, which was being planned as HSL's flagship facility. NewBridge's art collection was to be the first of its kind for a retirement community. In effect, it was the brainchild of both May and Fishman, both of whom believed that art would enrich the lives of residents and visitors; and I was given a budget to create such a collection.

This was a huge project, one that I could not have accomplished alone. I am deeply grateful to my friend Phyllis Robbins, a docent (now retired) at the Museum of Fine Arts in Boston, who was a major part of the process of identifying artists and choosing appropriate work.

Now, as a 96-year-old continuing volunteer, I'm pleased to see that the dream of a beautiful, art-enhanced facility for seniors has come true. As one walks along the corridors of the four continuing care sections of NewBridge, one can observe over 1,000 oil paintings, watercolors, sculptures, and pieces of fabric art.

I have often been asked why I accepted this assignment. I've answered that it was, for me, the fulfillment of my life's mission, to bring joy and pleasure to seniors. I had graduated from the University of Pennsylvania with a major in social work. After graduation, I developed a keen interest in aging and longevity. I realized that I very much liked older people and the idea of helping them in their senior years. Although I had no previous art training, I knew a lot about art from my life experiences. I had often visited art museums and began a personal study of art and its influence on one's well-being. I didn't realize, way back then, how this would prepare me for my future life efforts as a functioning partner in senior living.

I was a Bostonian, and I saw my opportunity to pursue an enriching experience in working to help older people. My mother introduced me to HSL. I envisioned a future of contributing to society in whatever ways opened to me.

Creating the NewBridge art collection became the answer. I could help residents and the family members who came to visit them to live with quality art objects such as they might have enjoyed in their own homes and the museums that they had visited.

NewBridge's art collection consists of original paintings—abstracts, landscapes, and creative designs—and sculptures and other art forms that I have added to over the years. These were purchased from both young and mature artists. There is no religious art, as part of the thinking in designing NewBridge was that it should be welcoming to all, no matter their religious orientation. Although I have personally selected every piece of art, I have involved my children and friends in the project for their enrichment and for ensuring the continuation and growth of the collection.

I have been repeatedly complimented not only for the quality of the art, but for how the pieces are positioned throughout the facility. I was privileged to study the original blueprints with Laurie Butler, the interior designer, before NewBridge was constructed, to determine possible locations for art materials. Residents have told me how beneficial they find it to be surrounded by such beautiful objects. Because all of the art remains in its same location, residents can rely on it to tell them where they are. One resident has told me that she never gets lost because she follows the artwork when she gets off the elevator or travels from one area to another.

An important decision that was made in hanging the art was that there is no identification of the artist adjacent to the work of art, just as there is no identification in one's home of any art piece. There are also no plaques or other information to distract the viewer from appreciating the artwork, and there is no financial information presented. The paintings are not for sale and are displayed as if they appeared in one's home. For those wanting more information about the artists and the specific works, there is an extensive catalog located in the residence library, as well as online at http://art.hebrewseniorlife.com.

I have often been asked why I originally started this NewBridge collection, and why I continue to monitor it. My answer has always been, "Because I enjoy it. It keeps me alive. It's part of my life."

Without a doubt, NewBridge's art collection is a great asset, positively affecting the mental well-being of all who experience it—residents, staff, and visitors alike. Even prospective residents applying for admission express admiration for the uniqueness of the art collection and the vast difference from the nursing home "warehouse" appearance of the past.

It is my firm belief that being involved with art and decorative objects will lengthen the lives of residents as they continue to explore the riches available to them within steps from where they live. By creating and curating the collection, I get to participate in that enrichment of lives.

Reflections for Readers

1. How does being surrounded by art contribute to a sense of well-being? Is this different for seniors than it would be for younger people? If so, why, and what are the differences?
2. How is the experience of looking at art different, in terms of being fulfilling, from the experience of making art?
3. Does looking at art give rise to wishes to create art? If so, how can retirement communities capitalize on that energy and desire, to engage seniors in art classes and workshops?
4. This (96-year-old) author felt a sense of fulfillment from creating an art collection. In what ways might other seniors be engaged to create something new, with a comparable sense of personal fulfillment?

CHAPTER 82

All Aboard!

Martin L. Aronson, Esq.
Trial Lawyer and Managing Partner, White Inker
Aronson PC, Boston, MA (retired)
New York, NY
Age 83

"All aboard!" While I'm talking about getting on board *the game of life*, I'm also talking literally about boarding ship . . . heading out on a glorious ocean cruise. It literally has changed my octogenarian life.

Relaxing on deck, reading, visiting interesting ports, anticipating the next fabulous meal? Although there is nothing wrong with that kind of vacation, that is not what I'm talking about. I'm getting at something much more creative. Let me explain.

In my mid-70s, long after I had retired from my career as a trial lawyer, I was enjoying the fruits of an ongoing education. You are probably familiar with lifelong learning programs offered by many universities. I joined one that's known as the Harvard Institute for Learning in Retirement (HILR). I took (and continue to take) courses that run the gamut: Shakespeare; Poetry; History of Jazz; Jane Austen; Memoir and Fiction Writing; Influence of WWII on the Development of Nationalism in India; Drama; and on and on. No exams, no papers. The only requirement: learning for the sake of learning. Courses are designed and led by our own members; not outside professors talking at us, but rather a system of peer learning.

I wanted to design a course. I struggled to come up with something out of the ordinary. I didn't want to research a traditional topic and present something, for example, on the history of the U.S. Constitution. Nothing wrong with that, but I wanted a more unusual course where I could combine fun with learning. To be successful, it would have to be a subject about which I was knowledgeable and passionate. Hours, days, weeks went by without the right idea surfacing.

"Patience!" I admonished myself. "It will come." Creativity is a mysterious, complex process that percolates and finally yields results, something meaningful. Voilà! It happened and it was so obvious.

"I've got it! I've got the formula," I burst out to my wife, Ellen. "I can put a course together that will combine my experience as a trial lawyer with my passion for classic courtroom movies."

"Go for it," Ellen encouraged.

"It'll be an interesting and entertaining way to teach some law . . . have enriching and meaningful discussions stimulated by exciting and interesting films," I enthusiastically added.

"Do you have any specific movies in mind?" Ellen asked.

"There are so many. *Twelve Angry Men; Witness for the Prosecution; To Kill a Mockingbird; The Verdict,* and a whole host of other silver screen courtroom dramas."

I named my course "*Courtroom Cinema.*" The format is straightforward: we watch a full-length movie for one class session, and the following class, we have a two-hour give-and-take discussion. Everyone is encouraged to exercise his/her thoughts, observations, opinions. Throughout the session, I weave in actual teaching about legal issues raised in the movie.

"So what did you think of Paul Newman's character, Frankie, in last week's film, *The Verdict*?" I asked the group. "I think he was a bum," answered one member. "But he redeemed himself, stopped the booze, and did a great job at the trial," was the retort of another member. "He was unethical," exclaimed another. "Why do you say that?" a group member chimed in. "Well, for one thing, he never told his client about the offer of settlement. What about that, Marty?" The window opened for me to "lecture" for a few minutes about ethics regarding a lawyer's obligations when negotiating a settlement. I think I've made my point.

Discussions are lively, stimulating, enriching, and fun! My peers enjoying this experience are seniors in their 70s, 80s, even 90s! But these are folks who want to be *"on board"* . . . who know that they may have slowed down a bit, but allow their wonderful youthful spirit to remain an integral part of their lives. Each of us needs a little jogging now and then to bring *it* all back . . . that inquisitive side of us filled with curiosity and energy. We just need to allow ourselves to have the courage to tap into that reservoir within our souls and brains, and *it* will come racing back.

Humility aside, the course became an instant hit and has been a staple in the HILR curriculum for many semesters. I get great satisfaction from writing recapitulations and a series of questions pertaining to each film that help guide our discussions. And the excitement that I experience during our give and take sessions brings out the "kid" in me . . . the very spirit I felt years ago when getting into a courtroom and advocating, indeed performing, before a jury.

So what has all of this got to do with cruising the oceans? I'm just about there. One late afternoon, after completing a writers' group session (yup, I'll get to that one, too), I walked into our apartment and saw an exclamation mark in Ellen's eyes.

"Marty, I was reading some of the 'Courtroom Cinema' evaluations written by your study group members. People *love* the course! We've got to do something with it." She paused. I frowned.

"Like take it on the road," Ellen said.

"Oh sure, *the road*," I responded sarcastically.

"Better yet," said Ellen, ignoring my negativity, "let's take it to sea."

I stood with my mouth open. I couldn't conceive of any possibility of expanding this program beyond a classroom on terra firma, particularly at my then-age of 78.

Yes, I confess. At that moment I allowed myself to feel old . . . too old to venture into something new. Ellen would have none of it. Sometimes we do need a little prodding . . . from our inner self or another person.

My wife became my agent. She called one of the elegant cruise lines, spoke with a vice president, described the course, and was told that it just might be of interest. Ellen, my daughters Tracey and Jenny, and I wrote a proposal (sometimes it takes a village). Within days, I had a telephone interview with the person in charge of engaging lecturers and entertainers. What a kick! At 78, there I was being interviewed for a new job! At the conclusion, I heard the words: "Sounds good. Let's give it a try." I'm sure that you can relate to my feeling like a guy in his 20s who had just been handed a dream job.

I'm now 83, and in a few months, Ellen and I will present our "Courtroom Cinema" program aboard a Silversea cruise for the fifth time!

Writing: A few words about this "advanced years" activity. During my prior life, I simply did not have the time to spend exercising a repressed desire: to write. Retirement opened that pathway. At HILR, I took courses in memoir and fiction writing, and then became part of a writers group. After reading one another's monthly offerings, we meet to discuss and critique our work . . . fiction, memoir, poetry. Writing for the sake of writing is another therapeutic, creative, and stimulating outlet. Try writing just a few paragraphs about your own life. You just may like it . . . feel a new awakening.

Each of us in our so-called senior years has much to express and offer.
I urge that we're better off not wallowing in our past, but staying focused on the present and being optimistic about the future. We simply have to give ourselves permission to realize that there's always a new *ship in life* to board. We just need to be open … to release that spirit and creativity within us … to step on board and cruise forward.

Reflections for Readers

1. This author combined his professional background with his creativity to organize an adult learning class that would "combine fun with learning." How might you undertake a comparable venture or encourage or help other seniors to do so?

2. How does participating in a lively learning experience provide a sense of fulfillment? Does it bring back "youthful spirit"?

3. Are we ever too old to venture into something new? Is this a matter of actual age, or of attitude?

4. What are some ways to unleash your creativity? Are there special techniques needed for doing this in older age?

5. This author suggests, "Try writing just a few paragraphs about your own life." Try doing just that, or expressing yourself in any other art form. How does it feel?

CHAPTER 83

Heal Yourself, Heal the World

Stanley P. Rosenzweig, PhD

Clinical Psychologist, Founder of the Massachusetts
School of Professional Psychology
(original name of William James College)
Dedham, MA

If I live a few more years, I will have achieved nine decades of living. I think it is legitimate to ask myself, "What have I learned during this time?" I was fortunate in coming from an intact family, with a father who was a decent earner during a period that was known as "the Great Depression." I was also fortunate in being able to get a respectable education with a number of advanced degrees. I was especially fortunate in being able to enter a profession for which I was appropriately suited and one which I am still able to pursue after 67 years. It is a profession working to understand human behavior and one dedicated to using the knowledge acquired to help individuals and populations function better. This brings me to one of the principles that has stood out in my learning and one that I wish to elucidate in this chapter. I will start with an attempt to give some background as to how I reached this point in my conceptualization, and conclude with some suggestions as to ways that we can constructively proceed.

Over the many years that I have been a practicing psychologist, my thoughts and orientation have changed or been modified many times over. The first orientation that I encountered in my training was the extremely exciting and seductive expositions that were found in the Freudian psychoanalytic view. In my earliest days in the field, that was the dominant view. However, as I advanced in my doctoral studies, I came across several faculty who were products of the Rogerian client-centered philosophy. In fact, I believe that one or two were directly trained by Carl Rogers in Chicago. As presented by his disciples and then reinforced by Rogers's own writings, this philosophy and the related therapeutic approach were very appealing and seemed to fit well with my own personality. I was reinforced in my devotion to this view of therapy when I was complimented by a Rogerian instructor when I presented segments of a few of my sessions.

As I progressed in my training, a new view of therapy was emerging. It was called *cognitive behavioral therapy* and drew heavily from learning theories. As the approach matured, its practitioners acknowledged the importance of some of the principles derived from the existing dynamic therapies. My initial reaction to cognitive behavioral therapy was highly skeptical, but as time went on, I began to incorporate some of their techniques (e.g., ways of extinguishing negative behaviors) into my psychotherapeutic endeavors. Gradually, as I matured as a therapist and widened the scope of patients I treated, I began to think of my psychotherapeutic approach as being integrative (i.e., blending the best of psychoanalytic theory, Rogerian principles, and cognitive behavioral techniques).

Admittedly, however, for a period of time, my therapeutic work was primarily based on the theoretical formulations of Carl Rogers, who was seen as a humanistic psychologist. He believed that therapy should focus on the present more than the past and that progress was made when the therapist provided a close personal relationship featuring warmth, genuineness, and understanding. In his view, clients typically were not functioning well because they were in a state of incongruence (i.e., there was a significant gap between the way they saw themselves and reality). It was necessary for the therapist to be congruent in the session. A significant tool in the treatment was the therapist clarifying and reflecting back the client's feelings. The therapist needed to hold the client in "unconditional positive regard" (i.e., be fully accepting).

While I held to the major principles in what was known as *client-centered therapy*, I shortly began to see that, in most cases, one has to go beyond them to achieve psychic healing. The therapy often needs to go back over significant early experiences to help the client see how feelings from the past, typically unconscious, were still influencing and guiding many of his or her current unproductive or aberrant behaviors. And there were times when destructive behaviors could most effectively be dealt with through a planned program based on cognition.

I continued to utilize this integrative approach for many years, with a reasonable amount of success until about 45 years ago, when I almost accidentally attended a conference featuring approaches primarily related to how the mind affects the body and vice versa. This point of view was typically referred to as a "holistic approach." Some of the leading proponents of this view were Bernie Siegel, Norman Cousins, Herbert Benson, O. Carl and Stephanie Simonton, and Joan Borysenko. I was introduced to guided imagery, meditation, the relaxation response, and mindfulness. My thinking and approaches began to expand. They were next significantly expanded when I began to integrate the principles which were first introduced to the behavioral sciences by Martin Seligman at the end of the 20th century, which fell under the heading of *Positive Psychology*.

Positive Psychology expands the role of the traditional mental health practitioner, going beyond helping individuals with emotional and behavioral problems to function in a healthier and more "normal" way, to include or even emphasize making ordinary people's lives richer and happier. The content of this approach, which includes meaningfulness, love, gratitude, and compassion, helps people flourish and become more fully functioning.

As I integrated these relatively new ideas into my thoughts and approaches, the emphases in my work began to change. I began to meditate on a regular basis 40 years ago, initially most influenced by Herbert Benson, as described in *The Relaxation Response* and further developed when I attended a training workshop directed by Benson and his disciples. Meditation almost immediately led to improvements in my physical and mental functioning.

In recent years, I became sensitized to one of the fundamental principles of Judaism, known as *Tikkun Olam,* generally translated as "Heal the World." What could be a more worthwhile goal than that? I gradually began to integrate that concept into my life and my work. While I was not consciously aware of "Heal the World" as a significant goal, when I think back, I recognize that that principle was always part of my value system. As a young adult, I became interested in organizations and tasks where the goal was to make our society a better place. I specifically became involved in an organization whose goal was to end prejudice. I remember writing two, 1-act plays for that group. I also remember organizing an interfaith group in the greater Boston area.

Once I recognized the value of "Heal the World," I became very impressed with its importance and impact. That is, until one day when I was trying to focus on that life goal when an inner voice from the deepest part of me said, "Yes, heal the world, but first heal yourself."

It all made so much sense to me and helped clarify the work I did and the way I led my life. While I might still call my approach "integrative," it is now richer and more inclusive. I have also now taught meditation in various settings, and I have produced a meditation CD, which many find to be useful. Since I now encourage all of my patients to meditate, I have observed much more rapid progress in their efforts to work through their problems.

I am so pleased that I have chosen a profession where the emphasis and goals are very allied with the concept of "Heal Yourself, Heal the World." As I look back on my life, as a person who is approaching his late 80s, I derive satisfaction from what I have accomplished both personally and professionally. And, while I feel content when I look back to where I have been, I am especially pleased at where I have come.

So, what can I contribute to others who give thought to their living to a ripe old age? My first notion is that what matters is not the number of years you have lived, but how you have helped yourself and helped others. In my lectures to various groups on the subject of "Positive Living," I have stressed various behaviors, which, on the basis of research studies and what I have personally observed, I have ranked in order. Those who know me would not be surprised that I have put meditation first. It is the single most powerful action that one can take that will improve his or her life. Second, I put exercise. It has only been in my later years that I have recognized the importance of regular exercise. It was probably 20 years ago when I first joined a gym, and I have been going regularly ever since then. The literature is now filled with studies as to how exercise improves your functioning, not only physically but mentally.

I will mention only a few other items on my list of behaviors basically within the grasp of most people, behaviors that can enrich your life and conceivably extend it. The next significant goal I stress is to have a supportive network of positive people. Other aspects of Positive Living include having an optimistic yet realistic outlook, maintaining a healthy diet, engaging in activities or endeavors that you find to be meaningful and self-enriching, working to bring out your creative impulses, and being cognitive of things in your life for which you are grateful and appreciative.

Yes, "Heal Yourself, Heal the World." Our society has a long way to go, but I wonder if paying attention to the major concept addressed in this chapter could make the journey more worthwhile and profitable to those involved in this lengthy course.

Reflections for Readers

1. This author has found his work to be a major source of fulfillment. How did his sense of fulfillment change over the course
of his career? Why did his changing emphases expand his sense
of fulfillment?
2. Fulfillment could be defined through this author's statement,
"While I feel content when I look back to where I have been, I
am especially pleased at where I have come." What would it take
for you to come to a similar conclusion about your own life? Is
this the sort of statement that people could make at all ages, or
is it something reserved for one's senior years?
3. Do you feel a sense of fulfillment from your own work similar
to what this author has found from his work? If not, what could
you do or change to make that be the case for you too?

Further Reading

Ben-Shahar, T. (2007). *Happier.* New York, NY: McGraw-Hill.

Benson, H. (1975). *The relaxation response.* New York, NY: William Morrow
and Company.

Benson, H., & Proctor, W. (2010). *Relaxation revolution.* New York, NY: Scribner.

Borysenko, J. (1987). *Minding the body, mending the mind.* Reading, MA:
Addison-Wesley.

Kabat-Zinn, J. (1994). *Wherever you go, there you are.* New York, NY: MJF Books.

Seligman, M. E. P. (2011). *Flourish.* New York, NY: Free Press.

Simonton, O. C., Matthews-Simonton, S., & Creighton, J. L. (1978). *Getting well
again.* New York, NY: Bantam Books.

CHAPTER 84

Why Live a Long Life?

Irving I. Silverman
Business Manager, Publication Division,
National Knitwear Association and
Proprietor of the Kosher Food and Jewish Life Expo (retired)
Dedham, MA
Age 97

I like being alive! At 97, I have already lived a long life—though I look forward to living more. I treasure every moment of my life, even the sad ones, even the mistakes I may have made, even the moments that have been hard to endure. Life is rich—there is still much I would like to accomplish, and that wish to do more, to experience more, forms the root of why I want to live a long(er) life.

I look forward to seeing my family grow. I like the idea of being a great-grandparent, not only for myself but also for honoring my first and second wives who contributed to that family and its ongoing expansion.

I want to reap the benefit of the advances in medical technology for myself, and I want to see other seniors benefit too.

I want to take advantage of my financial accomplishments to benefit the poor, the sick, and the citizens of less-developed countries. I believe that philanthropy is an important part of living a successful life, and I want to continue giving.

I believe in personal change, and that ideas of the past may no longer be relevant in today's changing world. I want to continue in life so I can continue learning and growing. I hope that I can see—and maybe help others toward—a recognition that although there is wisdom in the past, we may sometimes need to move in new directions, that what was said and determined a long time ago may not be relevant for today's living experiences. All of us who are living today can and should benefit from the wisdom and accomplishments of the past and be guided by the past, but should also be willing to embrace the present and optimistically look forward to the future. Living tomorrow can be even better than living today!

I would like to see an improvement in the civility of language in our country and in society. I'm disheartened by the tone of politics today. I would like to live long enough to see this change, to see people dialoguing with others about the issues of the day and coming to compromises that respect multiple perspectives.

I believe in pursuing both education and cultural accomplishment, and would like to foster ways for others to learn (not just the written word but how to improve the world we all live in) and to flourish artistically.

For me, living a long time would mean that I could see some of these thoughts come to fruition and the world become a healthier, happier, and more productive place for the next and succeeding generations.

Throughout my lifetime, I have always been impressed by older people—their accomplishments, their ability to overcome handicaps, and their capacities to pursue purposeful and happy lives. One of the things that I have found personally rewarding has been conducting oral history interviews with older men and women who had achieved successful careers, fulfilling communal service, and enriching family lives. I have learned so much from so many, and I want to go on learning more! My interviews with these fascinating individuals encouraged me to find new avenues of personal involvement, in spheres as diverse as philanthropy, political involvement, the investment of my assets, and the joy of spirituality. For me, conducting oral history interviews replaced pursuits I could not undertake because of my visual handicap; I have spent my years in doing what I *could* do and not being depressed by the difficulties of what I could *not* do.

Living long, and being actively creative, have enabled me to live a fulfilling life, concentrating on what I can accomplish and mentoring other people—adults and children both—to achieve their own successful aging and longevity. Life is worth living; that's my legacy, and my motivation to keep living as long as I possibly can.

Let me focus on the benefits of a *long* life: the chance to continue each day with the joy of accomplishment, acknowledgment, and friendship. Being able to make suitable choices, overcoming the worry of what displeases or hurts me, finding ways to live affirmatively and optimistically, and enjoying all the pleasures of happy, healthy living. Life may not be perfect, but it's so much better than the alternative!

Reflections for Readers

1. How does feeling excited and fulfilled in one's life lead to a desire for greater longevity?
2. What circumstances could make someone more or less interested in living long?
3. It is relatively easy for someone in good health to aspire to live long, but what about the person with significant health challenges?
4. What goals does living long make possible?

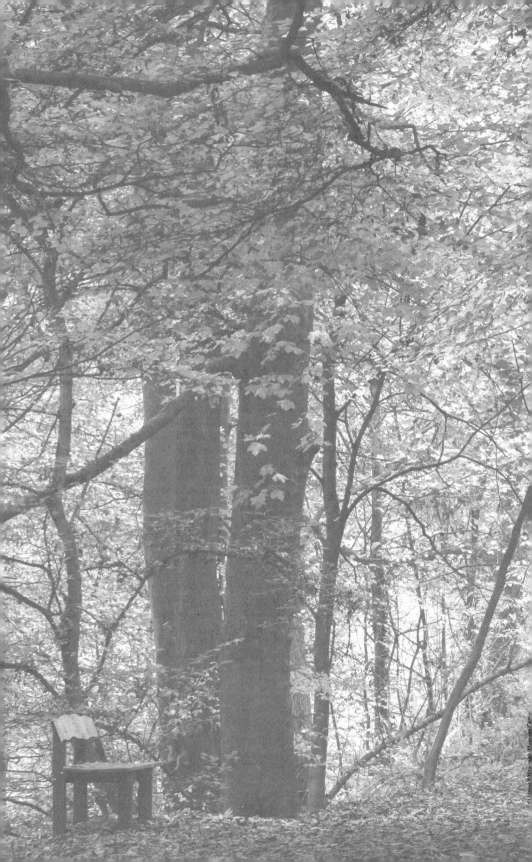

Religion, Prayer, and Spirituality

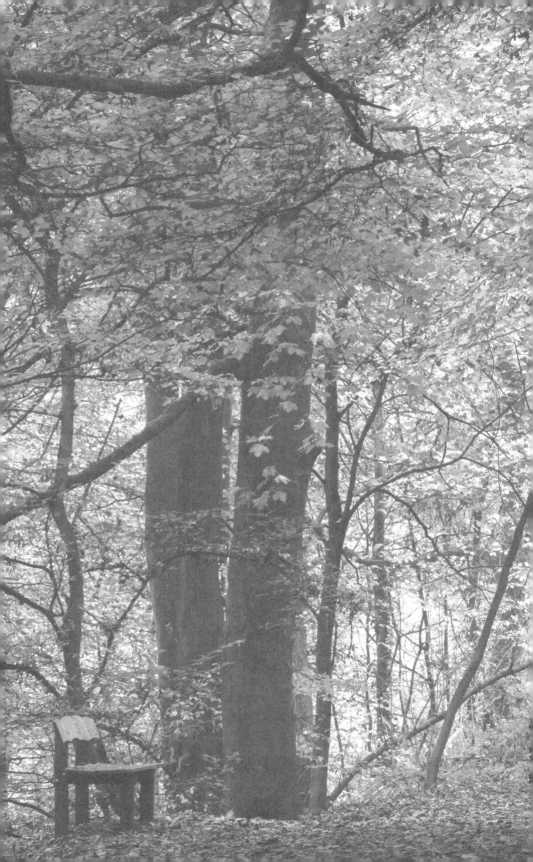

CHAPTER 85

Aging and Spirituality

Ricardo Bianco, PsyD
Assistant Professor, William James College
Newton, MA

Each person experiences transitions from childhood to adolescence, young adulthood, maturity, and finally old age. As we see life flowing like a river, in youth we are torrentlike, we live headlong. In maturity, we face the growing responsibilities of family and society. Next comes a period of deep reflection on the meaning of life—a time of wisdom and completion. Then comes the final summing up as, from the standpoint of old age, we look into the face of death (Ikeda, Simard, & Bourgeault, 2003). This is our inevitable trajectory through life; the beauty and wonders of our physical journey are so intense and captivating, no matter our cultural background, most of us will pose the more existential questions about the meaning of life (and death) only when we approach the last quarter of our material existence: maturity to "old" age.

Science is busy finding ways to cure all ailments, heal all disorders, mitigate all pains, extend life span, and improve quality of life in general to (ideally) all people. Thank God for science for creating the conditions where today we can say that 50 is the new 40, 60 is the new 50, and so on. However, we still continue to age, at different rates depending on one's lifestyle or access to resources; the body will eventually "fail" us and, inexorably, allow each and every one of us to step into the spiritual realm, meet our Maker.

Different cultures, different religious or spiritual beliefs offer us, for the most part, comforting news about what to expect when we make the transition. Yet, as we age, most of us will fear approaching the final days of our physical experience on Earth. At least 50% to 75% of older adults say that they experience fear or anxiety about death (Koenig, 1994). In addition, while in life the passing of a loved one is arguably one of the greatest catalysts to depression for those who survived, we end up living life desperately attempting to hold on to life itself: mourning our dead, our departed loved ones, and, at the same time, fearing joining them.

Spirituality may be understood or perceived as religion, but also as positive psychological or positive character traits. This could include having purpose and meaning in life, being connected with others, or experiencing peace, harmony, and well-being. Even those who deny any connection with spirituality claim that their lives have meaning and purpose, and that they are connected to others, practice forgiveness and gratitude, are altruistic, have times of great peacefulness, and hold high moral values—all traits that are subscribed to by all major religious traditions.

If then, in our common humanity, we experience a higher level of well-being or comfort when living a life embracing the traits listed above—once again, traits that are common to all humans—"religion" then becomes more of a political term because, even though the moral values and ways of (spiritual) life described by most major religious traditions are similar, we end up getting lost in the interpretations of rituals, self-interest, and ways to achieve an ultimate spiritual goal implicit in each particular religion. We spend most of our youth battling the wars of differences to prove the other dogma wrong, wasting precious time to celebrate and preserve life itself, to preserve our own well-being, and to age more graciously.

In fact, we start aging the moment we are born. The anatomical, cognitive, and intellectual developmental stages of human growth give us the illusion, for at least the first three or four decades into our lives, that we are invincible or that we are perhaps eternal. This belief becomes so ingrained, so impressed in our psyches, that the process of aging stays dormant in our subconscious, tricking us to believe there is a promise of eternal physical life. Consequently, we spend too much time abusing the capacities and limitations of our physical bodies, accelerating the process of aging to a degree where it becomes irreversible unduly too soon. In general, we put aside the religious and spiritual teachings of a well-balanced life in detriment of life itself.

The Western world gives too much emphasis to anti-aging attitudes; it is like a paranoid denial of the only phenomenon that is certain in life: aging. And many persons will finally turn to religious practices and spirituality when age becomes a factor, when sick, or when uncertainty, pain and disability, or some sort of loss of control befalls; in other words, at an older age, or typically at the last third of our life span. While it may be too late for some individuals, this consciousness shift or awakening is very beneficial to the process of aging.

Spirituality spreads beyond practices and rituals to encompass an individual's relationship to the transcendent and understanding of life. It is perceived as an acute consciousness that is autonomous of one's efforts and that intensifies awareness of self, others and the world (Lavretsky, 2010). It is in this process of manifesting our spirituality through religious beliefs and/or through a broader range of spiritual practices that we may find solace in the process of aging as conceptualized by Fowler (1991). He called the "Universalizing Faith" the stage where spirituality brings the idea of oneness with the power of being or divinity, willingness to promote justice in the world and fellowship with others, regardless of their faith stage or religious traditions.

This stage is achieved and can only be experienced outside of the limitations of dogmas and, at the same time, the path to achieve this state of consciousness is described and defined in most religious traditions. It is when religious traditions and self-awareness meet in the seat of the soul—whatever spiritual meaning we give to it, our intuition or intrinsic spiritual awareness; a phenomenon that must be innate so it can be applicable to all humans of all races and cultures.

Science is still in its infant stages to be able to grasp the complexities of the human mind, the brain, and other structures that may have the keys to a greater understanding of our aging process and spiritual experiences. However, many research studies have been demonstrating the benefits of and bringing transparency to the positive physical and psychological outcome when religious and spiritual practices are present in the individual's life as we age. For example, in a study by Harold G. Koenig (1998), he examined the prevalence of religious beliefs and practices among medically ill hospitalized older adults (n = 542). He found that over half (53%) of the sample reported attending religious services once per week or more; 59% prayed or studied the religious scriptures daily or more often; over 85% of patients held intrinsic religious attitudes; and over 40% spontaneously reported that their religious faith was the most important factor that enabled them to cope with life circumstances and the aging process.

Other benefits and positive outcomes in physical and mental health are also demonstrated in multiple other research studies. For example, spiritual practices are associated with slower progression of cognitive impairment with aging in older Mexican-Americans (Raji et al., 2007).

Spiritual practices were associated with longevity in a secular region in a 20-year follow-up of 734 Danish adults born in 1914 (La Cour, Avlund, & Schultz-Larsen, 2006). Similarly, nearly 2,000 individuals over the age of 70 who attended synagogue regularly were more likely than non-attendees to be alive 7 years later: 61% more likely to be alive versus 41% more likely to be alive for infrequent attendees (Litwin, 2007). Another study showed that religious and spiritual behaviors are associated with slower progression of Alzheimer's disease (Kaufman, Anaki, Binns, & Freedman, 2007). There are hundreds of other scientific publications demonstrating the beneficial link between spirituality and the aging process.

One of the most critical issues permeating the elderly population is suicide. We know that suicide rates are higher among the elderly population, especially men. Elderly white men over 60 years old have the highest rate (29 per 100,000) overall, and more than 47 per 100,000 among those over the age of 85 (Span, 2013). However, suicide rates are approximately 10 times higher for those individuals who do not attend to any kind of religious or spiritual practices (Martin, 1984).

Interestingly, when involving spirituality and the belief in life after death, as well as life before life, or reincarnation, other cultures that embrace this concept have an entirely different view and approach related to the aging process. Life span is viewed as a result of a "greater" continuum and, from a philosophical standpoint, what we are today is the result of our experiences of the past (including other lifetimes or past lives); therefore, what we are going to be in the future will be the result of what we are today, in the present moment. It is with this understanding, by welcoming the belief of cause and effect that we inflict upon the environment and the self, that individuals in these cultures embrace a more resilient attitude toward the aging process. Consequently, there is a greater acceptance of becoming old and a lesser degree of the anxieties and fears associated with the aging process and death itself. As a result, for example, the suicide rates and mental health issues among the population who subscribe to this spiritual viewpoint are lower than for the general population. Aging is achieved and experienced more gracefully.

In such cultures, religious and spiritual activities or interventions go beyond the benefits of attending religious practices or simply subscribing to a set of spiritual beliefs. From a philosophical and moral standpoint, life span and aging are processes on an eternal continuum. The spiritual becomes more tangible in the sense that the spiritual realm is the ultimate reality, not the physical experience alone. Consequently, there is a substantial difference in the emphasis on healing. Religious interventions are more structured, external, cognitive, ritualistic, and public, whereas spiritual interventions are more cross-cultural, transcendent, and experiential (Richards & Bergin, 1997). The brain and other structures appear to be built in such a way that they have an inherent tendency to search for sacred goals, objects, and healing.

Aging is very often associated with chronic illness and physical disability, as well as the mental and emotional distress connected with the aging process. Without a doubt, those are the most difficult days of our lives, as we gradually lose our independence and our capacity to continue expressing many of our passions in the physical realm. However, we are wired to experience the spiritual. Spirituality can enable the elder to transcend circumstances that cannot be altered, and it may teach truths about life that can be understood only by those who have experienced loss and suffering, yet have survived (Koenig, 1994).

In fact, it does not matter what religious or spiritual affiliation we chose to have, as determined by culture or birthright, or if we end up embracing something else completely different from a religious or spiritual standpoint. Quantum physics and other fields of science are slowly but surely meeting with the science of philosophy and the science of the spirit (and vice versa). We are finding that we are immersed in this everlasting ocean of energy. Spiritual practices do change the brain and other structures, and this may be why we benefit from the religious and spiritual connections as we age. We are all in this ocean.

The truth is independent of each one of us; however, at the same time and by design, the truth is in each and every one of us. I always think of this quote that says "the truth is in the limits of our own understanding"—as we expand our limitations; as we expand our knowledge and understanding of the Self, through spirituality and science; as we age and become more tolerant and wiser; let us touch the intangible and be one with Spirit.

Reflections for Readers

1. What purposes does the tendency toward life review and reflection serve in older age?
2. Does one's spirituality need to be connected with religion?
3. How might our aging connect us with a more universalist view of life?

References

Fowler, J. W. (1991). *Weaving the new creation: Stages of faith and the public church.* Eugene, OR: Wipf and Stock Publishers.

Ikeda, D., Simard, R., & Bourgeault, G. (2003). *On being human: Where ethics, medicine, and spirituality converge.* Santa Monica, CA: Middleway Press.

Kaufman R. J., Anaki, D., Binns, M., & Freedman, M. (2007). Cognitive decline in Alzheimer disease: Impact of spirituality, religiosity, and QOL. *Neurology, 68,* 1509–1514.

Koenig, H. G. (1994). *Aging and God: Spiritual pathways to mental health in midlife and later years.* Binghamton, NY: Haworth Press.

Koenig, H. G. (1998). Religious attitudes and practices of hospitalized medical ill older adults. *International Journal of Geriatric Psychiatry, 13,* 213–224.

La Cour, P., Avlund, K., & Schultz-Larsen, K. (2006). Religion and survival in a secular region. *Social Science & Medicine, 62,* 157–164.

Lavretsky, H. (2010). Spirituality and aging. *Aging Health, 6,* 749–769.

Litwin H. (2007). What really matters in the social network, mortality association? A multivariate examination among older Jewish-Israelis. *European Journal of Ageing, 4*(2), 71–82.

Martin, W. T. (1984). Religiosity and United States suicide rates. *Journal of Clinical Psychology, 40,* 1166–1169.

Raji, M. A., Reyes-Ortiz, C. A., Kuo, Y. F., Kyriakos, S., Markides, K. S., & Ottenbacher, K. J. (2007). Depressive symptoms and cognitive change in older Mexican-Americans. *Journal of Geriatric Psychiatry and Neurology, 20,* 145–152.

Richards, P. S., & Bergin, A. E. (1997). *A spiritual strategy for counseling and psychotherapy.* Washington, DC: American Psychological Association Press.

Span, P. (2013). Suicide rates are high among the elderly. The new old age: Caring and coping. *New York Times.* Retrieved from https://newoldage.blogs.nytimes.com/2013/08/07/high-suicide-rates-among-the-elderly/?_r=0

CHAPTER 86

Religion as a Resource for Comfort in Bereavement

Rachael Falk, MA
Fourth-year Doctoral student, Clinical Psychology
William James College
Newton, MA

It was early on a Monday morning that I received the ominous text message from my supervisor conveying the bad news: one of my patients was declining rapidly. This type of message had become all too familiar to me, as I had lost three other patients in the three weeks prior. I had known that this decline would be inevitable; after all, this patient was referred to me for psychological support services after his admission to the hospice care unit at a VA Medical Center.

I had quickly become very fond of this man, in large part because of his overwhelmingly positive and grateful outlook on his life and his acceptance of his impending death, despite a history of hardships. I would meet with him at his bedside, offering him a chance to review his life and find closure for any unfinished business. During one such visit, I asked him, "What provides you with this incredible strength and optimism?" The patient explained that his strong identity as a Christian provided him with constant support and comfort, even in the face of adverse circumstances.

Although the patient did not regularly attend church, he explained, he often prayed privately, and he felt a sense of spiritual closeness to God. On that Monday after receiving the message, I found the patient lying in his hospital bed, alive but unresponsive. I felt overwhelmed by sadness, yet comforted when I noticed that he lay clutching his favorite rosary beads, which remained wrapped around his hands, giving him hope and strength until his last breath.

One of the fundamental goals for psychotherapists is to improve the quality of life for those we encounter. We consider ourselves a source of healing and find it immensely important to support others while helping them to conduct their lives with dignity and respect. Likewise, these concepts can be examined within the context of religious schools of thought. For example, drawing from my personal religious background, Jewish customs have grown to reflect the value of community support and place high priority on comforting and healing the grieving.

There are many *mitzvot*, or commandments, in Judaism surrounding the rituals before and after death that provide therapeutic benefits to the bereaved. According to Rubin (2015), "The Jewish approach to death and mourning has been held up by some in the mental health field and elsewhere as a particularly sensitive way of assisting the bereaved to assimilate and accommodate to the loss of a highly significant person" (p. 80).

Even if you do not identify as Jewish or are an otherwise religious individual, you may have experienced some of these rituals firsthand. For example, if you have ever brought a customary meal of condolence to a *shiva*[1] house, exchanged memories of the deceased, or acted as a member of the *minyan*[2] so that the mourners could publicly recite the *Mourner's Kaddish* (mourning prayer), you have actively participated in religious rituals designed to bring community support to the bereaved.

This support can be invaluable to mourners, particularly older adults, who are relatively more vulnerable to the negative impacts of bereavement. Unfortunately, it is this same population that is most likely to experience frequent losses, often coupled with limited available social support. Depending on the severity of the loss, mourners may be faced with previously uncharted roles and responsibilities, health and mental health problems, and a sense of loneliness or isolation. It is important to consider the value that may be offered by involvement with—or rediscovery of—one's religious identity, particularly during times of transition.

Judaism offers one perspective by which to view rituals of mourning and their function in bereavement. These rituals serve to help the mourner face the loss, continually restructure and revisit memories of the deceased,

---

[1]*Shiva* is the weeklong mourning period following burial, in the Jewish tradition. During this interval, the mourners stay together in one home, and others bring them food and comfort.
[2]The *minyan* is a group of 10 people who, together, can say certain Jewish prayers that are not supposed to be recited alone.

and encourage social support from the community. However, all cultures have their own framework for treating the dying, the dead, and the bereaved. For example, Muslim families turn a dying individual's head so that it faces the direction of Mecca, and they whisper the call to prayer in his or her ear (Morgan, 2012). Japanese Buddhists emphasize direct, daily connection to the deceased and place memorial tablets on the altar to Buddha in their homes (Klass & Goss, 1999). In some Mediterranean cultures, widowed women often wear black clothing for the rest of their lives (McGoldrick et al., 1991).

In secular Western cultures, by contrast, there seems to be an emphasis on letting go, where the goal of bereavement is often to find closure and transition in social roles, rather than maintain ongoing connections to the deceased (Romanoff & Terenzio, 1998). In contemporary American culture, profound sadness is often perceived negatively. There exists no nationally sanctioned secular model for appropriate bereavement, and there is widespread discomfort with death (Goldberg, 1981).

Traditionally seen in organized religions, the use of ritualized behaviors is often overlooked. Rather than emphasizing letting go, they tend to focus on continued emotional connections between the living and the dead, as well as acceptance of the loss. Religious rituals may help mourners redefine a sense of self and examine how it is continuously shaped and reformed over time in relation to the deceased. Additionally, research has demonstrated that such rituals are beneficial even for those who do not otherwise actively practice their religion (Bosley & Cook, 1993). Rather, religion offers one possible resource for aging individuals that may be overlooked otherwise.

In his later life, my patient did not have any family or close friends. He had little money and few worldly possessions. He endured a lengthy battle with cancer and its accompanying pain and discomfort. On the surface, it may have seemed as though he lacked any resources to help maintain a sense of hope. Instead, this patient experienced a rich internal religious connection that provided him immeasurable strength while confronting great misfortune. As we age and often lose access to our usual support systems, it may be advantageous to touch base with one's faith, particularly during milestone points in life. Religion can provide spiritual comfort and community support from a network of like-minded individuals. Importantly, as with this patient, the benefits derived from faith do not necessitate church or synagogue attendance, but rather require only self-reflection about one's own personal beliefs.

Reflections for Readers

1. How might someone find comfort in religion or spirituality other than by attending religious services?
2. How might religious rituals aid mourners in experiencing their grief?
3. What effect would you think experiencing rituals would have on someone who is not religious? On someone of a different religious faith? Can you think of ways to make rituals more meaningful for such persons?
4. How does support from the community bring solace to mourners?
5. What can others do to support mourners in their grief? Are there special needs that seniors have?
6. Why might seniors be more vulnerable to the negative impacts of bereavement than younger people?
7. When a bereaved person has few natural supports—no family, or few friends—can the support of a community through ritual offer meaningful aid?

References

Bosley, G. M., & Cook, A. S. (1993). Therapeutic aspects of funeral ritual: A thematic analysis. *Journal of Family Psychotherapy, 4*(4), 69–83. doi:10.1300/j085VO4N04_04

Goldberg, H. S. (1981). Funeral and bereavement rituals of Kota Indians and Orthodox Jews. *Omega: Journal of Death and Dying, 12*(2), 117–128. doi:10.2190/BPHW-5NL1-V2PN-EOBR

Klass, D., & Goss, R. (1999). Spiritual bonds to the dead in cross-cultural and historical perspective: Comparative religion and modern grief. *Death Studies, 23,* 547–567.

McGoldrick, M., Hines, P., Garcia-Preto, N., Almeida, R., Rosen, E., & Lee, E. (1991). Mourning in different cultures. In *Living beyond loss: Death in the family* (pp. 176–206). New York, NY: W.W. Norton & Co.

Morgan, J. (2012). The religious point of view: Death in some major religious traditions. In K. Shulamith & F. Gunther (Eds.), *Confronting dying and death* (pp. 175–190). Hauppauge, NY: Nova Science.

Romanoff, B. D., & Terenzio, M. (1998). Rituals and the grieving process. *Death Studies, 22*(8), 697–711. doi:10.1080/074811898201227

Rubin, S. S. (2015). Loss and mourning in the Jewish tradition. *Omega: Journal of Death and Dying, 70*(1), 79–98. doi:10.2190/0M.70.1.h

Care of the Dying, Deceased, and Grieving

Father James Flavin

Director, Oblate Residence, Order of Mary Immaculate
Tewksbury, MA
Age 81

"Be careful, then, and be gentle about death,

For it is hard to die,

It is difficult to go through the door, even when it opens.

For the soul has a long journey after death."

—D. H. Lawrence, "All Souls' Day"

I have a friend whose thesis for a doctorate in ministry was entitled "After the Last Amen." It was an analysis of the variety of ways that friends, community, and the Church help the dying and also help grieving people process the loss, hurt, and bewilderment that comes with the death of a loved one.

The Church makes special effort to minister to the dying, the deceased, and to people's desire and need to care for the deceased by prayer and ritual. The Church's ministry seeks to create an environment for people to pray for the deceased and to support each other.

From the simple and even creative ways in which people care for the dying and for the grieving, there are three special, important Roman Catholic elements: the Sacrament of the Anointing of the Sick; the Vigil for the Deceased, or Wake Service; and the Funeral Mass for the Deceased. These elements are liturgical prayers, in that they are considered acts of official, public ministry, authorized by the Church, and are considered expressions of the community of the Church.

Sacrament of Anointing

In the 1970s, I worked as a hospital chaplain. One afternoon, I was walking in the corridor and a patient, from his bed, waved his hand to get my attention. He told me he wanted to talk with me the following day.

The next day I saw him, and he said, "I don't know if you remember me. One week ago, I was in the emergency room with a heart attack. I remember the doctors and nurses crowded around me working. Over the shoulder of one of the doctors, I saw you reach your arm in and anoint me with oil and say your prayer.

"When you touched me, the pain in my chest stopped and my body relaxed. My heart attack stopped, and I have been fine since then. The doctors have been observing me for a few days, and I am going home later today.

"I waited a week to tell you because I thought if I told you about what happened before a week was up, perhaps the effect of anointing would end, and my heart attack would return. Today a week has passed, so I think I am safe. Thank you for anointing me and praying for me."

It is rare that the Sacrament of Anointing has such a remarkable, visible effect. Most of the time, the anointing of the sick has an interior beneficial effect. The Sacrament of Anointing brings peace and comfort. It gives one the sense that God is touching the person's spirit.

Administering the Sacrament of the Sick is one of the effective, satisfying ministries of the Catholic Church. The priest touches the head of the sick person and anoints the forehead, saying, "Through this holy anointing may the Lord in his love and mercy help you with the grace of the Holy Spirit." The priest then anoints the palms of each hand saying, "May the Lord who frees you from sin save you and raise you up. Amen."

Over centuries, this sacrament of anointing was especially thought of as a ministry to those in the last phases of life. The practice of anointing was described as "the Last Rites of the Church" or "Extreme Unction." With the Vatican Council renewal of the Christian faith, the understanding of the Sacrament of Anointing was refocused and designated as a sacrament for all the seriously sick, for young people as well as for those burdened by the infirmities of old age and final illness.

The Church's understanding is that the Sacrament of Anointing the Sick was established by Jesus Christ himself. Like other sacraments such as Baptism, Confirmation, Eucharist, Matrimony, etc., anointing was established to bring God's grace to the person who is anointed. Passages in the New Testament refer to the practice of anointing. James 5:14, for example says, "Is anyone among you sick? They should call in the elders who will pray for them and anoint them with oil in the name of the Lord. This prayer, made in faith, will heal the sick person." Other Scripture passages, such as Romans 8:17 and Colossians 1:24, indicate that anointing the sick and dying has been a practice of the Church since its beginning.

The Vigil for the Deceased

The Vigil for the Deceased is an ancient practice of the Church. It provides an opportunity for the grieving and the larger community to gather in prayer and support on the day before the ceremony of the Funeral Mass. Different cultures care for the deceased and for grieving people in different ways. In Europe and North America, the Vigil for the Deceased, or Wake Service, is a principal way that the Church prays for the deceased and cares for the grieving community.

The Vigil for the Deceased, or Wake Service, is usually held in a funeral home or church on the evening before the funeral Mass. People assemble, the minister or priest performs the introductory rites and prayer, a Scripture is read, and reflection is given. When family members speak about the deceased, they have a unique ability to express the family's affection and love of the deceased. People then offer prayers and petitions for the deceased and for others. The minister or priest then reads a concluding prayer.

The Funeral Mass

The Funeral Mass takes place on the day of burial. The Mass is the central expression of the Catholic community's prayer for the deceased person. A funeral liturgy/ceremony can be performed without the celebration of the sacrament of the Eucharist—that is, the Mass. But if possible, the funeral ceremony, performed in a church with the celebration of Mass, is preferred. The Mass is the Church's highest form of prayer.

The funeral service, if possible, should be held in a church building. The church building is the place where a person was baptized a Christian. The church is the place where so much of Christian community life is centered. Usually, it is the most fitting place for people to gather to commend the deceased person to God the father, to acknowledge the deceased as one of their own, and to ask God to receive the deceased with the gift of unending life.

When possible, music and song accompany the funeral liturgy. Singing awakens the human spirit to be receptive to the spiritual world and its strength and comfort.

Scripture readings express the community's hope that they will reunite in God's kingdom. They also encourage people to faithfully witness to the Christian life. They speak of God's will that this world's suffering and death will release their hold on those whom God has called His own.

On the day of the funeral liturgy, the family and friends of the deceased person once again gather to pray and to thank God for Jesus Christ's resurrection and victory over death, in which we participate. The family and friends commend the deceased to God's compassion and mercy. The funeral also prays to God for strength for the family and friends at their time of grief.

The funeral Mass begins with an opening ritual, an opening prayer, Scripture readings, and a spoken reflection on the Scripture that is intended to console and strengthen the grieving. After the reflection or homily, people again respond with prayers and petitions for the dead, the bereaved, and for all the deceased.

The funeral Mass continues with celebration of the sacrament of the Eucharist; i.e., the consecration of bread and wine into the body and blood of Jesus Christ, and the sharing of the holy meal with the assembly. The Eucharist is especially a sign of spiritual unity with each other and with the deceased.

More than anything, the Mass commends the deceased to God's care. The Funeral Mass/liturgy ends with prayers of farewell. After the Mass, the procession to the place of burial is also a part of the formal liturgy.

Reflections for Readers

1. How do the various rituals of the Catholic Church help the dying? How do they help the bereaved? How would you compare these rituals to those of other faith traditions?

2. What do end-of-life and death rituals offer to those who want to help and support the dying person and his or her family and other mourners?

3. How might the performance of a religious ritual, such as anointing, ease a person's physical pain? Is this a function of belief or faith? In what other ways can such rituals bring comfort or peace?

CHAPTER 88

Looking at Aging from a Catholic Perspective

Sharon Gouveia, MA, MEd
Principal, Fontbonne Academy, Milton, MA (retired)
Dedham, MA
Age 73

Writing about aging from a Catholic perspective is a challenge for me. Not the Catholic part as much as the aging part and how to weave them both together. The first question I have to ask myself is, how did I get to be 73 so quickly? Where have the years gone, and what have I made of my life? How has my Catholic faith shaped my thoughts, my actions, and my words throughout my life?

Let me give you a brief summary of how I got to be my age. I consider myself blessed in that I came from an intact family, was a good student, went to college, taught school, married, had three children, went back to graduate school, and became an educational administrator in a Catholic school. We have had many opportunities for family gatherings, celebrations, travels, and basically, a good life. Our children married wonderful spouses and gave us 11 grandchildren. What more could I ask for?

Then my husband was diagnosed with Parkinson's disease, and life changed drastically for us. We sold our house and moved into a continuing care facility owned by Hebrew SeniorLife (HSL). I never imagined that I would spend my "golden" years in a residence with a Jewish majority. However, this was a gift, for the facility offers a wide range of services and activities that my husband and I take advantage of. The residents and staff are warm and friendly. I have learned so much about Judaism and have been able to share my faith with others. I have come to realize how much both religions have in common: a belief in the one God and a shared Scripture.

Church and prayer have always been a part of my life, from Sunday Mass and religion classes to a greater involvement in parish life as an adult. Like most people, my response to my faith has matured as I have aged. In childhood, I believed everything that I was taught. "Take it on faith" was the answer when the questions were beyond simple explanations. Traditions were important. Attendance at Sunday Mass was obligatory, as was abstaining from meat on Fridays. In public schools, without specifically seeking out children of other faiths, I had a circle of friends regardless of what religion we professed.

As I look back on those days, I realize how glad I am that Vatican II opened up the Church to a greater participation for laypeople. I do not mean to imply that I believe the Church is perfect. On the contrary, there are many Church positions that I disagree with and am hopeful that the Church will change its stance on them in the future. Yet, those "old" traditions gave me a foundation and helped form my conscience.

My childhood experiences formed a base of belief for my growth in faith and practice as an adult. I can build on these, disregarding those that I deem childish and allowing the true message of Christianity to be a part of my response as an adult. As I age, my life now deals with issues I never dreamed would be part of my future. I know that I have to be the "strong" one as I see the Parkinson's disease continue its devastating progression. Yet, through all of this, I know that I am not alone. In addition to my wonderful family and dear friends, I know that God is with me. When things get tough and more than I can deal with, I place them in God's hands and ask for help. I do not ignore my responsibility, but I move ahead and pray that I am doing what God wants me to do. This does not mean that once a tragedy or illness happens, we should give up. If we are able, we deal with life as it happens, using the resources that are available to us.

In the second half of life, my focus has changed. I no longer believe that I am an invincible young person always eager to take on life's challenges. Rather, I look forward to the future, not knowing what that will be. I realize that I am aging, but I will not let this process keep me from staying as active and healthy as I can. My husband and I participate in all that our bodies and minds allow us to do. Staying active has brought us both enjoyment and fulfillment.

This is true also of my spiritual life, spending time in prayer and learning more about not only my faith but other faiths as well. I know that Jesus teaches us to love God and to love our neighbor as ourselves (also true of Judaism and other world religions). How we do this is up to us. As the older generation, we have the experience, the knowledge, and the resources to set an example for our children and grandchildren and to try to make the world a better place. With the world in such turmoil, it is hard to imagine what one person can do to make it better. One answer is this: Simple acts of generosity and love toward one another can enrich the lives of those around us. At this point in our lives, we tend to take stock of what we have done in our prior years and try to make amends, if possible, for past grievances. We continue to look to the future but with the knowledge that most of our lives have already been lived. As Joan Chittister (2008) writes in her book *The Gift of Years*, "This is the period of spiritual reflection, of spiritual renewal in life. We have to come to grips with the person we have become and to find peace with ourselves."

One of the strengths of my faith for me as I age is a belief in an afterlife. Life on Earth is a journey toward the Kingdom of God. I do not mean that this Kingdom does not exist on this Earth, for we are called to live this message now while we are alive. Our deacon at Church used these words to describe how we are to live now to create that kingdom: "Get up in the morning. Do all the good that you can all day. Go to bed. Get up the next morning. Do all the good that you can. Go to bed. . . ." Sounds simple, but think of what those words challenge us to do. How much good can I do *every* day through my thoughts, my actions, and my words? Being human, I fail often in fulfilling these words, but I know that God is a merciful and forgiving God, who loves me unconditionally.

I have a friend who is dying of cancer. She has chosen to stop treatment and go into a hospice program. She is at peace with her decision. I am not sure what I would do if I were in a similar situation. I would hope that I would find strength and peace, knowing that death is a new birth from this life to the next. As we moved from our mothers' wombs into an unknown experience on Earth, at the end of our days on Earth, we move into a new life with the hope that we will be eternally with our loving God.

Reflections for Readers

1. This author stated that her faith matured with age. Is that generally true? What are other responses to faith as people get older? Do beliefs rigidify? Get abandoned? Get questioned?

2. How does the relationship with faith get renegotiated with advancing age? Does age lead to belief in an afterlife? Does it give new meanings to death and the end of one's days on Earth?

3. How might aging from a Catholic perspective be the same or different from other religious perspectives? From agnostic or atheistic perspectives?

4. How might this author's Catholic faith help her deal with a major life challenge, such as her husband's diagnosis of Parkinson's disease?

5. How might a professional consider someone's spiritual history in designing a treatment plan?

Reference

Chittister, J. (2008). *The gift of years: Getting older gracefully.* New York, NY: Blue Bridge Books.

CHAPTER 89

The Value of Prayer— A Christian Perspective and Beyond

Reverend Elizabeth E. Frigard, UCC
Interim Pastor, First Presbyterian Church
Big Flats, NY
Age 68

My reflection on the value of prayer begins from a Christian perspective, but truly its importance transcends faith tradition. It also transcends age. I might add that when it comes to aging, it is never a *them* and *us* scenario, but a *we* scenario. For any of us fortunate enough to live to a ripe age, we too may find a growing need and even dependence upon prayer.

We may ask, "What exactly is a prayer?" It can be a bit of a mystery. Very simply, it is a request or a petition for help, or an expression of thanks with the understanding or belief that someone, most often a divine entity, is there to listen, to care, and—we hope—to respond. Prayer is about relationship, and maybe most important, it is about creating an inner spiritual life. A healthy relationship with this inner world can lead to a better relationship with the outer world, regardless of our age. I suppose that what I am suggesting is that prayer can lead to peace.

As Christians, we are told, "Ask, and it will be given you; search and you will find; knock, and the door will be opened for you" (Matthew 7:7). The challenge is to believe in the promise that a loving God cares for us and that, indeed, life has meaning and that, in the end, all will be well.

Jesus modeled how we are to pray to a God whom he addressed as "Abba" or "Papa." He prayed short prayers and long prayers. He prayed for others, with others, and he prayed alone. He knew that not all prayers would be answered as we might wish. "Thy will," not "my will," he prayed in the garden of Gethsemane (Luke 22:42). But still he prayed.

In his letter of encouragement to his church in Thessalonica, the Apostle Paul urges the people, "Rejoice always, and pray without ceasing, give thanks in all circumstances, for this is the will of God in Christ Jesus for you" (1Thess. 5: 16–18).

As we age, our understanding of God may change. Instead of knowing God as a transcendent, more elusive entity, God may become more present, more personal, and thus the relationship more intimate. God is always ready and willing to hear our petitions and grant us the courage and the grace to live the best lives we can live at any stage, but as we age, our relationship can grow deeper and richer.

Prayer helps us to develop a deep inner life. It can be the root that keeps us grounded when the world around us is rapidly changing and, even at times, almost unrecognizable to us.

To say that growing old is not easy is most certainly an understatement. It is not only about the aches and pains that can come with age. It is about losses: the loss of some abilities, perhaps mental agility or physical strength; the loss of a sense of self or of a role that gave life purpose, meaning, and a reason for getting up in the morning. It is also about the loss of people, friends and family. Many of us as we advance in years lose spouses, siblings, and even children, not to mention friends. The other day, my mother, who just turned 100, reminded me that every single one of her friends of her generation is gone. At times, it can be difficult to keep one's spirits up under such realities, but prayers to a loving God always there to listen can provide assurance and comfort. God is also there to hear our prayers of gratitude, prayers that direct our attention away from the loss and toward those things for which we are grateful. Perhaps it is an appreciation for the gift of wisdom and perspective that comes with age, or something as simple as the way the sun shines through the window or the fresh scent of newly mown grass.

To have a God we can pray to for strength and courage is a gift of Hope. To have a generous God we can thank as we remember the blessings of our lives is a gift of Joy. To have a loyal God who never leaves our side is a gift of Peace. To have a loving God who promises that in the end all will be well is a gift of Love.

Of course not everyone has faith in a Divine Being or has developed a prayer life. My advice then is to focus on developing a spirituality of gratitude. Asking yourself each morning and each evening, "What in this life and in this world am I are grateful for?" is a good start. Reading poetry may also be helpful in this process. I also suggest spending time in Nature. I find that to be as close to heaven as I can imagine. These practices help us to develop humility, a key component in nurturing a sense of peace. Humility is not about lack of self-esteem, but it is about finding an interconnectedness with the world as we give up the need to protect and defend our ego. Humility gives us a healthy perspective on the world and our place in it. As we give up the illusion that we are in control, we may become less anxious and self-absorbed and less fearful of opening ourselves up to new relationships. Perhaps one of those relationships will be with that spiritual realm which lies deep within us. Who knows—it just may lead to prayer.

Reflections for Readers

1. Does prayer require belief in a divine entity?
2. How might one's relationship to God change with advancing age?
3. How might humility, gratitude, and acceptance support the individual facing the many vicissitudes of aging?
4. This author suggests that "developing a spirituality of gratitude" may be helpful, especially for people who do not have faith in a Divine Being; and she further suggests that reading poetry and spending time in nature may foster such a spirituality. Do you agree or disagree? Are there other practices that could help in developing a spirituality of gratitude?

CHAPTER **90**

Is Prayer Helpful in Your Life?

Gregory Ruffa
President, GRA Advertising
Plainfield, NJ
Age 91

I have wandered over the face of the Earth for more than 91 years. My earliest days of recollection are from about age 5 or 6. I served as an altar boy in St. Ann's Catholic Church. I loved hearing the organ playing and responding to the prayers and short passages. The resonating sounds vibrated to the most inner spirit in my body. What a great life it would be as a priest, saying morning Mass and hearing the penetrating music overwhelming the church.

That was it, I now knew that I would go to a seminary to make the priesthood my life's career. I asked Father Russo if priests married. He looked through me, and in a sharp note, he said NO! I had only one reaction: *I am not going to be a priest*. Why? All the teaching of my mother, who deeply influenced my early life, and had said, "We were put on Earth to have a family, to populate the Earth and live a holy life." I never forgot the words of my mother and the priest.

Through the Depression, times were tough, and with some care and saving, we survived. But my interests began to develop. I wanted to fly or become an artist, I loved to draw. One afternoon, I was making a painting and the radio blared out, President Franklin D. Roosevelt announced that the Japanese attacked Pearl Harbor, in Hawaii; "It was a day of infamy. . . ." Although I was painting, the war dictated my life, and the hand of God was felt. I knew that things would be different in our lives.

As my friends began leaving for their respective military service, I spoke with them and wished them well. First was the army, next were the drafted navy boys, then came the Marines; I bid them farewell too.

Every few days, they left, and I was still at the armory in Somerville, New Jersey, seeing them all off. I was approached by a good-looking Irish priest, Father Robert Graham, who asked me why I was still there. We were enlistees for what was then called the Army Air Corps, I said, and we were to leave the next week. Father Graham and I went to his church and said some prayers. Most I remembered, and I gave the Latin responses. From that day, he always wrote to me and some of his letters had $5 or $10 tucked inside. I was in pilot training and I prayed nightly, a habit that has stayed with me to this day.

The war ended and the world prayed for all those who did not return. But I also found myself praying for all those Japanese innocents who were killed at Hiroshima and Nagasaki. Had the war lasted a few weeks longer my group was on the schedule to go over there to join the fighter squadrons. The war ended with the Bomb. We shipped out to Buckley Field for transition, and later to Lowery Field, both in Denver. At discharge, we were offered increases in rank and pay to sign over for five years. With the smoke rising in Korea, I took the discharge to get on with my life.

Maybe This Is the Place to Stop and Think, What Is It All About?

The men whom I met in service were different by heritage, race, color, and religion. We spoke often about beliefs and how they began. We knew there were writings from the ancients teaching us our human behavior and our laws. Our families helped us take the right path in our beliefs and in our lives. We had agnostics and atheists who believed that God did not exist and there was another method that life was created: Darwin. He taught that our ancestors came from single-cell protozoa and then evolved into man. But I would ask, "Why isn't evolution still happening?" I know no way to believe in the development of humankind and our civilized world except through the early Commandments and teachings of the Church and prophets.

When I was in an astronomy class and the Big Bang theory was presented, with the myriad constellations and galaxies within our knowledge . . . was all that created by evolution as the historians tell us, about how our world began? Or was it spontaneous creation by the hand of God, Adam and Eve, the Ten Commandments, and our religion following Jesus?

The Hebrews had the Torah; the Muslims, the Koran; Orientals believed in Buddha, and so on. All of these in perspective are the same, leading us to a supernatural being that guides us and rewards us with eternal life and love.

I have my way of believing, as all others do. In every life and belief, some form of God is in our lives to believe in. Those who do not share this belief will find their own way out of what their vacuum holds for them.

Back to Reality

Soon I married, and we had Father Graham perform the marriage ceremony. I tried to join a group out of Newark Airport; they were looking for multi-engine pilots, but I was flying only single-engine aircraft. Bomber pilots needed no training; they got the jobs. I decided that I would try a New York art school and study there. As it happened, Father Graham and I would meet every Friday night to discuss the Church, world or local activities, and family while we drank Haig & Haig Pinch Bottle Scotch, only stopping when the bottle was empty. My work in art school was showing the effects of the alcohol; there always was prayer, he was a living God to me. I realized that our Friday pleasantries must end, or it would put an end to my art career. We parted, as friends forever.

I began my career in New York, but the commuting wasted three or more hours; it did give me time to say morning prayers and thanks for my career. Moving to a Newark agency was better for the commute, but the clientele was of a much lower level.

I worked for a printer in Plainfield, New Jersey, as a salesman. Pickings were slim in the late 1940s. I sold enough to hold my job, looking for art and advertising possibilities at the same time, feeling that there always was a divine hand guiding me.

It was winter. I was traveling down a back road that was covered with ice just before a traffic light. The brakes had no effect and I smashed into another car. The woman passenger slid off the seat and decorated her knee with five evenly spaced cuts that showed very little blood. That ended my job with the printer, and I was at liberty again. Now what? I looked for some guidance, but I was very worried. Married, living in an apartment and my wife was a clerk, making next to nothing, but more than I was earning.

I borrowed some money and bought a spiffy, brand new 1951 powder-blue Studebaker with a silver bullet nose that reminded me of my flying days. I solicited the *Fortune* 500 industries with some luck. My prayers were answered, along came PSE&G, the big power company in the state. They gave me all the opportunities that anyone could ask for. In time, we grew to a full-fledged ad agency, with 44 blue-chip accounts. We had a powerful art department, a three-man photo studio, typesetting, and a high-end printing company with a subsidiary mail-order company. I was blessed with a wonderful staff and my close advisor. None of this would have been possible without my constant faith and belief in God.

We don't appreciate fully the power of our prayers and our faith.

Reflections for Readers

1. What are some ways that one's faith or belief system develops over the life course?
2. Looking back, can you identify major decision points in your life that have been guided by your faith? How did faith—or lack of faith—influence your decisions?
3. What do you see as the purpose of prayer?
4. If you pray for something and don't get it, what does that mean? What does it mean if you *do* get what you prayed for? Is the purpose of prayer to get something you want, or is there a different purpose?

CHAPTER 91

Is There an Afterlife?

Stephen Colwell, MBA

Executive Director, NewBridge on the Charles
Dedham, MA

The Big Bang theory suggests that everything that ever existed was compressed into an area the size of a teaspoon. It contends that there was a spectacular moment of great expansion, a big bang, where everything that we know to exist became scattered throughout the universe. It is impossible to comprehend that every galaxy and every molecule once existed in the space of a teaspoon. Hell, it's difficult to conceive that there are as many suns as there are grains of sand on Earth.

This simply illustrates the limitations of our own understandings of the physical galaxy. We could, of course, go into our past. A hundred years ago, we knew nothing of DNA, little of relativity, and seriously doubted evolution. Now try to imagine that 100 years of time as a percentage of the 13 billion years that have elapsed since the Big Bang. As much as we do know, there is far more that we do not.

Answering the question, *Is there an afterlife?* is like Thomas Aquinas asking *How many angels can dance on the head of a pin?* Every view will be based on the backgrounds of those considering the afterlife. Scientists will tell you that there has been no *proof* of an afterlife, and therefore this can only be a wistful debate. Theologians can speak of how every major religion has some form of promise after death—often with the good getting rewarded and the bad being eternally punished. Agnostics and atheists will cynically point out that we were nothing before birth and we shall return to nothingness after death. Simply put, no one *knows* if there is something after we die.

Yet, there is something about the magnitude of the cosmos and the refinement of the basic components of life that is far beyond our abilities to fully understand our current existence. We know *that* we exist, but do not understand *how* we exist.

After we die, I know we continue to live in the memory of those who know us. Just as our parents and the culture around us have created our values, we each have contributed into the fabric of our families and friends. We have offered ourselves to the world and the world has moved ever so imperceptibly by our presence.

As John Donne so aptly noted:

> *No man is an island,*
>
> *Entire of itself.*
>
> *Every man is a piece of the continent,*
>
> *A part of the main.*
>
> *If a clod be washed away by the sea,*
>
> *Europe is the less,*
>
> *As well as if a promontory were.*
>
> *As well as if a manor of thy friend's*
>
> *Or of thine own were:*
>
> *Any man's death diminishes me,*
>
> *Because I am involved in mankind,*
>
> *And therefore never send to know for whom the bell tolls;*
>
> *It tolls for thee.*
>
> —John Donne, "No Man is an Island"

We cannot help but make a difference. Philosophers will ask whether our influence adds to or detracts from the world, but the effect is always evident. After we pass away, we continue to contribute to the memories of everyone we knew.

I have come to believe that the energy that makes us who we are never leaves. Also, I believe in a power that is as strong as what created the Big Bang. Some call this power God, others Allah, Jehovah, Vishnu, and thousands of other names. These have developed separately under different cultures and belief systems. They all share the same concept that man is humbled by the power of what we cannot comprehend and by the size of the universe and the complexity of the tiniest contributors to matter and energy.

In light of that, it seems incomprehensible that we simply fade to black when we die. I believe that our energy, our soul, is everlasting. What happens from there, I would never fathom a guess, but I sense it would be as great an adventure as life has been thus far.

Reflections for Readers

1. In what ways might we continue to live after our deaths?
2. How do we contribute to those we love even after we die?
3. There are mysteries that we as humans cannot resolve, questions that we can't answer. How might we cope with living with such ambiguities?

CHAPTER 92

What Is Heaven Like? Does It Exist? Will We Meet Our Loved Ones?

Stephen Colwell, MBA

Executive Director, NewBridge on the Charles
Dedham, MA

Death Cab for Cutie answers the questions in the title of this chapter in the song "I Will Follow You into the Dark":

> Love of mine
>
> Someday you will die
>
> But I'll be close behind
>
> I'll follow you into the dark.

Ben Gibbard (2005), the lyricist, completes the song with a chorus that simultaneously implies that there is a heaven but our souls' journey may not end there, and the journey needn't be traveled alone. He speaks in a tone of reassurance to an unknown friend who seems to be at the brink of death. He wants his friend to know that they will soon be together again. As hopeful as the song is, Gibbard acknowledges the ultimate leap of faith that everyone must have after our final breath leads us into the dark.

When asked to write this chapter, I was very hesitant to do so. There is no definitive answer to the questions posed. The simple answer is *who knows?* These questions lead more to a test of faith than of science even though nearly every major religion has a form of Heaven (Nirvana, Jannah,

Tian, Bhuva Laka, etc.). In every example, the "paradise" is similar—a place where suffering has come to an end.

To look into the question of heaven, a brief background on the human condition might be helpful. Mankind, despite our intelligence and sophistication, is first and foremost a biological life form. Life, when reduced to its most simple form, is about survival. People are known to suffer great difficulties in order to survive. We are not a species that gives up easily. Disease, loss of loves, and the aches and pains of aging are part of the human condition.

For most of us, the goal of maximizing pleasure and minimizing pain is part of our natural desires. As a species, we grew from hunter-gatherers to farmers; life hardly got any easier. But we did become more stationary. And our values started to be recorded for historians to ponder later. Notably, nearly every civilization created a spiritual view on the human endeavor. They all had a similar message, almost as if each civilization knew that man might start thinking too much of himself; and the message was this:

> We are part of a much larger universe. We cannot understand everything, so we must put our faith in God. He works in mysterious ways, and His will is always right even if we cannot understand it. If you do God's will, you will be rewarded after death.

Simplistically, was this a way to keep everyone in line? Or is there something greater in the human psyche that causes us all to realize there is something more out there? The fact that so many separate cultures created a greater deity (or deities) and a future after death leads me to believe that there might be something to our common thinking.

The image is ubiquitous but hard to envision: pearly gates, clouds to walk on, a paradise where all suffering has been eliminated. All pain is gone and love reigns supreme. For some, Saint Peter will guard the entrance. For others, you must cross a difficult bridge to get there. According to one description: A river, clear as crystal, will flow from the throne of God and of the Lamb down the middle of the city. On each side of the river, there will be a tree of life, yielding 12 kinds of fruit every month. The streets will be pure gold, like transparent glass. The walls of the city will be adorned with every kind of jewel: emerald, onyx, amethyst, topaz, etc. There will be no need for a sun or moon, and no need for a temple or church. The presence of the Lord will be its light.

Heaven sounds a bit like a perfect Earth, but the earthly prizes are not the best parts. Heaven seems to be a higher place of holiness—a paradise, where everyone will feel the warmth of love and eternal happiness.

Alternatively, Hell is a "lower place" where debauchery, pain, suffering, and chaos reign supreme—a concentration of the potential suffering that we might endure on Earth.

A friend of mine reposted the following quote on Facebook:

> "I try to do good in the world, not out of fear for hell or reward of heaven, but because it feels better not to be an asshole."

I wish I knew to whom to attribute this quote, but it seems to hit at the crux of the concept of heaven/hell or, at least, how the concept was first formed. An earthly reward at the expense of another hardly seems worth foregoing a chance for eternal bliss.

I cannot draw any conclusions on heaven for anyone but me. My faith determines the hope I may have for my existence beyond life. And yet, I am filled with doubt—*will I* see my loved ones again? Will we meet in the "blackest of rooms," i.e., after death? And what will that place *really* be like?

Hope and doubt prevail in these questions, and none of us will know for certain until we go.

Reflections for Readers

1. The central aspect of "heaven" or "paradise" in every major religious tradition is the same—that it represents an end to suffering and a place of love and eternal happiness. Is it possible to believe in a heaven without simultaneously positing a "lower place" of eternal punishment?
2. Is "heaven" an answer that we make up to comfort ourselves?
3. What trade-off would you be willing to make between suffering and continuing in life?
4. What value might someone gain by a belief in a divine deity? Does the answer to that question change with different formulations of the nature of that deity? Does the answer change at different stages of life?

Reference

Gibbard, B. (2005). I will follow you into the dark. On Death Cab for Cutie, *Plans*. United States: Atlantic Recording Corporation.

End-of-Life Issues and Care

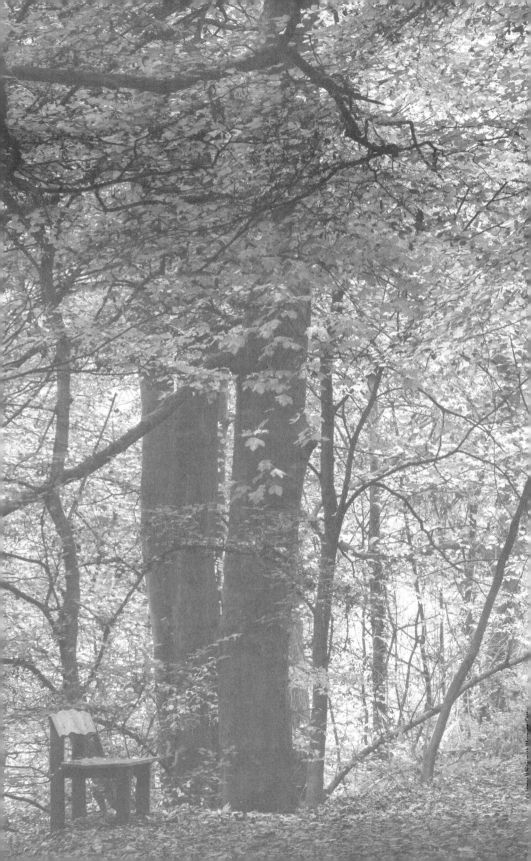

CHAPTER 93

Coping with Terminal Illness

Ellen Beth Siegel, JD, PsyD
Clinical Psychologist
Cambridge, MA

Many of my patients are dealing with chronic or terminal illness; this is more or less a specialty of mine. It is hard but rewarding work, as it takes me into the most intimate possible connection with patients. We talk about their lives in great detail—all that has been rewarding, all that they regret. What I aim for is bringing my patients to a sense of peace as they come to see the meaning in their own individual paths through life.

A few years ago, I had the privilege of working with Nadege,[1] a Muslim woman who had escaped from the war in Sudan with her two children. Her husband—who had abused her—had been killed before her eyes. She came to therapy to work on the good and the bad of her marriage, the complicated feelings surrounding her husband's death, and the struggle to make a new life in America. Shortly after we began working together, however, she began to experience severe pain in her rectum. She was diagnosed with colorectal cancer and told she had less than a year to live.

Many people confronted with such a diagnosis would go straight into denial or anger or some other nonproductive exercise. Nadege did not. She accepted that this would be her fate, but worried about her children. One was 19 and the other was in her early 20s; and according to my patient, they were too young to lose their mother after already having lost their father and their homeland.

Our work moved into how she should talk to her children—adults, but young adults—about her illness and her impending death. She wanted

---

[1] To protect confidentiality, the patient's name and certain identifying details have been changed.

to make sure they were prepared to live independently. She wanted to impress on them the importance of continuing their educations. She also wanted them to understand her wishes as she moved through her final stage of life. In particular, she wanted them to understand why she had signed a Do Not Resuscitate (DNR) order, and she wanted to know that they supported her decision not to prolong her life, which would have involved substantial pain and suffering. Above all, she wanted them to know the depth of her love for each of them.

Nadege's daughters, for their part, found it more difficult to accept their mother's impending death than Nadege did herself. They grasped at whatever they could find to keep her close to them: photographs, voice messages on their phones, articles of her clothing, written notes she had slipped under their pillows. They found it exceedingly difficult to talk to her in any direct way about her imminent death.

Not a religious woman, Nadege did not seek comfort in the Islamic faith in which she had been raised, or in religious ritual. She was too ill to have gone to a mosque in any event, and she was not interested in having an imam visit her. She drew comfort instead from believing that the cells of her body would return nutrients to the Earth that would enable other life to grow. This belief helped her feel that she was part of a larger whole.

Nadege's courage and concern for others in her illness were exemplary. She had moments of deep sadness, as when she pondered the fact that she would not live to see her daughters married or to know her future grandchildren. However, by and large, she kept her focus on the present, thinking mostly about helping her children as she moved through her final days.

She did not want to die. In spite of all she had suffered, she found joy in meeting the nurses taking care of her, talking to her children . . . and exploring her own life.

Nadege was still young when she died, just barely 50 years old. However, her journey to and through a terminal illness is one that seniors will eventually face; all of us will; we just don't know when. Some people, when faced with their own mortality, fall into depression. Some deny the truth of what is happening. Some become enraged. Some fill with self-pity, asking "Why me?" as if they were the only ones to be afflicted with mortality. And, as Elisabeth Kübler-Ross wrote, some try to bargain their way out of death, asking "if only" they could stay alive until some future event takes place. (Many of the "bargainers," if their wishes are fulfilled, rush to wish for something else, in an effort to escape from the overpoweringness of death.)

Nadege didn't bargain. She didn't deny and she didn't get angry. She didn't pity herself, though she was tremendously sad. Maybe because of the difficulties she had already faced in her life, maybe in spite of having had to face those difficulties, she accepted what was happening and used her remaining time to give as much as possible to those she loved, to prepare them for losing her and for living on without her. In that sense, she was a model for all of us.

Reflections for Readers

1. People facing terminal illnesses need to take care of themselves; they often also need to take care of family members, and the needs of family members are not necessarily the same as the needs of the sick person. In your opinion, how should a terminally ill person balance these possibly conflicting needs? How should the family members balance them?

2. While generally prioritizing her children's needs over her own, Nadege wanted something for herself: for her children not just to understand her decision not to prolong her life, but for them to *agree* with it. Why do you think having them agree with her decision was important to her? What did she stand to gain from such agreement?

3. Are there any ways that a terminally ill person can prepare his or her surviving children for the years ahead? What tangible resources might a person turn to?

4. What kinds of conversations would you recommend between a terminally ill patient and his or her family members?

5. Nadege found comfort not in religion per se, but in the belief that the elements of her body would return to nature, to nourish other life. Have you encountered this belief before? How do you think it would provide comfort compared to traditional Western religions?

94

A Meditation on Death and Aging

Jason M. Holland, PhD

Assistant Professor, William James College
Core Faculty, Geropsychology Concentration
Newton, MA

Conscious anxiety about death and dying is a relatively common human experience. From a developmental perspective, though, older adults tend to report less of it than others. Many indicate that they have simply accepted death or have come to terms with it in some way. And that certainly makes a good deal of sense. Much more so than for other age groups, older individuals are likely to have experienced multiple losses. Particularly among those in senior living environments, the death of friends, neighbors, and family members can become a regular affair. Thus, it's certainly reasonable to speculate that seniors may simply get better at managing anxiety about death with the repeated exposure that comes with having lived a full life.

At the level of thoughts and emotions, however, the picture becomes a bit more complex. Here, we find that the threat of repeated losses, whether of the interpersonal or health-related kind, can bring about major adjustments in coping. Remarkably, as friends and confidants across a lifetime begin to disappear, and as one's own health condition and ability to perform daily tasks is compromised, people still often seem to find creative and inspiring ways to accommodate the "new normal" that multiple losses impose. They may appropriately adjust their expectations or goals as a way of developing a healthy acceptance of personal limitations. For many, there may also be a greater propensity to look for the silver lining in stressful life events or even find some paradoxical and bittersweet humor in them. This phenomenon has been termed the *positivity effect*, which refers to older adults' tendency to favor positive over negative stimuli when processing information.

Although the existence of the positivity effect has been confirmed in multiple studies, its origins are still a source of great debate. Is it primarily due to neurological and vascular changes associated with aging? Or is there more of a psychosocial process going on—a kind of learning that takes place, leading one to conclude that life is short and we must look for the good in every moment? As a clinical psychologist, I am naturally biased toward the latter interpretation. Working on an inpatient hospice unit, I witnessed countless individuals who, despite the apparent hopelessness of their situation, dug deep within themselves to somehow make the very most of their final moments on Earth.

Roger was among the men and women that I encountered in hospice.[1] At age 67, he was diagnosed with lymphoma, and his health went steadily downhill from there. However, he still showed strong signs of life, even after learning that he likely had six months or less to live. I would find him outside, gathered with other patients smoking cigarettes, absorbed in conversation. He became a very popular guy on the unit. Though eventually confined to a wheelchair, he remained a significant presence, whether he was joking around in the hallway or rounding up a group for a spontaneous ice cream social.

Still, Roger raised concerns among many of the staff. He seemed to completely ignore his impending death. His remaining family only came to visit sporadically, seemingly because he preferred not to tell them just how dire his situation had become. Even though doctors and nurses explained to him numerous times that his condition was terminal and likely to progress quickly, it wasn't even entirely clear if Roger himself had fully digested that information. In fact, he was once overheard explaining on the phone that he was feeling much better now and was likely to be released from the hospital soon.

It was my job to go in and talk to Roger about this. He must have known it before I even walked through the door. Without breaking his gaze from the television hanging above his hospital bed, Roger cut to the chase. "I'm not going to talk about it," he said to me in a matter-of-fact tone.

My first reaction was to do what many therapists probably would in that moment. Rolling with the resistance, as some might say, I nudged him to go just a few inches further. "That's fair. I'm not going to make you talk about anything you don't want to. What would it be like, though, to

---

[1] To protect the identity of the client, names and some specific details have been altered here.

have an honest conversation with me about it—about what's going on with your health? What do you think might happen?"

He wasn't taking the bait. I had tried those therapist tricks on him before, and he saw it coming from a mile away. He looked me in the eyes and calmly but firmly asserted, "You can stay here and watch football with me in my room if you want, Doc. But if you keep pushing on this, I'm going to have to ask you to get out of here." I hadn't yet earned my PhD and appreciated the vote of confidence. With little other choice, I opted for football.

As I sat down, I realized it wasn't actually a live football game, but instead one of those NFL documentaries showing all of the glorious highlights of Super Bowls past. A scene from Super Bowl XXXIV played on the screen. It was an epic matchup between the Tennessee Titans and St. Louis Rams that was played only 30 days into the new millennium. Befitting of the first Super Bowl of the twenty-first century, the game ended with a miraculous, game-winning play by the Rams defense that has since been labeled "The Tackle." Watching it for the first time in nearly 10 years, I instinctively winced. Surprised by my reaction, Roger leaned over and asked, "Are you a football fan, Doc?"

I was (and remain) a football fan and remembered that Super Bowl very clearly. I grew up in Tennessee and had only recently moved to the West Coast to finish up my schooling. Like most Tennesseans on January 30, 2000, I was at home with my family watching the game. Our eyes were glued to the television set, as the Tennessee Titans quarterback, Steve McNair, took the final snap and completed a pass to Kevin Dyson, only two yards away from the goal line and a Super Bowl win.

As I recounted the story to Roger, I could see his eyes lighting up. Suddenly, I found myself on my feet, acting the scene out in front of his hospital bed as though it were a private stage. Using the curtain as a makeshift goal line, I reenacted Kevin Dyson's valiant but failed effort to reach the end zone and stretched my arms forward, holding an imaginary football that fell just inches short of its target. "It was absolute pandemonium in my house," I explained.

Contorting my face to convey the "weeping and gnashing of teeth" that took over my family that night, we burst into a spontaneous fit of laughter. And for a brief moment, I wasn't a therapist and he wasn't a terminally ill patient. We connected as human beings in a way that seemed to transcend the bleached walls of the hospital room.

Only days later, Roger's condition worsened, and it was determined that he could no longer make medical decisions for himself. His designated guardian was notified that death was imminent. As friends and family gathered around his bedside, there were tearful remembrances of Roger, intermixed with expressions of surprise and confusion about his choice to minimize his condition for so long. If only he knew our thoughts and could feel what we feel now, they seemed to be thinking, surely he would have made a different decision and been more forthcoming. At least that was the assumption at the time.

But that is an assumption of the living and the healthy. Although I imagine myself approaching my own death in a different way, I'm also hyperaware of the fact that a "good death" is highly subjective, not too unlike a "good life." What Roger knew, that no one else seemed to fully appreciate, was that he had made up his mind a long time ago about what he wanted to stand for and value in his life, as well as in his death. He couldn't be burdened with more bad news about his health. He was too busy connecting with other people and bringing out the best of them, just as he did with me that day in his hospital room.

When I catch myself contemplating death and a wave of terror comes upon me, my mind sometimes turns to Roger. Thinking about his friends and family holding hands and singing songs around his bedside, I wonder, "What would I want people to say about me on my deathbed?" Or put another way, "What do I really want to stand for in this world?" The answer is always a moving target. I never quite get there, falling inches short of the goal no matter how far I stretch my arms forward. Still, somewhere deep inside, I find a voice that tells me to keep pushing forward anyway, no matter how much the odds seem to be stacked against me.

Reflections for Readers

1. Why are older adults less anxious about death and dying than younger people?
2. Does death anxiety manifest in a different form for seniors than it does for younger age groups?
3. What strategies might someone use to cope with death anxiety?
4. In your opinion, what accounts for the "positivity effect"? Why?
5. In describing his interaction with a terminally ill patient, this author writes, "We connected as human beings in a way that seemed to transcend the bleached walls of the hospital room." Why was this important, and what healing did it permit?
6. The author describes a patient whose idea of "a good death" was one in which he focused on connecting with other people in the here and now and "couldn't be burdened with more bad news about his health." What would characterize "a good death" for you?

CHAPTER 95

A Time to Speak

Earl A. Grollman, PhD
Rabbi Emeritus, Beth El Temple Center
Belmont, MA
Age 91

Today, there is a surge of those living to 100 and even beyond. To be old today need not be synonymous with being weak, or frail, or helpless. It is estimated by the year 2030, 35% of the population of the western world will be older than 65 years of age.

The question: How to understand their needs?

A Time to Speak

> *To everything there is a season, a time to every purpose under the heaven. A time to be born, a time to die.*
>
> —Ecclesiastes 3:1

There is no doubt as to the inevitability of death—that our season will come. And no one is more aware of this inevitability than those who have reached the so-called golden years. They know that "young people can die, old people must die." Older people often want to discuss their thoughts of dying and death, but too often, we let them know that we are not ready for the conversation. Does any of this sound familiar?

Elderly Parent: "I hope I won't ever have to suffer like Uncle Jack."

Son/Daughter: "What are you talking about? You're in great health." (End of discussion.)

Elderly Parent: "You know I won't be here forever."

Son/Daughter: "You'll outlive all of us." (End of discussion.)

Elderly Parent: "I've been thinking about what I'd like for my funeral ..."

Son/Daughter: "Do we have to talk about this at dinner?" (End of discussion.)

We avoid the topic. Redirect the conversation. End the discussion. We think that by not talking about it, we can postpone his or her death. Our task is to move beyond denial into a realism of the inevitability of our loved one's death. Open conversation is a gift that we can grant elderly parents and ourselves. One woman recently told me that she asked her uncle, who was failing, about his wishes for his funeral. "I was afraid to talk about it. At first, anyway. Would it upset him (me) too much? But I learned so much from our talk. I found out about friends I never knew he had, music that I never knew he loved—I learned about what really matters to him. Since our talk, I feel a lot closer to him."

Act Now

END-OF-LIFE DECISIONS

Of the thousands of people who die each day, two-thirds will invoke end-of-life decisions. Now is the time to seek out information about advance directions from physicians, attorneys, hospitals and hospices. While many have considered the advantages of having such documents, only 15% to 20% are ever completed. But it might not be that simple. Beware: There is a crazy quilt of laws that vary not only from country to country, but from state to state and from province to province.

Whatever the geographical location, the challenges are similar. "How would our loved ones wish to be treated when they are physically or mentally unable to make vital decisions?" "Under what circumstances would they choose life-prolonging methods?" And most importantly, "What trusted individuals would they legally empower as their advocates were they so incapacitated?"

These questions are not only for the elderly. Can we talk?

LAST THOUGHTS AND WISHES

Dylan Thomas, the great Welsh poet famously wrote,

> Do not go gentle into that good night,
>
> Old age should burn and rave at close of day.

Even though this thought about the elderly and death was meant for his aging father, the poet could never bring himself to read the words to him. This poem has been read by countless strangers instead of the one old man for whom it had been written.

In addition to talking about the medical questions related to life-sustaining treatment, many seniors want to share their thoughts about the inevitable moment of their death. How often families tell me, "If only I knew what Dad wanted for his funeral arrangements. Now, it's too late."

Seize the teachable moment when you are now able. The opening may occur when you hear of someone with a protracted battle with an incurable disease or after attending the funeral of a relative or friend.

Dad, have you thought of . . .

- What specific place (i.e., house of worship)? Where would you like the service to be held?
- Alternative(s)?
- The particular funeral home you would choose?
- Preference as to clergy or other celebrants?
- Friends to be notified?
- Participating organizations—fraternal, military, or religious associations?
- Wishes for the body to be viewed? Yes? No?
- Favorite biblical or inspirational passages?
- Flowers desired? Yes? No?
- Hymns, musical selections?
- Pallbearers?
- Final disposition—grave, mausoleum, or crematory?
- Depiction of possible marker—Gravestone? Plaque? Other?
- If cremated, where would ashes be placed?
- Organ donation for medical use?
- List of family, friends, and colleagues to be notified?
- Memorial gifts?
- Other thoughts, wishes, and preferences?

You might try this conversation starter: "I know that you've been to lots of funerals. Describe the ones that really touched you; that you felt were the most meaningful. And, oh yes, the ones that you didn't like; maybe even hated. Tell me about those, too. Have you thought about what you might want?" Words often cascade freely and openly with their choices clearly stated. After the funeral, the highest praise: It's just what Dad wanted.

A Final Thought

The famed psychiatrist Dr. Elisabeth Kübler-Ross was asked in her book *Questions and Answers on Death and Dying,* "How do you, if you do, protect yourself emotionally in your relationship with terminally ill patients?" Her response: "I dare to get emotionally involved with them. This saves me the trouble of using half my energy to cover up my feelings."

Have I made my point? The elderly have feelings that we must recognize. And so do we—the caretakers and professionals who are there for them.

Reflections for Readers

1. For many, it is difficult to start a conversation about end of life issues, and yet such conversations are important as we reach later life, or as we deal with parents and other elders. How might a senior start such a conversation with family or friends? How might a family member or friend start such a conversation?

2. Once family members get past the denial that inhibits end-of-life discussions, what advantages might they gain from such conversations? What advantages might accrue to the senior to whom they are speaking?

3. What are the essential matters that should be included in end-of-life conversations?

96

Leaving Nothing Unfinished in Life and Death

Jason M. Holland, PhD

Assistant Professor, William James College

Core Faculty, Geropsychology Concentration

Newton, MA

On a recent trip to Prague, I had the opportunity to visit a museum devoted to the memorabilia and writing of Franz Kafka—one of the most significant existential thinkers of the twentieth century. Aside from reading a few pages of *Metamorphosis* (one of his most popular works) and watching a few minutes of Jeremy Irons's 1991 portrayal of the man, I really didn't know much about Kafka. But I entered with an open mind and heart to pay homage to this soul who inspired so many.

The museum was truly a tribute to Kafka's worldview, displaying rows of softly lit file drawers, interspersed with open, glass-covered drawers that contained pictures, handwritten notes, and other memorabilia from his life. This arrangement was perhaps a nod to Kafka's "double-life," as he put it, working in an office setting as an insurance attorney by day, and writing mind-bending masterpieces by night.

This frustration between the bureaucratic and mundane existence of Kafka's everyday life, coupled with his passion for free thought and self-expression, haunted him until his death from tuberculosis in 1924 at the age of 40. In his last letter, however, he seemed to gain some insight into this tension, which most often played out in long-standing conflicts with his father and the traditional values that he represented. As he began to soften toward his father, Kafka had a vision of a wall. But it was no longer seen as an impediment. He wrote, "It is not a shady wall; it is life, dear, sweet life pressed into wall form." Kafka could then see a city in the distance but had the sense that somehow he had arrived too early.

As a clinician and a human being, I've found that one of the most common concerns people express, both at younger and older life stages, is that they will in some way fail to fulfill their true destiny, neglect their most authentic passions, or fall short of their full potential in life. Like Kafka, they fear that they'll arrive too early at the city in the distance and leave something in their life unfinished, unsaid, or unresolved.

Dignity Therapy, developed by Dr. Harvey Chochinov (2012), is one way of eliciting conversations with people about the meaning they've made in their life, the lessons they've learned, and their deepest concerns for the future. In other words, it's a form of therapy that gets people to talk about the aspects of their lives that are most important. These conversations can cover a range of topics, but particularly at the end of life, they often center on those things that feel most unfinished, unsaid, or unresolved.

The ultimate aim of the therapy is to give people the space to have honest dialogues about what matters most to them and to record the lessons learned from a life for future generations. Since these topics are often emotionally charged and difficult to discuss, having some organization and structure, as in Dignity Therapy, is useful. Though initially developed for dying patients with a foreshortened future, the prompts and questions used in Dignity Therapy could be tremendously valuable for any person regardless of how long (or short) his or her future is perceived to be.

Typically, a skilled interviewer will walk patients and their family through the Dignity Therapy protocol. And it's worth noting here that it's only in this structured and manualized form that Dignity Therapy has been shown to improve mental health outcomes. Nevertheless, readers may still wish to consider the questions that are raised in Dignity Therapy, by themselves or with close confidants, simply for their own personal edification.

Paraphrasing and expanding upon the Dignity Therapy protocol, these questions include:

1. What do you most want to say to the people that you love in your life? What are your hopes and dreams for them? Pretend that this is the only moment that you have to say it to them. Tomorrow, or even in 10 minutes, it may be too late.
2. Now consider this: What might you have to lose or to gain by reaching out to the people you are thinking of and telling them how you feel? How might you phrase it to them in a way that minimizes any perceived risks and maximizes possibilities for connection and understanding?

3. When you think back across your entire life, what do you believe are the most important lessons that you've learned? Based on those lessons, what words of wisdom or advice do you have for the people in your life and for future generations? Some of these may be hard lessons, and careful phrasing of the message is crucial, especially if you plan to deliver it to an audience of more than one.

4. Taking stock of your life so far, what accomplishments are you most proud of? If you had to write your own eulogy today, what would you most want people to know about you? What have you stood for in your life? What stories and personal experiences best illustrate the values that you have embodied during your time on planet Earth?

The answers to such questions are, of course, highly subjective and personal. However, I believe that the goal is the same for all travelers. We must not leave anything on the table. Or else, like Kafka, we may arrive at our city in the distance before our time.

Reflections for Readers

1. Considering the themes that were raised in this essay, what do you most want to say to the people that you care about?

2. When you think about the values that matter most to you, how do your priorities in life shift or not shift? Viewed through this lens, are there aspects of your life that seem more or less important now than they did in the past?

3. How might you best convey the lessons you've learned in life to others? Is there a way to spread those messages with nothing but loving kindness, absent of all judgment or condemnation?

4. A major challenge as we near the end of life is to integrate and accept the life lived with the life intended. What can we bring to this developmental task to assist in negotiating it?

5. What are some important questions that can help guide this process?

6. What are some clinical mental health "tools" that can be helpful?

Reference

Chochinov, H. M. (2012). *Dignity therapy: Final words for final days*. New York: Oxford University Press.

CHAPTER 97

Making End-of-Life Decisions

Scott Mankowitz, MD

Emergency Department, East Orange General Hospital
East Orange, NJ

All life ends in death.

For most Americans, death happens within a healthcare facility. Approximately 44% of us will die in an acute care hospital, and 22% in a nursing home (Centers for Disease Control, 2016). What is fascinating is that when people are asked the question of where they would like to die, the overwhelming majority would prefer to die at home, surrounded by loved ones (Committee on Approaching Death: Addressing Key End of Life Issues & Institute of Medicine, 2015). Very few people would opt for a protracted hospital course or a long-term care facility with a ventilator and tube feedings. As a society, we treasure our autonomy and self-determination. What, then, created this discrepancy?

When patients are critically ill, their ability to make decisions is limited. In most cases, patients in the intensive care unit are unable to advocate for themselves, and medical decisions are made by family members, despite mounting evidence that families may not be aware of or agree with the patient's wishes.

Furthermore, all external incentives favor increasing the intensity of services provided. Physicians and hospitals are able to increase their reimbursement by providing diagnostic and therapeutic interventions. Family members often have unrealistic expectations about recovery, and even when they don't, they are incapacitated by the guilt surrounding allowing a loved one to die. They often prefer to "err on the side of caution" and "do everything" to prolong the dying process, rather than stand by and allow nature to take its course.

In my own experience, I am often faced with patients in the emergency department whose prospects of long-term survival are significantly limited. When I approach the family to discuss the possibility of withholding care, I try to convey that I am asking what the patient would have wanted had the patient had the opportunity to talk to me. I am specifically not asking what the family members would want. Usually, I ask a question like, "Do you think she would have wanted us to put her on a ventilator?" Very often, I encounter families who have not had a chance to process the full extent of the patient's illness. No matter how I phrase the question, I suspect the question they hear sounds more like "Would you like me to kill your grandmother?"

Restoring Patient Autonomy

So, what can be done to restore patient autonomy? How can people exert their will even if they are unable to verbalize it? A living will, also known as an *advance directive,* is a legal document prepared by an individual prior to becoming ill. In most cases, such documents include specific instructions regarding cardiopulmonary resuscitation (CPR), mechanical ventilation (e.g. ventilators), and artificial nutrition (e.g., feeding tubes). Most of them also grant a specific individual a power of attorney to make medical decisions for the patient in case the patient is unable to do so himself or herself. Implicit in this declaration is the assumption that the patient and the designee have discussed what kinds of treatments the patient would want in various circumstances.

Doctors have created specific terminology for people who do not want aggressive resuscitation. In 2005, the American Heart Association dropped the venerable *DNR* (i.e., Do Not Resuscitate) and adopted the more descriptive term *DNAR* (Do Not Attempt Resuscitation). It was believed that saying "DNAR" reduces the expectation that complete recovery is probable, and thereby facilitates more rational discussion. The newest term, *AND* (Allow Natural Death) perhaps makes the meaning even more clear (Breault, 2011).

Despite widespread education, only 26% of Americans have advance directives (Rao, Anderson, Lin, & Lauz, 2014). Moreover, even in those cases where the patient does have an advance directive, the patient's documents may not be available at the time of treatment, and all the previously described incentives take over. Many hospitals, for example, require a physician to specifically order that a patient be placed in DNAR status. Without this order, hospital policy mandates all resuscitative attempts, even in patients who have expressed otherwise.

This ethical conundrum led to the development of the Physician Order for Life-Sustaining Treatment (POLST) form. Essentially, this form is used in patients with significant illness, in cases where the patient and physician feel that aggressive resuscitation is unwarranted and probably futile. Unlike a living will, this document has the same force as a physician order and can be used in any setting, including a nursing home, hospital, or even an ambulance. On this form, patients can specify what sorts of life-sustaining treatments they want, such as comfort measures, DNAR, airway manipulations, full treatment, or other specifics. Most states have developed laws supporting POLST.

Symptom Control

The foregoing discussion has largely focused on what *not* to do. How to avoid the hospital. How to prevent CPR. The most important part of maintaining the dignity of a dying patient is expanding the services that *can* be provided to them. For this, we turn to hospice.

Hospice care is generally defined as shifting the priority in patient management from disease control to symptom control. Practically, it means that treating the pain and stress of serious illness is far more important than investigating a definitive cure. In the United States, Medicare beneficiaries are eligible for hospice when their physician believes that they have less than six months to live. Commercial insurers can extend this period even longer. Hospice care can be instituted in a hospital, a nursing home, a dedicated hospice institution, or at home.

In hospice-at-home programs, family members are incorporated into the care team. Every effort is made to keep the patient in a familiar, comfortable environment. When patients have pain or anxiety, family members can be trained to administer potent medications such as Valium or morphine to help ease the suffering. An on-call nurse or physician is available to help guide the family when they need advice or reassurance. Perhaps most important, the on-call provider can dissuade the family from calling an ambulance against the patient's wishes.

Have These Interventions Made a Difference?

Some of these evolutionary changes have begun to take hold. During the past decade, many deaths have shifted from acute care hospitals into nursing homes and other institutional settings, such as hospice (Teno et al., 2013). The goal for the next decade is to ensure that every death is met with the dignity that it deserves, in accordance with the patient's wishes.

Practical Advice

If you do not have an advance directive (even if you are completely healthy), it's probably a good idea to think about things that you would like to have done to you if you were in a position where you couldn't make your needs known. If your heart stops beating, would you want paramedics to perform chest compressions? Would you want a plastic tube inserted in your windpipe to breathe for you? How do you feel about artificial nutrition?

Preparing an advance directive is fairly straightforward, and a lawyer is not strictly necessary. There are many free or inexpensive options online. Be cautious when you pick a person to have power of attorney over you. In many states, the power of attorney holds more authority than your own expressed desires. For example, suppose that you have designated your brother as power of attorney, and you have specified in your living will that you do not want dialysis. If you are brought to the hospital unconscious, your brother can request dialysis on your behalf, regardless of the contents of your will.

Similarly, it doesn't make sense to keep your living will in a safety deposit box or in your lawyer's office. You should give a copy to your doctor and your family so that it will be available when needed.

If you are already ill, you should ask your doctor to fill out a POLST form for you; a sample POLST form appears as **Figure 97-1**. If you would feel more comfortable dying in your own home and have family support, consider hospice.

Reflections for Readers

1. Why might family members want doctors to "do everything" to prolong the life of a loved one? What if the person who is dying has different wishes? What if the dying person has never told anyone what he or she would want in terms of end-of-life care?

2. What would you suggest as ways to help families discuss end-of-life care?
3. Why do so few people have advance directives spelling out their wishes regarding end-of-life care? What can professionals and others do to increase this number?

HIPAA PERMITS DISCLOSURE OF POLST TO OTHER HEALTH CARE PROVIDERS AS NECESSARY

Physician Orders for Life-Sustaining Treatment

Last Name - First Name - Middle Initial	**FIRST** follow these orders, **THEN** contact physician, nurse practitioner or PA-C. The POLST form is always voluntary. The POLST is a set of medical orders intended to guide medical treatment based on a person's current medical condition and goals. Any section not completed implies full treatment for that section. Everyone shall be treated with dignity and respect.
Date of Birth Last 4 #SSN Gender M F	

Medical Conditions/Patient Goals:	Agency Info/Sticker

A
Check One

CARDIOPULMONARY RESUSCITATION (CPR): Person has no pulse and is not breathing.
☐ CPR/Attempt Resuscitation   ☐ DNAR/Do Not Attempt Resuscitation (Allow Natural Death)
Choosing DNAR will include appropriate comfort measures and may still include the range of treatments below. When not in cardiopulmonary arrest, go to part B.

B
Check One

MEDICAL INTERVENTIONS: Person has pulse and/or is breathing.

☐ **COMFORT MEASURES ONLY** Use medication by any route, positioning, wound care and other measures to relieve pain and suffering. Use oxygen, oral suction and manual treatment of airway obstruction as needed for comfort.   **Patient prefers no hospital transfer:** *EMS contact medical control to determine if transport indicated to provide adequate comfort.*

☐ **LIMITED ADDITIONAL INTERVENTIONS** Includes care described above. Use medical treatment, IV fluids and cardiac monitor as indicated. Do not use intubation or mechanical ventilation. May use less invasive airway support (e.g. CPAP, BiPAP).   **Transfer** *to hospital if indicated. Avoid intensive care if possible.*

☐ **FULL TREATMENT** Includes care described above. Use intubation, advanced airway interventions, mechanical ventilation, and cardioversion as indicated.   **Transfer** *to hospital if indicated. Includes intensive care.*

Additional Orders: (e.g. dialysis, etc.) _____

C
SIGNATURES: The signatures below verify that these orders are consistent with the patient's medical condition, known preferences and best known information. If signed by a surrogate, the patient must be decisionally incapacitated and the person signing is the legal surrogate.

Discussed with: ☐ Patient ☐ Parent of Minor ☐ Guardian with Health Care Authority ☐ Spouse/Other as authorized by RCW 7.70.065 ☐ Health Care Agent (DPOAHC)	PRINT — Physician/ARNP/PA-C Name	Phone Number
	✘ Physician/ARNP/PA-C Signature *(mandatory)*	Date *(mandatory)*
PRINT — Patient or Legal Surrogate Name		Phone Number
✘ Patient or Legal Surrogate Signature *(mandatory)*		Date *(mandatory)*

Person has: ☐ Health Care Directive (living will) ☐ Durable Power of Attorney for Health Care	**Encourage all advance care planning documents to accompany POLST**

SEND ORIGINAL FORM WITH PERSON WHENEVER TRANSFERRED OR DISCHARGED

Revised 4/2014   Photocopies and faxes of signed POLST forms are legal and valid. May make copies for records.
For more information on POLST visit www.wsma.org/polst.

Washington **WSMA**
State **Medical**
Association
Physician Driven
Patient Focused

Washington State Department of
Health

See back of form for non-emergency preferences ▶

FIGURE 97-1   POLST form

Courtesy of Washington State Medical Association.

HIPAA PERMITS DISCLOSURE OF POLST TO OTHER HEALTH CARE PROVIDERS AS NECESSARY

Other Contact Information (Optional)

Name of Guardian, Surrogate or other Contact Person	Relationship	Phone Number	
Name of Health Care Professional Preparing Form	Preparer Title	Phone Number	Date Prepared

D NON-EMERGENCY MEDICAL TREATMENT PREFERENCES

ANTIBIOTICS:

☐ No antibiotics. Use other measures to relieve symptoms. ☐ Use antibiotics if life can be prolonged.
☐ Determine use or limitation of antibiotics when infection occurs, with comfort as goal.

MEDICALLY ASSISTED NUTRITION:
Always offer food and liquids by mouth if feasible.

☐ No medically assisted nutrition by tube.

☐ Trial period of medically assisted nutrition by tube.
 (Goal: _____)
☐ Long-term medically assisted nutrition by tube.

ADDITIONAL ORDERS: (e.g. dialysis, blood products, implanted cardiac devices, etc. Attach additional orders if necessary.)

✗ Physician/ARNP/PA-C Signature	Date
✗ Patient or Legal Surrogate Signature	Date

DIRECTIONS FOR HEALTH CARE PROFESSIONALS

Completing POLST

- The POLST is usually for persons with serious illness or frailty.
- Completing a POLST form is always voluntary.
- The POLST must be completed by a health care provider based on the patient's preferences and medical condition.
- POLST must be signed by a physician/ARNP/PA-C and patient, or their surrogate, to be valid. Verbal orders are acceptable with follow-up signature by physician/ARNP/PA-C in accordance with facility/community policy.

Using POLST

Any incomplete section of POLST implies full treatment for that section.

This POLST is valid in all care settings including hospitals until replaced by new physician's orders.

The POLST is a set of medical orders. The most recent POLST replaces all previous orders.

The POLST does not replace an advance directive. An advance directive is encouraged for all competent adults regardless of their health status. An advance directive allows a person to document in detail his/her future health care instructions and/or name a surrogate decision maker to speak on his/her behalf. When available, all documents should be reviewed to ensure consistency, and the forms updated appropriately to resolve any conflicts.

SECTION A:
- No defibrillator should be used on a person who has chosen "Do Not Attempt Resuscitation."

SECTION B:
- When comfort cannot be achieved in the current setting, the person, including someone with "Comfort Measures Only," should be transferred to a setting able to provide comfort (e.g., treatment of a hip fracture).
- An IV medication to enhance comfort may be appropriate for a person who has chosen "Comfort Measures Only."
- Treatment of dehydration is a measure which may prolong life. A person who desires IV fluids should indicate "Limited Additional Interventions" or "Full Treatment."

SECTION D:
- Oral fluids and nutrition must always be offered if medically feasible.

Reviewing POLST

This POLST should be reviewed periodically whenever:
(1) The person is transferred from one care setting or care level to another, or
(2) There is a substantial change in the person's health status, or
(3) The person's treatment preferences change.

A competent adult, or the surrogate of a person who is not competent, can void the form and request alternative treatment.

To void this form, draw line through "Physician Orders" and write "VOID" in large letters. Any changes require a new POLST.

Review of this POLST Form

Review Date	Reviewer	Location of Review	Review Outcome	
			☐ No Change ☐ Form Voided	☐ New form completed
			☐ No Change ☐ Form Voided	☐ New form completed

SEND ORIGINAL FORM WITH PERSON WHENEVER TRANSFERRED OR DISCHARGED

Photocopies and faxes of signed POLST forms are legal and valid. May make copies for records.   OVER ▶
For more information on POLST visit www.wsma.org/polst.

FIGURE 97-1 *(continued)*

References

Breault, J. L. (2011). DNR, DNAR, or AND? Is language important? *Ochsner Journal, 11*(4), 302–306.

Centers for Disease Control. (2016). *CDC wonder.* Retrieved from https://wonder.cdc.gov/controller/datarequest/D76

Committee on Approaching Death: Addressing Key End of Life Issues, & Institute of Medicine. (2015). *Dying in America: Improving quality and honoring individual preferences near the end of life.* US: National Academies Press.

Rao, J. K., Anderson, L. A., Lin, F.-C., & Lauz, J. P. (2014). Completion of advance directives among U.S. consumers. *American Journal of Preventive Medicine, 46*, 65–70.

Teno, J. M., Gozalo, P. L., Bynum, J. P. W., Leland, N. E., Miller, S. C., Morden, N. E., . . ., Mor, V. (2013). Change in end-of-life care for Medicare beneficiaries: Site of death, place of care, and health care transitions in 2000, 2005, and 2009. *JAMA 309*, 470–477.

CHAPTER 98

Living Fully to the End of Life: The Hospice Choice

Roberta Horn, PsyD

Psychotherapist, Neponset Health Center (retired)

Quincy MA

Introduction

In 2013, it was estimated that there were 5800 hospice programs in the U.S., Puerto Rico, and Guam. The first American hospice was only established in 1973. Why was there such phenomenal growth of hospice care in only 40 years?

Hospitals, especially in the past, made dying a particularly harrowing experience. Typically, doctors tried in every way to keep patients alive, subjecting them to one test or treatment after another, often when all the patients wanted was to rest quietly, without pain and without bright lights in their faces.

Doctors and nurses were not trying to torture their patients; they were only doing what they had been trained to do: save lives. Keeping the morbidity or death rate low at the hospital was a cause for pride and even when the patient's quality of life was compromised, staff members felt virtuous. Hospitals today still often adhere to this aggressive-care approach but now terminal patients may choose to be transferred to hospice care, where the aim is to enhance quality of life and to allow a gentle death with little or no pain. Hospices do not attempt to cure; they provide palliative care, aimed at keeping patients comfortable for all their remaining time. Patients seeking hospice care are making the decision to end attempts at cure and to accept only comfort care.

It's important to recognize that hospice does not speed up or facilitate death but it also does not stop it. Death is seen as a natural stage in living and the goal is to make life enjoyable right up to the end. Jane, a former hospice nurse and later, hospice director, explains: "Death isn't a failure. Every living being dies. Hospice focuses on the quality of living, on providing safe passage and on caring for the survivors."

L's Story (Name changed to protect privacy)

L was a successful businesswoman who never married. She had many friends but lived alone. When, seemingly out of the blue, she was diagnosed with Stage 4 cancer and given the prognosis of weeks to live, she was immediately hospitalized. Just as quickly, she begged to be moved somewhere else, even though it was known as a "fine hospital." She was being awakened every time she tried to rest, she was brought food when she didn't want it and none when she did, and she disliked having different nurses every day (or so it seemed).

L became more and more exhausted and unhappy in the sterile hospital atmosphere and was finally moved to a nursing home that allowed hospice care. Even though she was dying, she thrived in the quiet, cozy atmosphere where she was allowed to have a cache of popsicles in the freezer to sooth her parched throat and as many visitors as she wanted, to read to her or just sit quietly. Her hospice nurse made regular visits and the nursing home staff honored the hospice philosophy. When her time came, L passed quietly, without pain, yet conscious of her surroundings.

B's Story (Name also changed)

Hospice utilizes both medical providers and volunteers. I was a hospice volunteer and then a hospice director in the time prior to my psychology studies. One of my patients, B, was an older man who was very afraid of death. As I sat with him, he began to share his concerns. He had had a falling out with his brother and the schism had already lasted for years. B couldn't accept the idea of his dying without apologizing to his brother. He had avoided doing so for years because he didn't know what to say and he feared being turned away. We talked and talked and finally he realized that he would not die in peace unless he made peace with his brother. He did make his apologies and both brothers ended up tearfully hugging, with lighter hearts.

B still had some dread around dying until I said to him, knowing that some people need permission to die, "It's all right for you to go." He passed away peacefully the next day. I get teary, even today, when

I think of him. Jane, the hospice nurse mentioned earlier, said, "Hospice was the best nursing I ever did" and I agree that it was also the best work I ever did because helping another person to have a peaceful death is an incredible gift. If you use hospice you will find dedicated, compassionate caregivers who value their patients and their work as much as Jane and I did.

The History of Hospice

The first modern hospice was established by Dame Cecily Saunders in England in 1948. Moved by Dame Saunders's work, Florence Weld, Dean of Yale School of Nursing, and her students opened the first U.S. hospice in Branford, Connecticut in 1973. Today the hospice concept has spread around the world, providing compassionate care to the terminally ill and bereavement support to survivors.

When Should Hospice Be Called?

Hospice works to keep terminal patients comfortable and can provide services not available through other means. Once a terminal illness is diagnosed and the doctor offers a prognosis of a maximum of six months of remaining life, there are advantages to contacting hospice as soon as possible. Conversations about entering hospice can begin even before the patient feels ready to move to hospice care. Opening such a conversation will allow the patient to quietly consider his or her wishes and to compare all the options. Understandably, it can be very hard emotionally to accept that the patient is approaching death, and in many cases there can be differences of opinion among family members about curative versus palliative care. Both the patient and the members of the family may need some time to absorb the situation; but the earlier hospice care can be initiated, the greater the likelihood of eliminating pain: it is much easier to avoid pain than it is to stop it. At the very least, patients should consider putting their names on a waiting list, in order to receive priority help if and when ready.

If the patient wants immediate hospice care even the earliest possible call could entail some delay in obtaining care. Anyone who has ever waited in a hospital hallway to be admitted to an E.R. can understand that an overloaded system cannot always provide service as quickly as one might wish. Given that, calling in hospice right away is sensible. The choice is always the patient's. Patients who change their minds and wish to return to curative care can make that election at any time.

Requirements for Hospice Care

Once a patient decides on hospice care, he or she will need to do the following:

- Obtain a document from a doctor stating that she or he has been diagnosed with a terminal illness and has a life expectancy of six months or less. (If the patient survives six months, the doctor can sign a new statement of terminal illness.)
- Sign a DNR (Do Not Resuscitate) or similar form (these forms are also known as Living Wills or Advance Directives).
- Commit that neither the patient nor any family member, or anyone else acting on their behalf, will call 911, as the care given by emergency and hospital personnel goes beyond palliative care.
- Frequently patients will also be asked to provide a Power of Attorney, a document turning decision-making over to another party. (Powers of Attorney are only used when the patient is physically or mentally unable to make decisions or handle details and paperwork involving health and welfare decisions. Powers of Attorney will not rescind the legal status of the DNR or Living Will.)
- Hospice will typically require that there be a family member or other primary caregiver in the home. (Although there are some residential hospices, most hospice care is provided in patients' homes.)

Other Family Concerns

An issue patients or family members often express is that they do not want the patient to become addicted to drugs. However, pain is the major issue for a terminally ill patient, not addiction. Another concern is that the patient may be "so drugged up" that she or he will not be able to interact with loved ones. Hospice philosophy puts strong value on the patient's ability to express love, heal old emotional wounds, adhere to spiritual or religious values, and express personal wishes. The hospice nurse will take all those needs into consideration and will adjust the medication in a way that balances the patient's comfort level with the need for conscious social interaction.

A very important factor concerning family disagreement is that someone who is dying urgently needs a calm and peaceful environment. In appropriate instances a doctor, nurse, or hospice representative will meet with family members without the patient, to advocate for the patient's right to make decisions and for the importance of quality of life during the patient's remaining time. All arguments should be banned in the patient's presence.

What Services Might Hospice Offer?

Hospice can provide:

- Medical equipment, such as hospital beds and commodes
- Medications
- Oxygen, if needed for breathing
- Nursing care (3 or more home visits/week)
- 24/7 on-call availability of medical personnel
- Easing of nausea
- Pain control
- Chaplain and/or social worker services (if desired)
- Compassionate support and a calming presence
- Grief counseling, including special grief camp programs for affected children and grief groups where survivors can share their issues and support each other
- Memorial services

Assisted Suicide, also referred to as Death with Dignity, is NOT supported or practiced by hospice.

Bereavement care is a major part of hospice work. In 1975, Elisabeth Kübler-Ross's book, *On Death and Dying*, was published. Dr. Kübler-Ross had interviewed 500 dying patients, then wrote about the stages of grieving. Understanding the stages of grieving has helped many bereaved families whose members have been told to "Let it go and get on with living." In truth, grieving is a very complicated issue that often requires the kind of support that hospice provides.

What Is the Role of the Hospice Volunteer?

Hospice volunteers offer non-medical support. A volunteer might read to the patient, pick up newspapers or toothpaste, or provide rides to and from medical appointments. The volunteer might be the good listener or the good conversationalist a patient needs, or might just sit quietly with the patient. She or he is a valuable team member.

Conclusion

Hospice offers compassionate care and support during a patient's final days, when there is still time to celebrate life and to work out difficult issues. As the brief stories of two hospice patients pointed out, hospice can help in many ways.

Seven Questions to Ask in Choosing a Hospice

1. Will the patient be cared for at home or in a residential hospice? If the latter, is the hospice located someplace convenient for family members and others to visit?
2. Which are the hospices in the area?
3. Will Medicare and supplemental insurance cover all the costs? (Some costs at for-profit hospices will not be covered.)
4. If the answer to #3 is No, will the care be affordable?
5. What services does each hospice offer?
6. If a hospice being considered is affiliated with a religious group, is its orientation one that feels comfortable and welcoming?
7. Do the patient and family members feel comfortable with the hospice staff members and volunteers they have met or spoken with?

Reflections for Readers

1. Given that hospice can provide so many services, and does a better job of keeping terminal patients comfortable than most hospitals will, why are so many people reluctant to call for hospice services until the final days of their illnesses?
2. What can be done to make it easier, emotionally, for terminal patients to connect with hospice earlier in their illnesses?
3. How might you deal with a situation where family members have different opinions about the care the terminal patient should have at the end of life?
4. Do you see addiction to pain medication as a problem for terminal patients? Why or why not?
5. What additional services do you think hospice should offer to the terminal patient and his or her family? Should services also be offered to friends?

CHAPTER 99

Old Age . . . A Mixture of Happy and Sad

Irving I. Silverman
Business Manager, Publication Division,
National Knitwear Association and
Proprietor of the Kosher Food and Jewish Life Expo (retired)
Dedham, MA
Age 97

Living in a retirement community is a new experience. One comes face to face with pleasant new happenings, such as constant invitations to attend and participate in birthday parties, anniversaries, and other family happenings involving new friends and acquaintances. In addition, because residents are often undergoing changes in their health condition and sometimes even passing on, there are sad occurrences too. All too often, present residents are advised of the death of a friend through a system of emails headed with the subject line "Sad News."

Because we're part of a community, we find ourselves desiring to participate in both types of personal experience. Attending a birthday party is a joyful event because it is another milestone in the ongoing process of life, another step forward in the pursuit of happiness. It's more than the pleasure of having a slice of birthday cake. It's a chance to meet with other residents and to exchange living experiences; it's the pleasure of creating new events to remember.

But then there comes a viewing of the "Sad News" subject line on your computer. You're pained to open it for fear of learning of the death of a good friend, someone you have become closely attached to, have had dinner engagements with often, have attended activities with, and have gotten to know a good deal about. When you open the message, you learn there will be a memorial service and a wake or *shiva*.[1] At first, you may hesitate to attend, for fear that it will recall for you so many of the pleasurable times that you experienced together. But you come to realize that life in a community does have these hills and valleys, and you have to, as a matter of respect and friendship, you *have* to participate. It's hard! But you do it out of both necessity and choice. In doing so, you may be reminded of your ongoing desire to experience many more joyful interactions with other residents. You want to spend time with them, living in the now as well as recalling the past. You catch your breath and meet with many of your friends; together, you attend either the birthday party or the memorial service.

And you move on, because life continues to give you these experiences of happiness and sadness. You learn from each other how to endure the bad and savor the good. You learn to acquire new strengths and new wisdoms to live purposefully in your community. By doing so, you strengthen yourself for whatever will come next and enable yourself to master the experiences as best you can. You're enriched by the camaraderie with your remaining friends and you learn how to treasure your memories, as well as how to move on to another day, another week, another year!

It's a lot better than many of your past years, where you might have lived alone, isolated from daily contact with family and friends, being bored with solitude. As part of a community, you accept both the happy events and the sad ones because they both occur with or without your choice. You find solace in memories. You find joy in the continued repetition of birthday parties and happy times together, and in the ability to share the sad events over which you have little or no control.

So, you move on, counting your blessings. Time marches on for you and your neighbors. You strengthen each other by continued togetherness. Tomorrow may be a day with less sad news and you develop the capacity to endure, even to prosper and grow. You weather the storms of sadness.

You've accomplished something else. You've enriched the lives of your remaining friends; you've continued to relish the good times that lie ahead. The mixture of happiness and sadness lies within our capacity to live—to deeply, truly, *live.*

---

[1] *Shiva* is the week-long mourning period following burial, in the Jewish tradition. During this interval, the mourners stay together in one home and others bring them food and comfort.

Reflections for Readers

1. Why might birthday celebrations sometimes seem like sad events rather than happy ones?
2. What internal and external resources can someone draw upon for help in facing "sad news" about the deaths of friends?
3. How does a sense of community help one face "sad news"?

CHAPTER 100

Death with Dignity

Ellen Beth Siegel, JD, PsyD
Clinical Psychologist
Cambridge, MA

Everyone dies.

We hope for peaceful deaths, preferably after long and fulfilling lives, but that's not the way it goes for everyone. Some people suffer terrible pain at the end of life, after it's already clear that there is no possible cure. The advent of the hospice movement has made it possible for many sick people to die in peace—the central mission of hospice is to provide palliative care so that the dying can live to their last moments with little or no pain. However, hospice does not offer all the relief that some people seek: some want the right to end their lives deliberately rather than enduring lingering deaths.

As of the date of this writing, six U.S. states and the District of Columbia have adopted so-called Death with Dignity laws that permit terminally ill individuals to obtain prescriptions for life-ending drugs. Oregon (1997), Washington (2009), Vermont (2013), and California (2015) have adopted Death with Dignity statutes; so has the District of Columbia (2016). Montana allows Death with Dignity pursuant to a 2009 court decision holding that the right to choose one's own death is a liberty right protected by Montana state statutes, specifically, the Montana Rights of the Terminally Ill Act, adopted in 1985; but at least one Justice stated that the decision should have been made on (state) constitutional grounds and not merely as a matter of legislative interpretation. Colorado adopted a Death with Dignity Act by public referendum in 2016.

Other states are interested in Death with Dignity too. A New Mexico court authorized Death with Dignity in 2014, but that decision is currently being appealed and is not yet in effect. Massachusetts tried to adopt Death with Dignity by referendum in 2012; the law failed by a slim margin after a massive publicity campaign was mounted against it by the Catholic Church and the Massachusetts Medical Society. All together, about 60 million Americans live in jurisdictions that already have Death with Dignity laws in effect.

Death with Dignity laws permit doctors to prescribe pain-relieving medication under stringent safeguards to terminally ill patients even if the medication is sufficient to cause death. Essentially, the laws declare that Death with Dignity is a valid medical procedure aimed at alleviating suffering, relieving doctors of the threat of being prosecuted or sued.

Death with Dignity laws are replete with safeguards. They only allow people who have been certified to have less than six months to live—the terminally ill—to elect to ask for or take life-ending drugs. To prevent acts by rogue doctors, this certification must be by at least two doctors. The patient has to affirmatively ask for the prescription; no one else can ask on his or her behalf. The request has to be made at least twice orally and at least once in writing, with witnesses who do not stand to profit from the patient's death. Furthermore, there has to be a determination that the patient is legally competent to make the request.

To further ensure that patients opting for such life-ending drugs are not being coerced, Death with Dignity laws require that the patient must take the medication independently; no one else can administer it to her or him.

Notably, Death with Dignity laws provide the option only to patients who are terminally ill. Doctors cannot write these prescriptions, for example, just because a depressed person wants to end his or her life, since depression is not a terminal illness.

Under these laws, if all the conditions have been met, a doctor who believes that he or she is acting ethically to prevent suffering can write a prescription to relieve the patient's pain, even if the medication being prescribed might end the patient's life. No doctor is required to write such a prescription; the laws simply say that, so long as all the conditions have been met, a doctor who does write such a prescription is not subject to criminal or civil action for doing so.

There is substantial disagreement among doctors about the ethics of Death with Dignity (which opponents frequently refer to by the alternate term "physician-assisted suicide"). Some doctors believe that any act that hastens a patient's death is a violation of the provision of the Hippocratic Oath: "First, do no harm." Other doctors believe that the Hippocratic Oath requires them to alleviate a patient's suffering, and that prescribing the pain medication called for by Death with Dignity laws is doing precisely that.

Death with Dignity has been in effect in Oregon since 1997 and has been studied there thoroughly. There are *no* reports of any patient being coerced to a premature death. In fact, 40% of the patients who request prescriptions never use them; having the option of controlling their own fates apparently gives them the comfort that they need. The experience in other states is comparable.

Why is it that—at least for some patients—hospice is not enough? Palliative care, the bailiwick of hospice, has vastly improved in recent years, but it still does not eliminate *all* pain for certain patients; and current medical technology is capable of keeping someone alive even after that person feels that his or her life is too compromised to be worth living. For some, there is a fervent wish to be in control, even in deciding when to die. And some people don't want to spend their hard-earned assets on end-of-life care that extends life without improving it; they would rather leave their money to family or to charity.

An individual who wants to control his or her death should make that wish clear by specifying in a living will or similar document what kinds of care he or she does or does not want. The document should answer such questions as "How long are you willing to tolerate suffering—and what kinds of suffering—if you are terminally ill?" Writing out your wishes will spare your family from uncertainty as to what you want. Once you have written all this out, as specifically as possible, on a form that is signed with witnesses and notarized, you can bring it to your doctor and ask point blank, "If I am terminally ill and ask you for barbiturates or similar painkilling drugs to end it all, would you be willing to prescribe them?" The fact is that some doctors have been doing this surreptitiously for years; Death with Dignity laws just bring this clandestine practice into the open and regulate it to prevent the possibility of abuse.

Even with Death with Dignity laws in place, not everyone will choose to ask for life-ending drugs. However, Death with Dignity laws do not force anyone—not patients, and not doctors—to do anything. Each person can act in accordance with his or her own conscience and wishes. And—if the option to control their deaths would provide comfort to some, what is the reason for denying that comfort to those who want it?

Reflections for Readers

1. Death with Dignity legislation aims to give people who are terminally ill the right to end their lives on their own terms. Why is it so difficult to get such legislation passed? What are the countervailing factors?

2. If you oppose Death with Dignity legislation, do you have any alternative ideas for ensuring that the dignity of the dying is preserved in their last weeks and months?

3. Those opposed to Death with Dignity frequently refer to it as "physician-assisted suicide." What comes to mind as you compare these two different names?

4. What kind of legislation would be ideal in terms of helping people die with dignity? What safeguards are important?

5. Should Death with Dignity legislation be expanded to cover patients who are severely and chronically ill, but not terminal? Many such patients live with great pain. What risks would be associated with extending the Death with Dignity concept in this way?

PART **XVII**
Coping with Losses

CHAPTER 101

Loss of a Spouse: Claire

Charles L. Blauer
Chairman of the Board, Blauer Manufacturing Co., Inc.
Dedham, MA
Age 87

How do you describe, in words only, the grievous loss of a spouse? Simple, you can't. After being married to my beautiful Claire for sixty-four years and four months, there is no way to describe the sense of loss, the tears, the torture of watching your beloved fail over a period of four years and four months while in an Alzheimer's unit—a locked household—in a long-term-care center.

She walked into the unit on her own. She was able to eat and drink by herself. She was continent when she arrived. She greeted her aides as they welcomed her. It was the beginning of a long, and heart breaking, steady degeneration. She never uttered words such as "Why me?" She never said "Take me out of here." She simply complied with what they asked of her, and was stoic. I knew and I could feel the terrible depression in which she was wrapped. Occasionally she cried when I was with her. When I stupidly said, "Why are you crying?" she simply looked at me.

The progression of the disease was unending. Day after day, it went on. In just a short period of time, she was incontinent. Anybody would be so if they were one of 14 residents who are attended by only four staff members. They cannot get to you when you need to relieve yourself. You have no choice but to be incontinent, even if you are not. Next was the loss of ability to walk—just a few months after walking in unaided! Unbelievably, I noted one day that she looked like she wanted to get out of her wheelchair. We summoned physical therapy (PT), and along with the therapist, I was able to get her back walking without assistance for a rather long distance! A small victory over the disease? Not really; over a short period of time, she needed more and more help, as she could not move her feet in the normal heel-toe progression. They forbade me to help her walk or encourage her to do so. Another loss.

Oh, I tried desperately to slow the progression of the disease. I was with her for lunch virtually every day. Before lunch, I exercised her in the chair. With her cooperation, I was able to move every joint in her arms and legs. After the exercise session, it was into her room, where I combed and brushed her hair in the way that she liked to do it herself. Rearranging what the well-meaning staff had disarrayed. Then I applied some of her favorite blusher, as well as her lipstick. She pursed her lips in anticipation of the lipstick. She wanted to look her best. Now it was time for me to wheel her though the corridors of independent living, where we had been able to live for two years. In that period, she had made a number of friends. Even as they saw me talking to her and trying to stimulate her, they would say "Hello, Claire." Occasionally, they would get a smile and a return hello.

Then it was back to her household for lunch. Try as I could, she would eat only a little of the food from me. However, her principal aide, a saint of a woman, could get her to eat a substantial amount of food. Even as I thought that I had achieved some sort of success, I was failing. As time went on, she ate less and less. Even her cherished ice cream did not stimulate an eating response as it once had.

Still, I was undeterred. I was fighting as hard as I could to keep her going. I knew all the time that she would have signed any paper that would have allowed some way, some person, to end her life. My good friend, the rabbi, told me that she was staying alive because of me. She was living because she knew how much I loved her. What could I do? How do you not stand by the love of your life, your best friend, the mother of your six children, your tennis, golf, and skiing buddy? An especially gifted teacher who taught reading and math to kids with learning disabilities? An outrageously gifted cook, who could simply open a refrigerator, scan the contents, and whip up a meal in no time? No, there was no way that I would ever abandon her, as she would never abandon me.

So, after dinner, it was back to her unit, where I would take her into a living room area that had a couch. With a little assistance from her, I would move her from the wheelchair onto the couch, where I could hold her in my arms. There we sat, with her head nestled into my chest. I know that she liked that part of the day with me. Because I had insisted that she be the last person who went to bed for the night, we could sit until about 8:30 p.m. I kissed her once again, told her I would be back the next morning, and the days started again—one after another.

To no avail. The disease never lets up. The monthly meetings with the staff and attending physician were only more sadness. She was declining rapidly. There was no need for any medications. She was pocketing her food in her cheeks and not swallowing. Her drinking of liquids caused some aspiration, which produced coughing fits to eject the water from where it shouldn't be.

It was my routine to work out at the gym on Monday, Wednesday, and Friday mornings until 11:00 a.m. From there, it was time to see Claire. In this particular week, my daughter was visiting overnight, and she, too, was in the gym. She advised me that she wanted to just check on Claire, and I told her I would be along in a few more minutes. Suddenly, I looked up and my daughter was urging me to get to the unit as Claire was dying. I raced there, only to be about a minute or two late. She had passed. I cried and flung myself on her to kiss her. It was too late for me. She had a death mask on her face that I will never forget. I closed her eyes and closed her slack-jawed mouth. I didn't know what to do but weep and weep. I couldn't let her go, but I knew that she was at peace and that she would never have to endure the indignities that go along with the disease.

It has been one year, one month, and one day since my beloved left me. I speak to her every night when I go to sleep. I relate the day's activities. I tell her how much I miss her, and how empty the bed is. How empty the days are without her. How there is no one to turn to while watching either a terribly sad movie or TV program or a great comedy. No one to be with in the movie theater, where she always insisted that I buy her a big box of popcorn, with lots of butter. No one to be with me as I head towards the last years of my life. We were supposed to go together. But she left me by myself.

Reflections for Readers

1. What does Alzheimer's take away from the person with the disease? What does it take from family members?

2. It is terribly difficult for a spouse—or any family member, for that matter—to watch a loved one slip away as he or she descends into Alzheimer's. What coping strategies can you suggest? How can family members deal with their pain?

3. Conventional wisdom has it that the person with Alzheimer's does not know what is happening and therefore does not suffer. However, as this author describes his wife's degeneration, she appears to have moments of lucidity, stoicism, and sadness. If

you have had experience with Alzheimer's patients, what is your impression of their awareness of their condition?

4. This author acknowledged that his spouse "would have signed any paper that would have allowed some way, some person, to end her life"—yet for him to have done anything other than "fighting as hard as [he] could to keep her going" would have felt like he was abandoning her. What can be done to help in situations where the sick person's wishes may not be the same as the wishes of family members?

5. After someone dies from a long and debilitating illness, she or he is at peace—but the survivors continue in pain. How to reconcile relief, that this loved person is no longer suffering, with one's own feelings of devastation?

6. What resources would you suggest to comfort surviving family members after a death?

CHAPTER **102**

When You Lose a Spouse: Wayne

Reverend Elizabeth E. Frigard, UCC
Interim Pastor, First Presbyterian Church
Big Flats, NY
Age 68

My husband died on August 11, 2002. It was a Sunday. We would ordinarily have attended church, but we stayed home to get some chores done and to order paint from a store in Catalina, Arizona. The paint was for a townhome that we had recently purchased in Tucson. Our oldest son had attended the university there, and we had fallen in love with the desert southwest and thought that in time it would be a good place to move, not to retire, but just for a slower paced life. Wayne was an attorney for a law firm in Boston and dealt not only with stress on the job, but with a daily commute through the "Big Dig," a seemingly interminable and massive construction project.

It seemed like a good time to consider a change. Two of our three sons were finished with school. The youngest would soon be entering his senior year at a college in North Carolina. Our life was opening up.

That Sunday was a hot and humid day, but Wayne was set on playing golf with his friend Dick. That evening, Dick and his wife June, one of my best friends, were coming for dinner. I was going to try out a new recipe and we would, of course, eat on the screened-in porch.

It was a little after noontime, and I was upstairs when Wayne called out to say that he was leaving. I wished him a good game. And I heard the door close.

I picked up around the house and headed out to TJ Maxx and the grocery store. I returned home at about 3:30 p.m. to find two cars in the drive. One was June's. Standing next to the other vehicle, an SUV, was a young man I did not recognize, but whom I later learned was an off-duty police officer.

June walked up to meet my car. I could tell by the look on her face that something was terribly wrong. I asked, "One of the boys?" She said. "No." "Wayne?" I asked. She said, "Yes." "Gone?" I asked. She said, "Yes." My legs went out from under me and I fell into her arms. I felt as though I had been severed—half of me was gone, how could I ever stand? Thus began the journey into widowhood and finding another way of being with the man whom 31 years before, I had chosen as my life partner.

We had met while working on Cape Cod the summer before our senior year in college. His school was all men, mine was all women, but both were in New York State and not too far from each other. We were engaged that November.

Our marriage was good—more than good, we were a team. We loved and respected each other. We fit together so well. You could say that we complemented each other. We had the same values. Family always came first. When the boys were young, he chose corporate law with more family-friendly hours so he could coach each of their soccer teams. We both were concerned with peace and justice issues and were active members of our church. And we both loved to entertain our friends and we loved to dance.

Wayne was also my most fervent supporter. When I began my poetry workshop business, he cheered me on and helped to edit my books. He bought me books by such poets as Mary Oliver and Billy Collins, and we read them together, and he listened to each poem I ever wrote. And his advice was always, "Keep writing; do what you do!" Who was I, and what was I to do, now that he was gone?

An autopsy determined the cause of death to have been hemorrhagic plaque, which had broken off and clogged an artery. A month before, I had encouraged him to ask his doctor to run some tests. I was concerned that something might be wrong. His neck and wrist had bothered him, and his face looked as though he might be retaining fluid. His father had died at 60 years of age from what was called a heart attack. But Wayne's doctor assured him that tests were not needed, he was fine. His cholesterol and blood pressure were good. In his chart, the doctor had written. "Great for a man of 54." But now he was gone, and not only was I dealing with my grief, I was furious with his doctor and worried for my sons' future health.

Wayne was physically gone, but I felt his presence in both dreams and in a mystical sense. I have read of "Big Dreams," which psychologists believe are ways that our minds help us to cope with a loss. I, for one, understand them to be much more than a mere coping mechanism.

The term I use to describe the week after his death is "excruciatingly beautiful." The support we received was indescribable, the care that surrounded us seamless and loving. The memorial service was beautiful and meaningful and packed to overflowing, not surprising for a man who died in midlife stride.

Then it was over. Aaron went back to Boston, Sam to California, and Nate to North Carolina. Rumi, our beloved Australian Shepherd, and I were left to piece together a life. Friends were around, but they had their own lives. What was I to do with mine and who was I now? And what to do with Arizona?

Suddenly I found myself inundated with paperwork. I had not known how complicated death can be. Within a couple of weeks, I continued with my workshops. I functioned in the outside world and cried when I returned home. I found grief to be profound sadness, but also rage, anger, and frustration that no matter what you do, you cannot bring your loved one back.

October came. In a meeting with the lawyers, I was advised not to keep both houses. Suddenly, my path became clear. I would sell the house in Massachusetts and move to Tucson. It was a busy fall, dismantling the home we had lived in for 24 years, deciding what to take with me, what to sell, and what to give away. My decision felt right. I was continuing with our plans. The boys seemed fine with my moving, but friends were concerned, reminding me of the advice given to widows and widowers not to make any big changes for the first year. I was not to be dissuaded. The prospect of escaping a long, gray, cold, and snowy Northeast winter made my decision that much easier.

On January 3, 2003, in a light snow, Sam, Rumi, and I headed west. Sam would fly back to California from Tucson. I settled in, making my new home my own. On my little street, I made new friends and numerous friends from back east came to visit. I found a church and attended a Widow-to-Widow support group. I also entered a two-year program to become a spiritual director and began leading poetry programs. I spent a great deal of time writing, reflecting upon my experience and my grief, and communicating with Wayne. I also spent hours hiking in Sabino Canyon, our favorite place to visit in Tucson.

In May 2007, shortly after a day with a therapy horse in Sonoita, I heeded the call that had been beckoning to me for some time, and applied to Andover Newton Theological School in Newton, Massachusetts. Through the horse, I had come to recognize the grief that I was still feeling and that was holding me back. I called my sister, who agreed to take dear Rumi, and in September of that year, I moved into a studio apartment on campus which was to be my home for the next three years.

I believe that Wayne was a major factor in my decision, that he was urging me forward, cheering me on, giving me both courage and confidence. In a sense I have felt that I am living for both of us.

I graduated in 2010 and returned to Tucson. Then, in 2013, our grandson was born in western Massachusetts. The moment I learned that Nate and Jen were expecting, I began a book for the then-unnamed child, telling him/her all about this world and life and about the family, including, of course, stories of the dear grandfather he or she would never know. I do feel profound sadness that Wayne will never hold his grandson and that Noah will never know his Grandpa Wayne.

In April 2013, Noah's birth brought me back East, not just to visit, as had been my intention, but to stay, though I have kept my home, my refuge, in Tucson. I am now living in a small city in upstate New York, the city in which I was born and raised and in which my sister and mother live. I am also serving as pastor of a Presbyterian church in the next town.

I feel that Wayne is still with me and will continue to be so. I have never considered marrying again. In a sense, I still feel married. At times, the years that we have been apart feel like a day. I do pray that someday, in some realm, we will meet again. In one of those dreams right after his death, we were in a crowded theater and became separated from one another. As he was being pushed along in front of me, he looked back over his shoulder and said, "It's ok, I'm just going on ahead." In my heart, I do believe that it is true.

My life is not what I had hoped it might be at the age of 68. I have been alone now for 14 years, but my life has meaning, purpose, good friendships, a beautiful grandson, and I had 31 years in a loving marriage with Wayne. I'll take that.

Reflections for Readers

1. When a spouse or other loved one dies suddenly, there is no time to prepare, no possibility of last words—just an ending. What resources would be helpful for a person faced with such a loss?
2. What particular worries afflict the survivor of a sudden loss? This author writes of concerns for the health of her sons, but are there other concerns that arise too? How are survivors to manage them?

3. Survivors of loss not infrequently describe dreams or hallucination-like waking experiences of the deceased being physically present. How would you deal with someone accounting such an experience? Would you consider such experiences as positive or negative events?

4. What do you think this author found "excruciatingly beautiful" about the week following her husband's death?

103

When an Elderly Parent Dies: Impact on Adult Children

Earl A. Grollman, PhD

Rabbi Emeritus, Beth El Temple Center

Belmont, MA

Age 91

Adult children are intellectually aware of the real possibility of a parent's death. Yet deep down, we can't shake the assumption that perhaps, in our case, an exception will be made. We are never prepared for the inevitable moment of farewell. No matter what the age or circumstances, when parents die, their children are bereaved—feeling partially robbed of their identity. (Incidentally, the word *bereaved* comes from the Old English word *berafien*, which means "to rob.") Grief is a natural and profound reaction to their loss.

Parents are an integral part of our existence. We would never have known life without them. There is a cohistory of caring, mutuality, and interdependence. Our mother was "bone of our bone, flesh of our flesh"; we were the center of her world as she was a center of ours. The death of our father may be the death of our protector, our confidant, someone compelling in our lives. Even if the relationships were not always congenial, says A. Lakner in his book, *When a Parent Dies*, "an emotional umbilical chord [sic] is cut and can never be replaced." Suffice it to say, after parents die, their children's lives will never be the same.

When friends hear of the death of a parent, they may instinctively ask, "How old was he?" "How old was she?" Are they measuring how close they may be to their own death? Or are they trying to determine how much grief the mourner should endure, based upon how long someone has lived, as if there were such a formula? So often friends (who really do want to help) offer platitudes such as: "Well, she did live a long life."

At a vulnerable time, when the bereaved sorely need consolation and support, they are often put in the untenable position of having to defend their normal emotions or to unwisely bottle them up inside. But consider the quote from the poet Sherman Alexie: "When anybody loses a parent, it hurts the same if you were only five years old . . . or thirty-five years old. All of us are always five years old in the presence and the absence of our parents." Acknowledging these intense feelings of anguish is a monumental step in the healing process—learning to let go of what was and to live with what is.

Adult children may bear an additional loss that is illustrated in this ancient Chassidic story:

> There was an 85 year old man whose 103 year old father had just died after a long and productive life. In their efforts to console his grief, the son's friends reminded him of the rich and blessed life that his father had lived. The bereaved son looked up, eyes filled with tears, and said, "Though my heart aches for my father, that is not the only reason why I weep. I weep because yesterday I was a son. Today I am just an old man."

We don't have to be 85 years of age before we become aware of the fragility of life. The death of a parent reminds us of our impending mortality. How many times have you heard people say, "I am now the older generation. I'm next in line for the grave"?

> All persons are mortal:
> I am a person.
> Therefore, I am mortal.
> (Do you believe it?)

> With the death of elderly parents
> you may begin to realize
> that good health is not permanent.

> The slogan
> "Today is the first day
> of the rest of your life"
> is but a half-truth.

> Now you know the other half.
> "Today may also be
> the last day you'll ever get.
> No one knows about tomorrow."

The philosopher Moses Maimonides urges us to become reconciled to our limitations here on Earth. He explains how the realization of life's brevity could at the same time invest life with enduring significance. "People complain that life is too limited. The truth—while life is not endless, we live as though we had eternity at our disposal; we waste too much of life." The problem is not that we are allotted an uncertain life span, but rather that we are extravagant in spending it.

We can either squander time or sanctify it. The personal tragedy, the waste, lies in what we can do with time but do not—the life we do not give; the happiness we do not earn; the kindness we neglect to bestow; the gratitude we have not expressed; the noble thoughts and deeds we would realize if we truly live life today.

Rather than "falling into old age," the death of a parent can prompt us to transform our lives by moving beyond denial into a realization of the inevitability of our own death. We are prompted to rethink our own priorities, to refine our goals and redefine our future as we consider the following questions:

How can I be a more compassionate and loving member of my family?
How can I help my neighbors, my community, and humankind?
How can I create living memorials for my beloved parents?
How may I live my remaining years more meaningfully?
What memories will I leave behind?

Pondering these ultimate questions may help us to make our lives more purposeful and precious, offering us an opportunity to create a legacy. I love the words of the philosopher Cornel West: "To live is to wrestle with despair, yet never to allow despair to have the last word."

Reflections for Readers

1. Adults who have lived their whole lives—maybe even into their own senior years—with living parents may feel lost when a parent dies, even though intellectually, they know that death is inevitable—yet others may shrug off the loss of an elderly parent as being in the natural course, not requiring much in the way of comforting. How can an adult bereaved child ask for or find consolation and support?

2. What is the significance to a bereaved adult child that he or she is no longer someone's child?
3. How might we use the death of a parent, and the corresponding realization of our own mortality, as a stimulus to rethink our priorities, to live our limited life spans with less of what this author calls "waste"?

CHAPTER 104

The Lonelinesses of Long-Distance Elders

Clark C. Abt, PhD

Founder and Chairman Emeritus, Abt Associates, Inc.

Cambridge, MA

Age 87

This chapter is about the lonelinesses of long-distance elders, and how elders can overcome these situations and feelings by keeping on going with interesting people and activities. While not a memoir, the observations and advice are based on my own experiences as a moderately healthy elder in his late 80s.

What are "long-distance" elders? In the last 25 years, particularly in large, developed countries undergoing increasing urbanization and family mobility and dispersion, many if not most elders no longer live within walking distance of their parents, children, grandchildren, siblings, or other close relatives. The increasing geographic dispersion of families creates several types of lonelinesses, even for married elders: loneliness of place and location, loneliness of lost family proximity, loneliness of lost friends, loneliness of lost loves, loneliness of lost work, loneliness of lost capacities and competencies, loneliness of lost freedoms, and—encompassing all of these—loneliness of lost social and cultural context.

Loneliness of place and location is suffered both by leaving the old familiar neighborhood (as when elders move to a retirement community or warmer area), and by the people and shops and activities of the old neighborhood changing or moving away (because of gentrification or urban neglect and abandonment). The elders abandon their familiar long-term home neighborhood, or it abandons them by declining (or even upscaling) local shops and services. It is also the loneliness of age segregation, lacking contact with adult children and grandchildren.

Antidotes to lonelinesses of place include avoidance of late-in-life moves to remote and unfamiliar locations and age-segregated communities (whether retirement homes or Miami Beach). Elderly singles—widows, widowers, divorced, never married—need to locate with a diversely aged group with which they can identify, through similar education, work histories, class, taste, or preferred activities.

Lonelinesses of lost family members can sometimes be compensated for by spending time with close friends or even by starting another family by marriage or (informal or legal) adoption.

Lonelinesses of lost friends of similar age can be compensated for by making new friends with compatible cultural, athletic, or political interests and similar ages or up to a generation younger, located nearby. All cities and towns have multiage affinity groups, which can be a source of new friends. And to overcome shyness, remember that if you want a friend, be one.

Loneliness of lost loves—sexual, romantic, sentimental, platonic— depending on one's physical and emotional and social capacities—can often be compensated for by sublimation into literary, musical, philosophic, and scientific activities and interests. Vicarious reexperiences of lost loves recalled in music, arts, films, and literary romances, even in writing wish-fulfilling fictive "memoirs," can allow the bravely imaginative to reexperience the emotional and esthetic essences of lost loves. The empathic passions of viewing and listening to romantic opera, musicals, and movies can reduce the loneliness of lost loves, with the silver lining consciousness of it feeling better to have loved and lost—and perhaps even lost with some relief—than to never have loved at all.

The loneliness of lost work—especially of work that one loved or depended on for income and companionship—is especially widespread among the still-active and healthy elderly who have been forced into retirement. With longevity outrunning retirement age by one, two, and sometimes even three decades, there is an increasing need and opportunity for second or third careers, hobbies, charitable vocations, even child-rearing by grandparents. Freud said somewhere that the two most important things in life are love and work. Love is most crucial in childhood and youth, and work is most important in maturity. The intellectual, emotional, and economic satisfactions of work and its stimulating companionship can often be re-created by charitable activities, including tutoring, teaching, and mentoring poor kids in schools, homes, and hospitals. Learning and applying new skills, from knitting and carpentry to playing a new musical instrument, gardening, writing, etc., can bring many of the satisfactions and companionships of lost work.

The loneliness of lost capabilities, for many elders who still are in reasonably good physical and mental health, is one of the most painful. Speedy multitasking becomes difficult. Hearing a single conversation clearly amid noisy party or restaurant background noise becomes difficult. Walking is slower. Patience is limited, as is energy. Athletic speed, vigor, and endurance are all reduced. "Holding one's water" through a two-hour lecture, drive, or night's sleep is difficult. Peripheral vision is reduced, and response to sudden brightness of oncoming traffic or tunnel emergence is slowed.

All these and other lost or reduced capabilities tend to result in the loneliness of lost freedoms. This is especially painful for those who have been fortunate enough to have enjoyed many freedoms, having had enough time, money, skill, and education for adventure travel in fast and interesting company worldwide. Elders become more physically and financially risk-averse. The antidote is to keep doing what you have enjoyed doing, while acknowledging and accepting the limitations of even a healthy older age. As Dylan Thomas advised, "Do not go gentle into that good night . . . rage, rage against the dying of the light." And if you don't want to retire, rewire into adjacent satisfying work. Work and love are where you find them.

Reflections for Readers

1. Loneliness emerges from loss. Loss is the backdrop of old age. How might we assuage or compensate for this natural accrual of losses?
2. Taking risks can be dangerous. Yet, taking risk is essential for growth, meaning, and a sense of living a life that matters. What, then, is "reasonable risk" in old age?
3. This author proposes multiple strategies for dealing with the "lonelinesses" he describes. What additional strategies can you suggest?

PART XVIII
How Do We Want to Be Remembered?

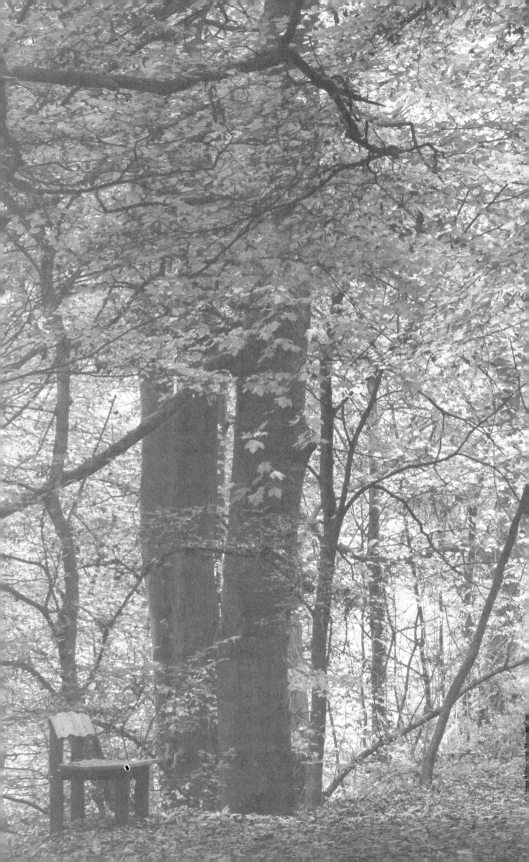

CHAPTER 105

Writing Your Own Memoir

Irving I. Silverman
Business Manager, Publication Division,
National Knitwear Association and
Proprietor of the Kosher Food and Jewish Life Expo (retired)
Dedham, MA
Age 97

Everyone's life is important and should be remembered, acknowledged, and recorded. But all too often, elderly people don't realize the importance of writing their own memoirs, for their own benefit and the benefit of their children, grandchildren, and future generations.

Sometimes they mistakenly think that writing a memoir is an expression of ego, to be avoided. That's not true. Especially when no biographer has come forth to write the history of a person's life, people should do it themselves.

Here are some steps to help you begin the process. Start by making a few important decisions. Are you willing to be totally truthful? Are you willing—and able—to go back to the earliest stages of your life? Go through your memorabilia box. Find items that will help you recall the important details of your life, all the successes, even the experiences that may not have been successful but are still part of your memories and worth recording.

Perhaps you can start by making notes along the following lines. Think in terms of blocks of time: your birth and childhood; your education; your work experiences; your marriage; the births of your children and grandchildren; your "achievement milestones." Recognize that your memoir does not necessarily have to be in chronological order. As Gertrude Stein wrote, "Think in terms of the flow of thoughts, ideas, and recollections."

A memoir does not have to be written in one sitting—and probably should not be, as writing it can be an important and growthful process for you as an author. The writing can be done in stages, and it can be edited as you go along and even reedited. But don't hesitate to begin! There's nothing wrong if you choose to enlist the cooperation of your siblings, relatives, and friends to help you recall items that you may only dimly remember.

Think positively about the purpose of your memoir. First, it can be therapeutic for you to revisit your life experiences. Second, your children, and especially your grandchildren, will want to know about you, who you are, and what distinguishes you from everyone else. You may not be writing your memoir for publication. It still is a very important document. Don't think negatively about the effort. Obliterate the thought that you're writing your eulogy and your obituary. Hopefully that's far in the future.

Even if you write it in successive stages, write it for preservation. You may want to save each successive step in the writing of your memoir, to be edited by you and others if you choose. This may very well be one of the most important documents you will have written in your lifetime. Your life is worth remembering. It's also worth recording.

Reflections for Readers

1. What can an elder give to his or her loved ones through writing a memoir?
2. What benefits can an elder derive for himself or herself through the process of creating a memoir?
3. Are there benefits to elders or to their loved ones if what is written as a memoir is untrue?
4. What audience do you have in mind as you consider writing a memoir?

CHAPTER 106

Remembering Our Loved Ones

Janet Gottler, LICSW
Social Worker, NewBridge on the Charles
Dedham, MA

Tear after tear is falling. My rigid heart is tenderly unmanned. What I possess seems something far away, and what had disappeared proves real.

—Goethe, *Faust.*

Grief is an inevitable, universal experience. Throughout our lives, we face ongoing transitions, both developmental and traumatic. We grieve our yesterdays and anticipate losses to come. One of the most profound experiences of grief is the death of a loved one, and the stronger our attachment, the greater our grief (Wong, 2008). When we are confronted with these losses, we are challenged to create new meaning and new identity, and to develop new skills.

Through the process of grieving, we start to regain our equilibrium and fill the void after a loss. We reorganize our lives and routines; we may sort out confused and conflicting emotions; we reach out for support and to share our stories and feelings with others. For a time, we may question our own identity and life's purpose. In addition, through the transformative process of grieving, we may try out new experiences and relationships, revise our own priorities and life goals, and transform our pain into creative works.

Under the best of circumstances, our narratives of grief and loss may lead to transformation and growth, even contributing to the greater social good. Grief may mobilize mourners by helping us to turn passivity into activity, or it may lead to altruism. Grief and loss may lead to a mourner's desire to do for others what was not done for him or her (Berzoff, 2006).

Research on successful aging indicates that many older adults have an extraordinary capacity to be resilient in the face of loss. According to a University of Arizona report called "Resilience in Aging" (Edwards, Hall, & Zautra, 2012), accepting one's own aging is an important element that builds emotional resilience. I would add that older adults who accept the inevitable losses of friends and loved ones demonstrate resilience and adaptation in the face of these events. The "paradox of old age" is that in spite of losses and physical declines experienced in later life, older adults report feeling content and have lower rates of psychopathology than the general population.

Say not in grief he is no more, but live in thankfulness that he was.
—Hebrew proverb

One lives in the hope of becoming a memory.
—Antonio Porchia

While we can ultimately make an adjustment to a profound loss, the ritual of remembering and commemoration is a vital part of integrating our lost loved one into our new experience. Some of our losses are communal as well as individual losses, and we may participate in commemorations such as Memorial Day or Veterans Day rituals, Holocaust remembrances, or in community healing remembrances, such as after the Marathon bombings in Boston.

People who have experienced traumatic losses may transform their experience into social justice projects or other works toward a common good. We think about efforts of Mothers Against Drunk Driving (MADD) and Mothers Against Gun Violence as efforts to transform personal pain into action to prevent this suffering from ever happening to others. Older adults who suffered losses during the Holocaust or who have witnessed other genocides have taken on the task of speaking at schools and colleges, to educate the next generations to "never again" allow these inhumanities to occur.

When I give, I start to be alive.

—Anonymous

Individuals and families can incorporate a range of practices and rituals to remember their loved ones and to commemorate their lives, their values, and their legacies. Some of the ways that we can remember the lives of our loved ones include the following:

- Creating something meaningful to honor a loved one
- Finishing a project that your loved one was working on

- Sharing a meal together on his or her birthday and sharing favorite foods and memories
- Naming a newborn after the deceased family member and sharing stories of this person's qualities and values to emulate
- Explaining to children whom they were named for and why
- Sharing rituals around the anniversary of a loved one's death; lighting candles is one such ritual, common to a number of religions, as are gifts of charity in the person's honor
- Investing in a project that would have meaning to our loved one's values and life, such as naming a building or place for a loved one
- Donating to a charity or fund or creating a charitable fund in our loved one's honor
- Endowing scholarships
- Writing a person's history or biography or sharing an oral history to be passed down to younger members of the family
- Creating a scrapbook of pictures or videos to share and pass on
- Carrying on activities that reflect the values and legacy of our loved one
- Creating rituals of remembrance at anniversary times and birthdays to share stories, visit the grave, bring flowers, make charitable donations
- Visiting or spending time at a place that was meaningful to your loved one
- Reaching out to someone else who is going through a loss to provide support and understanding

The process of remembering and of commemoration is part of our ongoing healing and our continuing relationship with those we have loved and who will always be a part of our lives.

When someone you love becomes a memory, the memory becomes a treasure.

—Anonymous

There beneath the light of the moon we sang a love song that ended too soon.
The moon descended and I found with the break of dawn,
The song is ended but the melody lingers on . . .

—Irving Berlin

Reflections for Readers

1. How does accepting one's own aging contribute to building emotional resilience?
2. Does accepting the losses of friends and loved ones similarly build resilience and adaptation? How?
3. What is required to transform feeling grief into the active process of grieving?
4. What can mourners do to transform their grief into something growthful, societally beneficial, or both?
5. Is it possible to grieve "too long"?

References

Berzoff, J. (2006). Narratives of grief and their potential for transformation. *Palliative Support Care, 4*(2), 121–127. doi:10.1017/S1478951506060172

Edwards, E., Hall, J., & Zautra, A. (2012). Resilience in aging. *Eldercare.* Retrieved from https://nursingandhealth.asu.edu/sites/default/files/resilience-in -aging.pdf

Wong, P. T. (2008). Transformation of grief through meaning: Meaning-centered counseling for bereavement. In A. Tomer, G. T. Eliason, & P. T. Wong (Eds.), *Existential and spiritual issues in death attitudes* (pp. 375–396). New York, NY: Psychology Press.

CHAPTER 107

How Will I Be Remembered?

Peggy E. Chait
Wall Street Principal and Compliance Consultant,
and creative writer
New York, NY

I can't recall at what point I began to think about, ponder, or even care about how I would be remembered. Life was in the here and now. In the earlier days of my life, I was like so many others; I never thought about getting older, about the meaning of life, about what I might accomplish or not, and certainly I was not concerned in the least about how I would be remembered. Life was in the moment, transitory, and without too much self-introspection. However, I was aware of how others, especially the older generation, were often consumed with their legacy and how they would be remembered in times to come.

How I will be remembered is in good part the way that I understand others to perceive me. What I think about myself may be true or self-delusional, or somewhere in-between. I know how I would *like* to be remembered, which might be quite different from how I will actually be remembered. I believe that how I would be remembered by others would differ greatly at each stage of my life.

If you were to ask my early childhood friends how they would remember me, I think their most vivid memory would revolve around one very distinguishing fact: my parents were divorced. Clearly, this would not be particularly memorable in 2017, but in 1967, it was an aberration and something I was ashamed of. My mother wouldn't allow my sister or me to tell anyone, but eventually it was discovered that we no longer had a father living in our house. I knew that people judged us, mocked us, pitied us, and remembered us for that reason. There was no other divorced household in the neighborhood where I lived. I was also known to be a sickly kid. My childhood friends would remember this as correlated with the depression that I experienced after my parent's divorce. Would I wish to be remembered by these events? Probably not, but how we wish to be remembered may not be the way we would be remembered.

How we want to be remembered must be answered on so many levels. There is the physical level, the intellectual level, the spiritual level, the emotional level, and perhaps the material level as well. How one wants to be remembered is often related to how individuals define themselves. The qualities that others define you by are not always the qualities you may wish to be defined by or remembered for. Sometimes though, we are most defined through life's challenges.

I began working on Wall Street when I was 21 years old. I did not have a degree in economics or finance; rather, I had a creative writing degree. I went to work at one of the world's largest brokerage houses, not because I was at all interested in it, but because I needed a job to support myself. I worked in an environment that was extremely sexist and where women were not treated equally and oftentimes not respectfully. I worked with some of the biggest accounts on Wall Street. Despite not having taken math since the 11th grade, I was able to learn the business and gained respect in the industry.

In the 1980s, I became the Chief Financial Officer and Chief Compliance Officer for a New York Stock Exchange firm, with an office overlooking Park Avenue. I had overcome many of the challenges of being a woman in a male-dominated industry. I would like to be remembered for my ability to have done so, not so much because of what I achieved, but because of how I achieved it, and the fact that it allowed me to be independent and the sole financial support for my children later in my life.

Life was a big adventure when I was in my 20s, and I lived it with great joy and zeal. I dated quite a bit, had long- and short-term relationships, and had a fully encompassing life. Reflecting upon it now, I would probably say that I was somewhat wild. At the end of that decade, I married a man whom I loved. He was boyishly good-looking, incredibly cultured and intelligent, and was a doctor in the making. He also had a psychiatric illness, which he informed me of after our third date. After some trepidation about moving forward in our relationship, I decided to look beyond the known facts and think positively about the power of love. We married, and for many years and in many ways, we had an "enviable" life. He had success in his career, we had two beautiful children together, a home in the suburbs, and enough money to live comfortably. Until we didn't.

With increasing responsibilities and pressure at work and at home with a wife and two children, my husband was beginning to spiral downward. Despite all that I tried to do to prevent it, and despite all the love that I had for him, I was powerless. He was hospitalized again, but for a longer period of time than ever before, and when he was discharged, he wasn't really stable enough to return home. I had decided that it was in the interest of our children, his welfare, and my own, that we separate. Eventually, with our support, he was able to reconstruct his career and his life and move forward. Unfortunately, this wasn't a long-term success. On a March morning, while visiting my elderly sick father in Florida, I received a phone call that would change my life, his life, and the lives of our children. My former husband had been arrested, and the arrest was publicized on the front page of the Long Island newspaper. His actions were a reaction to his father's death, causing him to be manic. The children and I were thrown into a world that was foreign to us. Criminal attorneys, jail visitations, gawking neighbors, and cruel children became a part of our existence. I championed his cause at every turn, while working to keep a somewhat stable and always loving home for our children.

During these turbulent years, we also sustained other immense losses. My father, my mother-in-law, my stepmother, and my mother all passed away within 16 months of each other. Losing my mother to an accident was the last injury that I thought I could sustain. Despite feeling at times that I wouldn't have the strength to continue, I taught my children about loyalty, love, family, survival, and binding together to get through even the most challenging of times. Although there were times of extreme emotional fragility for me, I tried to remain positive and have a sense of humor. I turned a horrific experience into one from which the children and I learned to be compassionate and strong. I learned to defend and protect the ones that I loved with fierceness and unyielding determination. I would want to, and believe that I would, be remembered for my strength during this period in my life.

I have always considered myself to be a nonconformist. I have never fit into any particular type of mold or stereotype, whether it be of a "Jewish-American girl," a "Wall Street" type, or a New Yorker. I never looked to others for my cues nor followed others to gain my identity. One of my greatest joys in life has been the ability to travel and to experience it in a way that most other women have not. When I was younger, I had no fear of traveling alone, and pride myself for having done so. I went to Mexico, the Canary Islands, Europe, and South America by myself. I was proud of being able to navigate the globe without relying upon anyone else to do so.

Even when I wasn't traveling alone, I chose to travel to locations that weren't typically visited by my peers. I went to climb the ruins of Tikal in the Guatemalan jungle during its civil war, visited jungles and ruins in remote villages in Mexico, visited the Straits of Magellan in Patagonia, and had my honeymoon in Costa Rica in 1991, when it was hardly visited. I have inculcated my children into the joys of travel and have recently taken them to Cartagena, Colombia, which is not a particularly popular tourist site for Americans. My sense of adventure, lack of fear (whether wisely based or not), open-mindedness, and global awareness are characteristics that I would hope to be remembered for.

I want to be recognized for the immense and intense love that I have for my children and my devotion to them as a mostly single mother. Of any of my accomplishments that others might admire, the one that is most meaningful to me would be my legacy as a mother. I cherish my children and hope that the values I have instilled in them will be the same values and legacy that my parents instilled in me. These are the values of education, open-mindedness, kindness, compassion, justice, and devotion to family. My hope is that my children will always cherish the times that we have shared together and remember me and my influence on them in a positive fashion. I am certain that they remember my idiosyncrasies, such as making them dance to the Beatles and to disco music and my forthright discussions about life and love.

As I look at the clock feverishly moving forward, I think about my own mortality and how it is no longer just a hazy dream set well in the future. I think about how I can make the most of every day, and focus on the positive aspects of life and love and the elements over which I can yield control. I am attempting to let go of the annoyances that invade my thought processes at times, as they are not really integral to my survival or the survival of those I love. I remember to be gracious to others and to be grateful, so grateful. I open my home and my heart to my friends and family and my children's friends, and I have been rewarded in doing so.

How will I be remembered? I'll probably be remembered for my green eyes, high cheekbones (thank you, mom!) and a mop of very curly hair (thank you, dad!). I hope to be remembered as a good listener, a confidante, and a good, loyal friend, daughter, sister, and mother. I hope to be remembered as a very hardworking, loyal, tenacious individual. I hope that people will remember my "zaniness" (again, thank you for the label, mom!), my love of music and of playing the piano, of cultures, of all people, of travel, of writing, of laughing, of justice and peace. I would like to be remembered as having made some impact on those who loved and trusted me. Most of all, I would like to be remembered in my children's minds and hearts and those of my family and friends. I have lived well and loved well and there is no sadness that should be associated with that. When I reside in the "ectoplasm," in the spiritual world, in heaven, or wherever my soul will lie, I would like to imagine that when I am remembered, people will smile, shake their head, laugh, or even get slightly moist around their eyes when they think of me. Then I'll know that I'm still with them.

Reflections for Readers

1. What steps can someone take to ensure that how she or he wants to be remembered is how she or he *is* remembered?
2. In what ways might how one wants to be remembered change over the life span?
3. In terms of how you want to be remembered, how much importance do you put on the physical level, the intellectual level, the spiritual level, the emotional level, and the material level? Are there other levels to be considered as well?
4. This author has laid out the ways that she would like to be remembered. Try writing a comparable statement for yourself.

CHAPTER 108

My Generations of Women

Talya Oded, MS
Director of Student Advancement and College Guidance,
Margolin Hebrew Academy/Feinstone Yeshiva of the South
Memphis, TN

The women in my family die young. My mother, herself already riddled with cancer, called me to come and see my first dead body, my grandmother's. We stood together, gazing at my grandmother's peaceful face. My mother kept saying, over and again, "She is so beautiful." And she was. At 74, her proud Hungarian face had barely a wrinkle, and her blonde hair had faded into a light gray that still retained its fullness and style. My mother's hair had already fallen out—chemotherapy is the cruelest therapy—but when I gazed down upon my grandmother's face, I recognized the woman I had always known. Squeezing my mother's hand and gently stroking my grandmother's still-warm arm, I thought about life and aging; death seemed an afterthought. That moment, three generations of women—my women and our generations—was all too fleeting.

Within a year, my mother was dead and my daughter, her namesake, would not be born for another three. I carry the generations now, and I strive to give my daughter the gift of old age, my old age, in the hopes that I will live to participate in another moment of grandmother, mother, and daughter, this time with me as the grandmother. My goal, don't die young, propels me forward toward aging. Having surpassed my mother by almost two years and still holding strong, I wrestle with getting older, with the full knowledge that I am *it*; I will be the model for aging for my daughter. Given that my daughter has never known her grandmother and has had little experience with older women in her family, I feel compelled to grow old with grace and dignity—not for my sake, but for hers.

Those of us hitting middle age are poised to live longer, healthier lives, if only we get the balance right. Eat more whole grains, walk daily, don't drink milk, do drink red wine, limit animal fats, do strengthening exercises, get enough sleep, avoid stress, hug someone you love, play games, sing songs. The never-ending barrage of tips for how to live a long life overwhelms and intimidates me. What if I get it wrong? What if I unwittingly contribute to my own hasty demise? More important, what will my daughter think of aging if I botch it up and age poorly? The possibilities are endless; aging has become a malleable process and perhaps I can shape it in my own image. With scientific knowledge and self-awareness, I can try to maintain some control. I read voraciously and journal often. I try to learn a word a day and walk around the block three times each evening. I limit my fat intake, go for annual check-ups, and pray daily. I know when I need to get more sleep (I snap at my husband) and I shut my phone off when necessary. In short, I try to find the balance that works for me. On a good day, I convince myself my efforts are working; at other times, I know it is a haughty folly to think I can change my destiny. Yet, I keep up the facade and plod along, grateful for every day past 48. My mother died 15 days after she turned 48.

Years pass, and I must reconcile with this new, older version of myself. Have I changed? Will I change? A happy person remains happy; depressed spirits find little solace in old age. I remember my mother and grandmother and how their strengths grew as they aged, but their weaknesses, those quirks of personality, became equally powerful. My grandmother remained judgmental to her last day, questioning and critically assaying her daughter and granddaughter's choices. My mother greeted each person as her best friend, warmly smiling at them and immediately making them feel special. Yet she also required total devotion and 100% commitment from her daughter. She almost suffocated me and I ran away, losing precious years because I could not embrace her totally. Only too late did I realize that her love for me sustained her and filled her life; she was not asking for anything in return but my presence. Now that she is no longer in my life, her absence has become a part of my essence. I now demand devotion from my own daughter, thriving on our relationship, yet fearful I will push her away.

Was I always this way? Deep down, I wonder if I am drawing my daughter closer in some bittersweet homage to my mother. While my daughter and I always had an organically close relationship, there has been a paradigm shift. "I hope you have a daughter who is just like you." My mother's voice echoes sonorously in my head and I see her, hands on hips, fiercely commanding me. My mother's wish has come true; does this mean I am becoming more like her as a result? Did she bless or curse me? Did she know, then, that she wouldn't be here to guide me or to answer questions about what it means to raise a child into adulthood?

We will be old for many more years than we are young; we should prepare appropriately. So, who will teach me how to grow old? I am acutely aware that there is no one to show me the way. Therefore, I spend my days reflecting on who I will become rather than embracing who I am today. Because I carry the weight of three generations, I think about how my unborn grandchildren will perceive me. I hope I can stave off the encroachment of age; I hope I remember stories to tell them.

When I speak to my daughter and find I am complaining about my aches and pains, does she shrug off the words as melodramatic hyperbole, or does she hear my subtle warning that health must be guarded and protected? For all that I have told my daughter about her grandmother and great-grandmother, I have never been able to tell her about that moment when I stood at the foot of the bed that my grandmother died in. In my mind's eye, I am back in that room, and I know they are urging me to heed the warning that health is not a guarantee. I pray I can keep my vitality in ways they were denied.

One day, I hope to stand with my generations of women, those who will follow me, preserving the memory of those women who, though they could not teach me how to grow old, taught me how to live instead.

Reflections for Readers

1. What responsibility do we have to serve as role models for aging to the rising generations?
2. In what ways are our essential personalities revealed "ever more clearly" as we age?
3. When we lose people we are close to, we often take on their characteristics. Is this to preserve them for ourselves, or to make them visible to the generations that follow?

CHAPTER 109

On Old Age, Friendship, and Loss

Glorianne Wittes, LICSW
Social Worker (retired) and artist
Dedham, MA

Almost seven years ago, I moved from the condo that my late husband and I had shared and loved in Sarasota, Florida, to NewBridge on the Charles in Dedham, Massachusetts. This was my first move as a widow, and it was to new territory, where I knew nobody. That was to change quickly through meeting my next-door neighbor, Eve, the Auntie Mame of NewBridge, who knew everyone and who included me in her life. We ate together almost every Friday night, and at her table, I met many residents who became friends.

As my chronic dizziness problem progressed and it became difficult for me to make and honor engagements, she never failed to check in with me on Friday mornings to confirm or cancel our Friday night appointment and to see if I needed anything. She was always available to me, but she never imposed herself on me and respected the privacy that I craved when my dizziness laid me low. We sometimes exchanged emails when we hadn't been together, especially interesting pieces we had received on the Internet.

It was from my wonderful friend that I received the latest news of NewBridge happenings and people, but she never shared it as malicious gossip. Eve served as our Floor Leader and as a member of NILMA, our residents' council, where she was very productive. She also sat on the Dedham Town Council, where she did us proud. The colorful scarves that she knit for friends were seen all over NewBridge, and those she knit for me will always keep my body and my soul warm.

Three Fridays ago, Eve called to cancel our dinner. This time, it was she who was not well, though she would not say what was wrong. Everyone was concerned about her, since she had been nowhere in sight and had spoken with no one about what was bothering her.

Last week, I sent her a bouquet of flowers through my aide, who was greeted at the door by someone from hospice who told her Eve was not well and not up to company. I was shocked as was everyone else. Hospice! That meant bad news. My anxiety mounted. I ate with others on the next two Friday nights, and we all expressed our concerns for her. Dinner was not the same without her.

On Monday afternoon, I went next door to deliver some cookies to her family and to find out how my dear friend was doing, and was told the horrifying news that she was no longer with us. She had died earlier that morning, the victim of a returned lymphoma, a vicious one that she had decided not to treat.

She wanted to be back with her late and beloved husband. Her daughter was just like her mother, concerned about me. She insisted on walking me back to my apartment, as she saw by my face how shocked and grief-stricken I was by her news.

Shortly before Eve took sick, I read an email on the NBOC Resident Google group. It was from Ellie, another of my dear friends here, who had become very ill a few weeks earlier. She wanted to let her friends know that she was terminal and to express her great appreciation for their friendship and concern. Ellie is an amazing woman, dynamic in her incredible softness, intelligence, artistry (she had put together a gorgeous collection of pop-up books that were exhibited in the Danforth Museum), and was a devoted friend to many. She was my movie mate, dinner companion, and confidante. The bravery she has modeled for me—for all of us—is second to none. Even in her extreme illness, she still thought of her friends and wanted to be in touch in the best way she knew how.

The news of Ellie's terminal illness put me in a blue funk, from which I had not recovered when Eve suddenly died. I felt weepy, listless, and withdrawn. Death and illness are frequent visitors to senior living facilities, where the mass of the elderly is not offset by large numbers of younger healthy people. I dreaded the next email notice that would notify us "with great sadness" that still another resident had died as so many had in the weeks and months before.

"I am because you are"—an African quotation. With the death of each friend, we lose a piece of ourselves that cannot be replaced. This is especially true in senior living facilities, where a shared sense of place and belonging builds relatively quickly in the course of dining, playing, sharing, and yes, mourning together. We bond, we grieve even without knowing each other well. We seek and give comfort to one another.

We are more than neighbors; we are friends of a very special sort. Some of this is summed up by the comment of a resident who noted the absence of a neighbor from many events. "I have nothing in common with her," she said, "yet I worry about her. I must look in on her to see if she's okay."

Old age brings loss. But it also can bring wisdom, the wisdom to reach out for comfort when one needs it and to receive it when it is offered. In my youth, I valued independence and autonomy. In my old age of increased frailty, I am able to acknowledge what I need from family and friends and revel in what I am still able to give. NewBridge has provided me with many vehicles and opportunities for both, for which I will be eternally grateful.

At this moment, as I ponder about the meaning of old age, I recognize that it is not primarily about loss unless one makes that its sole meaning. It's about how one's shape of existence ends and how we make a transition to another shape and being in the world. My husband and I both thrived on life as an adventure, where spontaneity was more the rule than the exception. Today, it is difficult for me to live that way.

I now have to create for myself new kinds of adventures if I am to LIVE my life rather than BE LIVED by it. I don't want to be a passive beneficiary or victim of my inherited body and genes. My task now is to find out how to adapt to my current shape of existence with appropriate excitement and muscular expressions; how to engage in the creative activity I love best without being hampered by reduced energy and mobility. I want to create new shapes and behaviors for living that are not trying to duplicate or maintain the past, but rather are enabling me to engage in what is present and what is forming in the next phase of my life.

Stanley Keleman, an eminent psychologist, defines old age as a time for a metabolic ripening, a continuum of slow pulses displacing the need to race towards peaks of instant expression. It is time, in our ripe old age, to live the waxing and waning, the swells and troughs of desire and contact which deepen our contact with ourselves and with others. Yes. I will continue to experience loss, but I will also continue to experience friendship and discovery until my last breath.

Reflections for Readers

1. There is a vulnerability attached to making friends in our later years, when we are extra-aware that the relationships may be fleeting. What is required to open ourselves to that vulnerability? How do such late-in-life friendships affect our life experience?

2. What does the African proverb "I am because you are" mean to you?

3. How can grieving with others build new friendship bonds?

4. This author writes, "Old age brings loss. But it also can bring the wisdom to reach out for comfort when one needs it and to receive it when it is offered. In my youth, I valued independence and autonomy. In my old age of increased frailty, I am able to acknowledge what I need from family and friends and revel in what I am still able to give." How do you see the value of independence and autonomy changing as we age?

5. According to this author, old age "is not primarily about loss unless one makes that its sole meaning." How do you understand this statement? Do you agree or disagree?

6. What advice would you give a senior to help him or her deal with the illness or death of a friend?

PART **XIX**
Wisdom

© James Whitesmith/Moment/Getty

CHAPTER 110

Mental Health as I Age

Reverend John MacDuffie

Pastor, Central Congregational Church, Eastport, ME (retired)

Bernard, ME

Age 85

I am a Caucasian male who spent a long career in Protestant parish ministry, raised a family of four children with my first wife of 56 years, and remarried after being widowed, and am continuing a style of life which seems to undergird mental health, inner peace, good relationships with people of all ages, and a general contentment—for all of which I am deeply grateful!

I can introduce the two simple principles of my successful philosophy of life with a couple of personal stories.

I remember well hearing my mother, then widowed and in her 70s, remarking about one of her activities during her time as a widow and trying to assuage her loneliness as much as possible, doing good works. She said "I go to see Nellie Dorr at the nursing home every Wednesday at 2:30 in the afternoon." At the time, Nellie was also a widow, had advanced in age and disability to the point where she could no longer live alone, and greatly appreciated my mother's friendship. In further conversation, Mum said, "Everybody needs something to look forward to." That weekly visit, not random but on a certain day at a certain time, was Nellie's anchor to reality and a much-anticipated pleasure. I found later that there were several others to whom my mother brought that special blessing.

My daughter Margi is a professional violinist who has lived and worked in Germany ever since finishing her studies. She has played in the same symphony orchestra for 35 years. It has been a fulfilling experience for her as a musician and as a person. A few months ago, this orchestra began a new life as part of a merger with another German ensemble in a fairly distant city. There are now 200 or so players to make up a performing unit of 100 or so at any given time. So out of, say, two dozen second violins, any random dozen might be making music together on a concert program during a number of rehearsals and performances. It is a challenging time for the entire orchestra.

Recently, Margi sent a message home after an eight-day concert tour in several Spanish cities. She said that one of the things that she had enjoyed was sharing delicious Spanish food with her section colleagues as they became better acquainted during free time. I asked in a return message, "How about your music-making? Are you satisfied with the quality of your playing as a section?" Part of her reply was this: "We do not sound as well as we need to—that will take time. But we second violins are making better progress than the firsts—because we have always had to know how to listen to each other. They seem to prefer to listen to just themselves."

Now, not being much of a musician myself beyond singing in amateur church choirs, I can have only a limited understanding of what a professional instrumentalist might mean by such a sentiment. The nearest I can come to it would be realizing that since I do not actually read music, the only way I can sing tenor in a group singing two or three other parts is by letting my ear guide me to the degree of harmony that my part is producing in the total effect. So I, too, must listen to those around me, following the advice all of us preachers have heard from our teachers and mentors, which says, "Since you have two ears and only one mouth, just remember how much of the time you ought to be talking!"

So now to the two main elements of my philosophy of life, which I believe have been of inestimable value as I have aged. All my life, I have engaged in a practice that I suppose most people might describe as "dreaming." I think I'd prefer to call it "imagining," or even "fantasizing." Going to sleep at night has never been hard because in earlier years, I would read myself to sleep, even to the extent of hiding under the covers with a flashlight so my mother would think I had turned off the light at the required time. I devoured adventure stories, almost exclusively involving ships or boats of some kind. And when I finally did shut off the light, my brain was full of pictures of those adventures in which I always found myself an active participant.

As I grew older, the stuff of imaginary adventures took the form of things that I could actually picture myself doing in real life—and again, boats were almost always at focal points of desire and intention. "Everybody needs something to look forward to," my Mum would say—and what I imagined while falling asleep at night was always the essence of what I looked forward to in an ideal life scenario. I didn't remember the events of the day that was past unless the awareness of something pleasant fueled the determination to do it again, or to do it even more successfully. It was future hope, not past review that nourished me. It still happens as I move more slowly and carefully, now, toward the next milestone, which will carry the numerals 86.

One thing I have realized is this: the dreams, the imaginations, the fantasies of my nights now do not hark back to swashbuckling adventures on the high seas or anything like the stuff of an adolescent boy's creations. If I were still trying to do that, I'm sure that the result would not be peaceful contentment in any form, but regret and sadness that these things could never come again. Instead, my dreams plan how I will make just some modest progress in the rehabilitation of an old boat out in my shop, knowing that for some tasks I will need the help of a young neighbor who seems always happy to give me a hand today so I can move ahead under my own steam tomorrow. What I can look forward to is realistic, doable, within my capabilities that are much more limited than what I pictured even a few years ago. This follows my mother's example: she might have taken Nellie Dorr out for a ride of a Wednesday afternoon four or five years ago; now she brings a small bouquet of flowers she picked at Nellie's old house, and they talk of the days when her children were still at home, her husband still working to bring in his modest paycheck, some good times with the neighbors they enjoyed on holidays.

The other mainstay is harder to remember, the wisdom of it harder to apply. To talk half as much as I listen, especially if I am with a Nellie Dorr, or even someone closer to my own age such as my brother, is a challenge. Without really wanting to, or realizing that I am acting like a first violin, more interested in my own sound than anyone else's—I'm talking too much and listening too little! And as I am doing it, that is when I am disliking myself for that very behavior—because, of course, I am remembering how someone did the same thing to me when I wanted to talk and be listened to!

In this case, pleasure and contentment are harder to come by, but when the greater effort is made and I hear some new ideas, some interesting reflections, some unexpected truths as I listen, it is so rewarding! I find myself coming home to my wife and telling her what treasures I received from my time listening instead of talking. Being a preacher, I of course reflect that one of my most cherished commandments is "Love your neighbor." And as I think about sermons I have prepared, I know that I have tried to give to others the advice that I am now trying to remember and to apply in my own life. It even occurs to me that once I gave this very title to a sermon: "The Blessedness of Playing Second Fiddle."

It occurs to me that I am really very lucky. I have one source of contentment that actually comes easily, as it is a lifelong habit, and its rewards are almost automatic, so long as I can keep on imagining a pleasurable project for tomorrow. The other blessing comes only if I can remember a more challenging rule, and apply the necessary insight and self-control to obey it: to listen twice as much as I talk!

Reflections for Readers

1. What can someone do to give a loved one a regular "something to look forward to"?
2. Why is listening to others more important than listening to oneself?
3. In terms of emotional nourishment, what can be gained from past review, and what can be gained from future hope?
4. How do one's future hopes change over one's life span?

CHAPTER 111

Sharing Experiences Through Talking

John Averell, PhD
Physicist, Polaroid Corporation (retired)
Dedham, MA
Age 82

Sharing—that is the important word in the title of this piece. Humans have progressed in societies. People need people. When they don't want to communicate with others, or perhaps more accurately, are not able to communicate properly, we call that "autism." The term encompasses such a wide spectrum of diagnostics that I hesitate to offer this definition, but for me it seems appropriate.

I'm sure that our human ancestors shared many things—food, shelter, artistic items, and audible communication like warnings, hand motions, grunts, such as nonhuman animals also share. But the development of language of sufficient complexity to share experiences was a breakout step for *Homo sapiens.* Here are some of the reasons why sharing experiences was and is so important:

- New, useful tools and how to make them could be shown, explained, and taught to others in detail.
- Much more complex details could be discussed interactively, question-and-answer style.
- Ideas could be exchanged, enlarged upon, and developed into abstract concepts that had the power to improve society as a whole.
- Personal exchanges between people could develop that would help one or both to improve their lives.

This last point is what today is so important to us. Many people are very private. The problem is that this may lead to isolation and depression. Here are a few quotes, proverbs, and biblical passages that show the importance of sharing:

A burden shared is a burden halved.

A burden shared is a burden lifted.

Carry each other's burdens, and in this way you will fulfill the law of Christ.

—Galatians 6:2

I remember that as I grew older, there came a time when I was the only person left in my generation from my thin line of Averells. There was no one left to ask about the experiences of my father, my mother, my Aunt Dorothy. Even my younger brother had passed away earlier. I had only my memories and a lot of photographs with small notes on them. I have realized how important it is to talk with your sons, daughters, and grandchildren about your own experiences while you can, even if they don't ask. The era of oral traditions has faded.

Here at NewBridge, one of my activities is as editor of the *Bridge Journal* quarterly. Many, really most, of our stories are written accounts of our own experiences, the very information exchange that should occur with family. A number of our authors were wise enough to write these experiences down throughout life. But many have to be dredged out of memory and written down. In my experience, everyone I have talked with here has a story to tell, and everyone is interested in the stories that our neighbors have shared. I encourage everyone to share their own experiences with younger family, both through talking and writing them down, so that succeeding generations will know and remember you.

Each day at NewBridge, we walk past our neighbors, and the invariable question is "How are you?" This invitation to share our experiences of the day is, almost invariably, about our health. Sometimes we just say, "Fine. How are you?" But really, most of us truly do care about each other. Stopping for a few minutes and discussing what is going on in our lives may be about our latest family visit, our visit to the doctor, our continuing back problems, our recent trip—that host of limited experiences that we share now as we move through old, and older, age.

Other opportunities have become available at NewBridge. Programs have included presentations by residents about personal life histories and expertise. In the so-called Men's Club programs, which now are open to all, we have heard interesting talks about things that we never would have known about. I am thankful for all the amazing careers that so many of our fellow residents have had. Other programs featured panel discussions about chosen topics. The shared experiences of each participant added to our own new understanding. You can see these personal presentations on our NBOC website: NewbridgeResidents.org, and click on Presentations/Public.

Although my little essay on this subject is a "looking back" piece, I hope that readers who are much younger will not miss the opportunities to share their experiences through talking. Texting and Facebook and Twitter are not the same, but perhaps that is because I am older myself.

Do yourself, your friends, your family a favor: *talk* about your experiences.

Reflections for Readers

1. This author sets out several reasons why sharing through talking is societally and personally valuable. What other reasons would you add to his list?
2. Why is it important for elders to share their life experiences with younger family members and friends?
3. What is the role of relationships and sharing in older adulthood?
4. What might get in the way of having honest dialogue with others?
5. What are the benefits of talking about your problems? What risks, if any, do you perceive?
6. In senior living communities, what resources can be made available to encourage seniors to record and share their life experiences?

CHAPTER 112

Development of a Positive Outlook

Virginia Pratt Agar
Early Childhood Educator (retired)
Bernard, ME

Optimism

Through faith and spiritual practices, I am able to move into a more optimistic, hopeful state of being. Saying yes to life's opportunities; trying not to be "stuck" in certain lifestyle choices or situations; being brave to go forward with what one loves, really cares about, and values.

Health

To seek whatever will help me to be more "healthy." For mental health, trying to combat loneliness and isolation with physical exercise, community endeavors, socializing with family and neighborhood, being part of groups committed to purposeful ideals. In addition, trying to minimize stress, resting and eating well, and including in our lives what really matters to us: love of what we really care about. Health is about paying attention to our physical selves.

From my Christian perspective, there is a prayer that I love called "A Morning Resolve" from a booklet called *Forward, Day by Day*:

I will try this day to live a simple, sincere, and serene life, repelling promptly every thought of discontent, anxiety, discouragement, impurity, and self-seeking; cultivating cheerfulness, magnanimity, charity, and the habit of holy silence; exercising economy in expenditure, generosity in giving, carefulness in conversation, diligence in appointed service, fidelity to every trust, and a child-like faith in God.

In particular I will try to be faithful in those habits of prayer, work, study, physical exercise, eating and sleep which I believe the Holy Spirit has shown me to be right.

And as I cannot in my own strength do this, nor even with a hope of success attempt it, I look to thee, O Lord God, my Father, in Jesus my Savior, and ask for the gift of the Holy Spirit.[1]

This prayer really sums up what I *try* to do/be.

Our Legacy

What do we want people to remember about us at our funerals? What I love and cared about, my relationships, my family, my animals, my communities that I lived in, my endeavors of relationship-building and attempted beautification of what was around me.

Life is a ribbon of the unknown. I am the opposite of the "whatever" attitude; I believe that with diligent focus on what matters to you, you can have a sense of control, mastery, and pure enjoyment that contributes to a "positive outlook."

Reflections for Readers

1. Does optimism come harder or easier as one ages?
2. How does maintaining good health contribute to having a positive outlook? How does having a positive outlook contribute to good health?
3. This author cited a prayer she finds helpful and inspiring in her day-to-day life. Is prayer something you also find helpful and inspiring? How do you react to this particular prayer?
4. Why is leaving a legacy to family and friends such an important value, especially as we get older?
5. What is the legacy you would want to leave to loved ones? To the world at large?

---

[1]"A Morning Resolve" is reprinted with permission from Forward Movement, www.forwardmovement.org

CHAPTER **113**

Words to Live By: Today, Tomorrow, and the Future—My Final Legacy at the Age of 97

Irving I. Silverman
Business Manager, Publication Division,
National Knitwear Association and
Proprietor of the Kosher Food and Jewish Life Expo (retired)
Dedham, MA
Age 97

Who am I? What do I believe in? What do I still want to accomplish? What have I already accomplished? What do I hope for the world?

I have a lot to say in these final words . . . though I confess that writing this chapter is a challenge. To encapsulate a lifetime of living, dreaming, hoping, loving, achieving, and advising, though hard, is an important part of fulfilling my mission to create something of value to my children, my family, and my readers.

Principles

I have already lived a long and successful life, fulfilling most of what I intended to achieve in both my working career and my volunteer activities. I have engaged actively with many individuals and organizations and have always observed my self-created guidelines of behavior. I've made many decisions, maintaining what I believe to be the highest level of integrity and honesty. I've worked hard, whether I was being compensated financially or not. I have tried to be a role model for others. These actions reflect values I have, things I believe in.

I believe in kindness, that the world offers kindness to me and that I can offer the same to all. There are many sick and unhappy people in the world who need to be helped, and I can offer help, at least to some of them.

I believe in the power of the human will. My mantra is, "If I will it, it will get done." Being motivated and working hard are the keys.

I believe in education. Against all odds, I managed to get through school despite my visual handicap; I went on to college and graduated with honors.

Parenthood

As a workaholic, I left much of the parenting of my children to my first and second wives, who indulged my behavior. I often missed the pleasure of dinners and weekend activities. However, I made sure that I would always be with my family for Sabbath dinners and other family events and celebrations.

I was the father who was always present when I needed to be. Thankfully, I feel that I have fulfilled my parenting role successfully. When my first wife, Henrietta, died in 1956, leaving me with two young children, I had to go on as a single parent. When I married Nancy, my second wife, and acquired her two children, I adopted the principle of having a truly blended family and never succumbing to the mistaken thought of "my children" and "her children." That was something very important to me, and it still is.

I regard my children, grandchildren, and now my great grandchild as my proudest achievements. I look to them to carry on my legacy.

Politics

I believe in being a good citizen; this is part of what I conceive of in terms of being a role model for my children, other family members, and the society in which I live.

I believe in treating everyone with respect and dignity. I was a good employer and a good employee for every enterprise with which I was involved. That came from a core belief that everyone was equal.

Perseverance

I learned the art of perseverance at a very early age. Being handicapped visually impressed upon me that I had to try harder. I got my first medal for perseverance when I graduated from my elementary sight conservation class.

I have succeeded and failed in many respects, both academically and careerwise. But I developed the capacity of bouncing back and overcoming any difficulties that I encountered. I learned the advantage of not saying "no" when a job had to be done. A case in point: I endeavored to create an organization and a project that had never been done before, a Kosher Food Expo. Nine out of ten advisors whom I consulted said, "Don't do it. It will fail!" But I did it, and it succeeded.

I have faced difficult times, even tragedies like the deaths of each of my wives, and I have found my way to new beginnings. I have overcome poverty and physical handicaps—my vision problems from birth and my hearing difficulties in older age—and have found ways to advance myself in spite of everything.

Even this book, which has been "in the works" for almost two years, is an example of perseverance.

Prayer

I have always been an adherent of the practice of prayer. I personally pray frequently. Sometimes it's to ask for God's help in achieving the successful outcome of a difficult circumstance. Other times, I pray to achieve comfort and the resolution of something that troubles me or someone else who needs help. Prayer helps me get through the challenges life brings.

As I come to the close of this book, I wish to include a special prayer that inspires me and I hope that it inspires you also:

> Master of the Universe, I hereby forgive anyone who angered or antagonized me or sinned against me—whether physically or financially or through disrespect, or in any other matter affecting me; whether involuntarily or willfully, carelessly or deliberately; whether by word or by deed. I forgive every person: let no one incur punishment because of me.

Reflections for Readers

1. What is the value—to yourself, to your loved ones, to a wider circle such as your community or the world—in spelling out "words to live by"?

2. Do you conceive of "words to live by" as aspirational? Do you see them as "This is who I am"? Are they guidance for yourself or for others?

3. What are your reactions to this author's "words to live by"?

4. If you were writing your own "words to live by," what would they be?

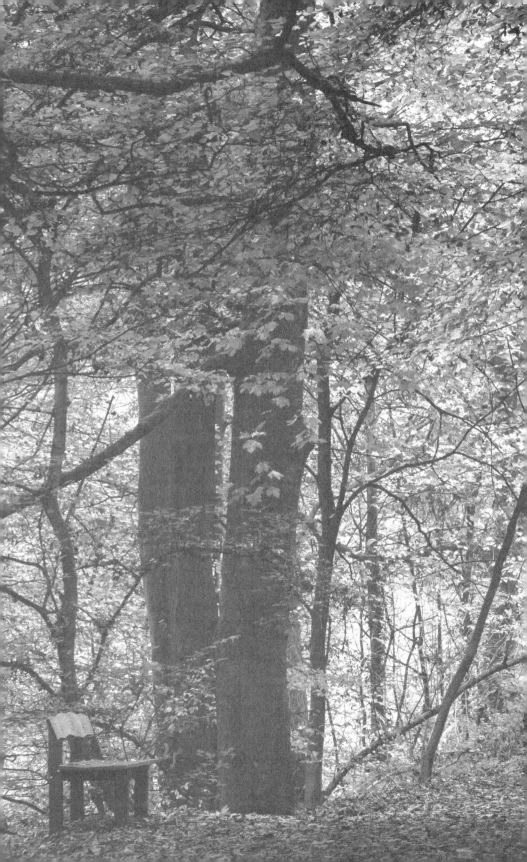

AGHE Competencies

Gerontology Competencies for Undergraduate and Graduate Education

Contributors

We would like to extend our deep thanks to the many chapter authors who generously shared their insights to help create this book.

Clark C. Abt, PhD, is an engineer, educator, social scientist, entrepreneur, and environmentalist (in that order). Involuntarily retired at 76 as Chairman Emeritus, former Chief Executive Officer, and founder of Abt Associates Inc., he has pursued a third career teaching at Boston University, Franklin Institute of Technology, Cambridge College, Harvard University Extension School, Brandeis University, and Harvard Institute for Learning in Retirement, and volunteering as a senior tutor at a Boston public high school. Dr. Abt (MIT PhD, 1965) authored 10 books and many papers, among them *Serious Games*, *The Social Audit for Management*, *AIDS and the Courts*, *The Termination of a Nuclear War*, *Disarmament as a Strategy*, and *The Social Costs of Cancer*. He continues to take courses ranging from cosmology to Shakespeare and hosts a biweekly memoir-writing group. At 87, he has given up flying, skiing, and sailing, but still plays tennis and harpsichord.

Virginia Pratt Agar grew up in an upper-middle-class family in Andover, Massachusetts, and followed the path of what she was "supposed to do": get an education, get married, and have a family—a recipe to which she added her own unique salt and pepper. It was not until her young adulthood that she learned about suffering. She earned a BS in early childhood education from Wheelock College in 1964, has worked at an assortment of preschools and Head Start programs, and is now retired but attending to four grandchildren, three of whom are in the early childhood stage. She is 74 years old.

Clara Melendres Apodaca, former First Lady of New Mexico and a patron of the arts, was General Assistant to the Chairman of the Democratic National Committee and served in the Clinton administration and as New Mexico Cabinet Secretary of the Department of Cultural Affairs. She is the former President and Chief Executive Officer of the National Hispanic Cultural Center Foundation. She also served as Commissioner on the DC Commission of the Arts and Humanities and was selected for *100 Influentials* by *Hispanic Business* magazine. Age 82, she is the mother of five children and has ten grandchildren.

Carolyn Arnish, PharmD, RPh, grew up in Needham, Massachusetts. During her senior year of high school at Ursuline Academy, she started working at Wardle's Pharmacy in Dedham, where she met Leanne Jasset. She attended a six-year Doctor of Pharmacy program at the Massachusetts College of Pharmacy and Health Sciences in Boston, continuing to work with Leanne during school breaks. She graduated with her PharmD in 2014, and then completed a residency in Clinical Veterinary Pharmacy in North Carolina. After returning to Massachusetts, Carolyn worked for two veterinary compounding pharmacies before ending up back "home" with Leanne Jasset at Dedham Pharmacy. She regards both geriatric and veterinary care (although very different) as her callings and passions.

Martin L. Aronson, Esq., a graduate of Dartmouth College and Boston College Law School, was a trial lawyer and managing partner of a Boston litigation firm, White Inker Aronson P.C. He taught two courses as an Adjunct Professor at Boston College Law School for 40 years, is a past President of the Massachusetts chapter of the American Board of Trial Advocates, and was designated as a Massachusetts Super Lawyer (awarded to the top 5% of all practicing attorneys) by *Boston* magazine. After retiring, Marty served as a mediator for several years. He teaches a course entitled "Courtroom Cinema" at the Harvard Institute for Learning in Retirement, and also presents that program on Silversea cruises. He is the father of two adult daughters and grandfather of four. He and his wife, Ellen, reside in Manhattan, and he is 83 years old.

John Averell, PhD, spent his early years in Darien, Connecticut, going to church as an evangelical Protestant, participating in music, and editing the yearbook in high school. He met his first wife at Wheaton College (Illinois), continued in music and religious activities, and obtained a degree in Physics. He then earned a PhD in Physics at Harvard, married, had three children, and worked in defense and at Polaroid. Computers were his tools from 1960 on. After the death of his first wife in 1981, he ceased religious activities, remarried, and continued in his careers until retirement in 2000. He and his wife, Shirley, moved to NewBridge in 2010, where he remains active in music and writing. John is 82.

Stephanie Batista, MA, has a Master's in Counseling Psychology and a second Master's in Professional Psychology. She is in her third year at William James College in the doctoral program in Clinical Psychology.

Ricardo Bianco, PsyD, is an Assistant Professor at William James College in Newton, Massachusetts, where he serves as the Director of the Counseling in Health and Behavioral Medicine program. His primary expertise is in the areas of primary care/medical settings and health psychology, behavioral medicine, multicultural issues, and general mental health. He utilizes an integrative bio-psycho-social-spiritual approach in the process of assessing and treating a variety of behavioral health problems, both in his teaching and in his clinical work.

Charles L. Blauer earned his BS in zoology from the University of Massachusetts (Amherst) in 1951. After serving in the Air Force for two years, he went to work for Pitman-Moore Companyas an Ethical Medical Sales Representative, leaving there to join Blauer Mfg. Co., Inc. in 1958. He became President of that company in 1986 and currently serves as Chairman of the Board. Charles is 87.

Eli Botkin, MS, earned his BS in engineering physics from New York University and his MS in physics from California Institute of Technology. He began his career as Section Head, Orbital Mechanics Section, at Hughes Aircraft Co. in California, and then moved to Grumman Aircraft Co. in New York as Principal Engineer in the Controls Section. While at Grumman, he was part of the team that designed and built the lunar module that put men on the moon. Subsequently, he designed the Satellite Attack Warning System (SAWS), a computer-installed mathematical algorithm needed to be deployed by the North American Aerospace Defense Command (NORAD) to safeguard U.S. satellites from hostile activity. Eli is 91.

Diana Hope Bronner, MEd, started teaching in Miami, Florida, after getting her undergraduate degree at the University of Miami. She was caught up in the pains of integration during a very difficult time, especially for rookie teachers. She eventually returned to school, earning a Master's in Education in Learning Disabilities, and began teaching other teachers to work with special needs children in both the United States and Canada. She retired from teaching at age 48 and has never looked back. The joy of her life has been living near her son and daughter-in-law and watching her grandchildren, now 19 and 22, grow up. Almost 79, she would like to think that she has made a difference in the world and will continue to do so through the ongoing good deeds of her family.

Peggy E. Chait was brought up in the suburbs of New York City and attended NYC public schools and Queens College, where she obtained her degree in English/Creative Writing. Having to earn an income and not having a patron to support her in her creative journey, she found herself working on Wall Street, where she has remained since her college graduation. She has two extremely intelligent, beautiful, and compassionate children, both of whom have attended Macaulay Honors College of the City University of New York, following in the footsteps of their mom and their grandmother. Life comes full circle.

Stephen Colwell, MBA, is the Executive Director of NewBridge on the Charles. As such, he is responsible for overseeing NewBridge's campus and facilities, activities, programming, and services to residents. Steve has over 24 years of experience within the hospitality industry, working in front office and food and beverage offices at Sheraton and Hilton hotels, as well as having hotelwide responsibilities as a general manager. Most recently, he worked as the Executive Director at Cabot Park Village, a senior living community in Newton, Massachusetts. He earned his BS from Cornell University's School of Hotel Administration and his MBA from the University of Rochester.

Nicholas A. Covino, PsyD, has been the President of William James College since July 2002. For 20 years, Dr. Covino was a psychologist at the Beth Israel Deaconess Medical Center (serving for most of this period as Director of Training, and then Director of the Psychology Division) and Assistant Professor at Harvard Medical School. Trained in psychoanalysis and behavioral medicine, Dr. Covino's clinical work has been both in long-term psychotherapy and symptom-focused interventions with medical patients. Dr. Covino received his doctorate in psychology from the University of Denver and completed a fellowship at the Harvard Health Plan. He is a member of the Boston Psychoanalytic Society and Institute and the past president of the Society for Clinical and Experimental Hypnosis.

Muriel Trask Davisson-Fahey, PhD, was born and raised in Tremont, Maine, the oldest of five children, daughter of a lobster fisherman and a teacher. She is a seventh-generation native of the Tremont area, descended from original settlers. She graduated from Southwest Harbor

High School, earned her AB *cum laude* in zoology from Mount Holyoke College and her PhD in genetics from The Pennsylvania State University. Her 41-year research career was at The Jackson Laboratory in Bar Harbor, Maine, where she retired as Professor Emerita in 2012. She divides her time between Tremont, Maine, and New Orleans, Louisiana, and is 75 years old.

Rabbi Judi Ehrlich is a rabbi and a certified Interfaith Chaplain at New-Bridge on the Charles, a Hebrew SeniorLife continuous care retirement community in Dedham, Massachusetts. She provides spiritual care to seniors, their families, and staff, teaches Bible and Judaica classes, leads services, and facilitates interfaith dialogue. Prior to becoming a rabbi, Judi earned a Master's degree in Counseling Psychology and worked as a Jewish matchmaker, directing a nonprofit introduction service for 14 years. Born in South Africa, Judi lived in Israel for 12 years and immigrated to the United States with her husband and children in 1984.

Richard Payne Evans, EdM, a graduate of Boston University and Harvard University, is a retired management consultant and teacher of organizational behavior (Northeastern University and Fitchburg State College). He worked in human resources at Raytheon, Simplex, and Honeywell and was a member of both the human resources staff and the consulting staff at Arthur D. Little Company. In retirement, he joined Harvard Institute of Learning in Retirement (HILR) where he served a term as cochair of the Admissions Committee, as well as taking and leading courses. Richard is 80 years old.

Rachael Falk, MA, a fourth-year doctoral student in Clinical Psychology at William James College (WJC), graduated *summa cum laude* from UMass Amherst and received her Master's degree in Professional Psychology from WJC. She has trained at Emerson College's Counseling and Psychological Services; the Bedford VA Medical Center (Geropsychology Program); McLean Hospital (Anxiety Mastery Program); and Ethos Elder Protective Services. She plans to pursue a career primarily serving older adults. Her doctoral project is entitled "How Jewish Rituals of Mourning Affect Bereavement Outcomes for Widowed Older Adults."

Caryn B. Finard amazed her parents from the moment of her birth, when they discovered they had (fraternal) twins. Though very different, Caryn and her sister are a lifelong source of love and support to each other. She graduated from the University of Bridgeport with a bachelor's degree in Special Education. For many years, she stayed at home to raise two daughters, of whom she is enormously proud. In addition to writing for this book, Caryn enjoys writing poetry.

Father James Flavin has been a Catholic priest for 52 years. He was born in Quincy, Massachusetts, and attended the Oblate Seminary and Catholic University in Washington, D.C., from 1955 to 1964. He also attended Harvard Divinity School and earned a doctorate in ministry from St. Mary's University in Baltimore, Maryland. He is a member of The Oblates of Mary Immaculate, a missionary order headquartered in Rome, with about 4000 members. Father Flavin is the Director of The Oblate Residence, a residence for 35 elderly, infirm, and retired priests and brothers in Tewksbury, Massachusetts. With characteristic modesty, he also confirms that he has "written a couple of books." Father Flavin is 81.

Reverend Elizabeth E. Frigard is a minister ordained in the United Church of Christ and currently serving as an Interim Pastor in a Presbyterian church in upstate New York. For 15 years, she led poetry programs in adult care facilities in the Boston area and published several books encouraging the use of poetry with the aging. Following the death of her husband in 2002, she moved to Tucson, Arizona. In 2007, feeling the call of the ministry, she returned east to attend Andover Newton Theological School in Newton, Massachusetts. Beth has three sons and one young grandson. She is 68.

Judith S. Goldstein, PhD, founded Humanity in Action in 1997 and has served as its Executive Director ever since. Under Judith's leadership, Humanity in Action has organized educational programs on international affairs, diversity, and human rights in Bosnia and Herzegovina, Denmark, France, Germany, Greece, Poland, the Netherlands, and the United States. She received her PhD in history from Columbia University and was a Woodrow Wilson Scholar for her MA studies. Judith has written several books and articles about European and American history, art, and landscape architecture. She is a member of the Council on Foreign Relations and several boards and advisory groups. Judith is 76.

Janet Gottler, LICSW, is a Social Worker at NewBridge on the Charles, a continuing care retirement community of Hebrew SeniorLife in Dedham, Massachusetts. She has provided supportive services for their Independent Living Residence since 2012. Prior to this, she was the

Director of Long-Term-Care Programs at Kit Clark Senior Services, a multiservice, multicultural senior agency in Dorchester, Massachusetts. In that capacity, she managed multilingual adult day health and dementia day programs and home care programs that supported elders aging in their community. Janet served as President of the Massachusetts Adult Day Services Association from 2006 to 2008.

Sharon M. Gouveia, MA, MEd, was born in Lowell, Massachusetts. She graduated from Emmanuel College in Boston and completed a Master's in Spanish, including study at the University of Madrid, Spain. She also received a Master's in Educational Administration and served as Principal at the Fontbonne Academy in Milton. She was a founding member of the Catholic Educator's Collaborative at Stonehill College. Since retiring, she has volunteered at Mt. Auburn Hospital and on the Advisory Committee for The Women's Table, an outreach to women sponsored by the Sisters of Saint Joseph, and remains active at St. Paul's Church in Cambridge. She currently resides with her husband, Bill, in Dedham, Massachusetts. Sharon has 3 children and 11 wonderful grandchildren and is 73 years old.

William A. Gouveia, MS, served as Director of Pharmacy at Tufts Medical Center for 34 years before retiring. Throughout his career, he was involved in the American Society of Health-System Pharmacists and numerous international pharmacy organizations. He served on the board of the Accreditation Council for Pharmaceutical Education and received an honorary Doctor of Humane Letters degree from Western University of Health Sciences, Pomona, CA. He has published extensively on hospital pharmacy here and abroad and is a recognized leader and trendsetter in the field of pharmacy practice. He currently resides at NewBridge on the Charles with his wife, Sharon. At age 74, Bill is the proud father of three children and "Papa" to 11 grandchildren.

Leonard J. Green served two years in the U.S. Air Force as a Budget and Accounting Officer after graduating from Boston University with a major in accounting. He worked for several engineering firms, rising to Vice President for Contracts for The Analytic Sciences Corporation (TASC), a highly regarded firm with 3000 employees whose work was primarily for the U.S. government. After 18 years there, he retired— and immediately began working part time for Procurement Technical Assistance Center (PTAC), a government-funded organization that offers free assistance to companies looking to sell products or services to governmental entities. Len continues as a Procurement Advisor to the Massachusetts PTAC, working 20 hours a week as a productive, happy retiree. He is 84.

Susan H. Green, MBA, earned a BA from Wellesley and an MBA from Simmons, and then worked with the Massachusetts Association of School Business Officials, handling financial software for 16 years, marketing, selling, teaching, and enjoying a busy life while raising three children. Her busy life now includes time spent with four grandchildren; keeping up with friends and family; attending theater, lectures, and concerts; and taking courses. Writing for pleasure is a new skill. Susan is 83.

Earl A. Grollman, PhD, a pioneer in the field of crisis intervention, is Rabbi Emeritus, Beth El Temple Center, Belmont, Massachusetts. A certified death educator and counselor, he was cited as "Hero of The Heartland" for his work with the families and volunteers of the Oklahoma City bombing. Dr. Grollman has spoken at many colleges, clergy institutes, seminaries, and medical forums, and has addressed such groups as Compassionate Friends, Mothers Against Drunk Driving, and Widows Personal Services. He has appeared on *The Oprah Winfrey Show, All Things Considered,* and *Mister Rogers' Neighborhood,* and was featured on National Public Radio's *End of Life* series in their roundtable discussion on grief and bereavement. He is a recipient of the Death Education Award by the Association for Death Education and Counseling and many other awards, and his books on coping with bereavement have sold over 750,000 copies. He is 91.

Emily Grossman, MSW, CMC, is a Life Care Manager with LifeCare Advocates of Newton, Massachusetts. She is the former Associate Director of Home Care for a home health agency and has consulted to home care agencies, the Combined Jewish Philanthropies Task Force on Jewish Aging, and the Massachusetts Executive Office of Elder Affairs. She is the Treasurer of the New England Chapter of Aging Life Care Association. Emily has a Care Manager Certification from the National Academy of Certified Care Managers. She holds a BA in Community Health and Classical Studies from Tufts University and an MSW with a Clinical Concentration in Older Adults from Boston College.

Jason M. Holland, PhD, is a licensed Clinical Psychologist and Assistant Professor at William James College. He earned his doctorate in Clinical Psychology in 2008 from the University of Memphis after completing an internship at the Palo Alto VA (PAVA), specializing in geropsychology. After graduation, he worked as a postdoctoral fellow at PAVA and Stanford University. His program of research focuses on stressful late-life transitions, such as bereavement, caregiving, and coping with debilitating illness. Dr. Holland has published more than 60 peer-reviewed articles on these topics and currently serves as the Associate Editor of the journal *Death Studies.*

Roberta Horn, PsyD, is the proud mother of three and a loving grandmother of six. Her role model was her intrepid grandmother, who provided for a family of seven throughout the Depression, encouraged a love of reading, and inspired Dr. Horn to complete Bachelor's, Master's and Doctor of Psychology degrees in middle age following careers in photography and hospice care and management. Dr. Horn holds degrees from the University of California at Berkeley, the New School for Social Research, and William James College (formerly the Massachusetts School of Professional Psychology). The most meaningful work of her life has been helping abused children, burn victims, and terminally ill adults.

Leanne Jasset, RPh, began working at the soda fountain in her neighborhood pharmacy at age 13. That began a lifelong love of pharmacy. She graduated from the Massachusetts College of Pharmacy in 1978 with a Bachelor of Science in Pharmacy degree, and opened her own store, Dedham Pharmacy & Medical Supply, in 2016. Leanne's love for community work, especially with the elderly, shows through in her 20-year history of working on the Dedham Council on Aging and advocating for senior programming and benefits. She is currently the Chairperson of the Dedham Board of Health and the Dedham Council on Aging and the Co-Chair of the Dedham Coalition for Drug and Alcohol Awareness.

Ruth Kandel, MD, is a graduate of Albert Einstein College of Medicine and a board-certified geriatrician. She was an Assistant Professor at Harvard Medical School and directed the outpatient Memory Disorders Clinic at Hebrew Rehabilitation Center until her retirement in December 2016. Dr. Kandel also had a primary care clinic at NewBridge on the Charles. Her research projects primarily focused on infection control or dementia in long-term-care residents. She teaches about cognitive issues with aging and dementia in academic settings, as well as in the community.

Brenda Keegan, PhD, graduated from Wellesley College, completed substantial coursework in educational leadership at the University of

Pennsylvania, and earned her PhD in English literature from the University of Rochester. Moving frequently to support her husband's career, she taught English at several high schools and colleges, then served as Assistant Dean at SUNY/Empire State College and Director of Curriculum in the Bridgewater schools (where she created the nationally recognized Challenging Thinking Potential program). She then returned to her career of choice as Head of the English Department at Newton North High School, later becoming Principal of Newton South High School and (until her retirement) Deputy Superintendent of the Newton schools. Since her retirement, she has taught prospective English teachers at Brandeis, volunteered with inner-city students, and served as Principal of General Studies at Torah Academy. She travels frequently to Colorado and Tennessee to visit her two children and six grandchildren.

Melissa M. Kelley, PhD, is Associate Professor of Pastoral Care and Counseling at the Boston College School of Theology and Ministry. Previously, she was on the faculty of Weston Jesuit School of Theology in Cambridge, Massachusetts. Dr. Kelley earned her PhD in Pastoral Psychology from Boston University and is a fellow and nationally certified pastoral counselor through the American Association of Pastoral Counselors. She is also a Fellow in Thanatology: Death, Dying, and Bereavement through the Association for Death Education and Counseling, the primary organization in the country for bereavement researchers, educators, and clinicians. She is the author of *Grief: Contemporary Theory and the Practice of Ministry*, published in 2010 by Augsburg Fortress Press.

Laura Lee, MS, OTR/L, CHT, received her Master's degree in Occupational Therapy from Thomas Jefferson University in Philadelphia in 1996. In 2001, Laura obtained a certificate in lymphedema management and received her certification from the Hand Therapy Certification Commission in 2003. She has been affiliated with Hebrew SeniorLife since 1997, with a special interest in geriatric-related conditions affecting the upper extremity and function. Laura has also pursued advanced clinical practice within the area of Driving and Community Mobility. She is a member of the Massachusetts Occupational Therapy Association, American Occupational Therapy Association, and the American Society of Hand Therapists.

Liane Reif Lehrer, PhD, was born in Vienna in 1934 and escaped to New York in 1941. She is a graduate of Barnard College and University of California, Berkeley (earning a PhD in chemistry). Throughout her professional career, she worked as a Principal Investigator in nonprofit retina research (Mass Eye and Ear, Schepens Eye Research Institute); as Assistant and then Associate Professor, Harvard Medical School; as Director of the Office of Academic Affairs, Harvard Medical School; and as President of Erimon Associates. She has written three books and given grant writing workshops to other scientists. Married with two children and one grandchild, she has lifelong interests in teaching, poetry, writing, and dancing. She wrote the poem in this book in 1982. Liane is 82.

Sherwin (Sam) Lehrer, PhD, earned his BS in chemistry from University of Pittsburgh and his PhD, also in chemistry, from University of California, Berkeley. After a stint as a Research Scientist at MIT Lincoln Laboratory, he and his wife, Liane, traveled extensively for a year. Through most of his career, he was a Principal Investigator, conducting nonprofit basic research in muscle biophysics (Retina Foundation and Boston Biomedical Research Institute, 1966–2014). He also served as a Principal Research Associate at Harvard Medical School (1970–2014) and as Fogarty International Fellow, Kings College, London (1978–1979). He has published over 100 peer-reviewed articles. Married with two children and one grandchild, at age 82, Sam remains active as a photographer, bicyclist, and ballroom dancer.

Maurice Lesses, Esq., was born in Boston 84 years ago and raised in Newton, Massachusetts, settling in Cambridge, Massachusetts, in 1955. A graduate of Harvard College and Harvard Law School, he became active in Cambridge civic affairs and politics during the 1960s, managing several political campaigns, running for City Council, and serving on the Cambridge Board of Zoning Appeals. In his late 30s, he learned to play banjo, and at about 48, he began the fiddle, playing old-time Appalachian square dance/fiddle tunes and jamming regularly with local musicians. He has three children, two grandchildren, a great grandson, and two stepchildren. His first wife died in 1981, and in 1996, he married his second wife, Eve.

Nan Lincoln has been a newspaper reporter since 1986; she also writes features for magazines including *Down East, Yankee,* and *Reader's Digest.* She is the author of two books, *The Summer of Cecily* (about raising a harbor seal pup) and *Cecily's Summer* (a children's picture book on the same subject). She has received state, New England, national, and international awards for her work. Now at age 70, she writes primarily arts-related features and reviews for the *Mount Desert Islander* and the

Ellsworth American, two of the top-rated weekly newspapers in New England. She lives in Bass Harbor, Maine, and is busy building a new house and working on another book. Nan is 70 years old.

Mariah MacKenzie was born in Lexington, Massachusetts, but spent much of her youth in the suburbs north of Chicago. She is now a senior at Needham High School, Needham, Massachusetts. Mariah loves music, art, and literature and participates in her high school band and a community orchestra. She plans to continue her education at George Washington University beginning in the fall of 2017 to study political science and education, so she can one day help to improve the educational system in the United States.

John N. MacDuffie was born in 1931 and is a resident of Bernard, Maine. After graduating from Bates College, he earned a Master's of Divinity from Oberlin College's Graduate School of Theology. He was ordained to the ministry of the United Church of Christ in 1958, and since then has served as the Pastor of various churches in Ohio and, more recently, in Maine. His most recent position was as Pastor of the Central Congregational Church in Eastport, Maine, where he served until 2014. He is 85.

Scott Mankowitz, MD, earned his BS from Cornell and his MD from the State University of New York Downstate Medical Center College of Medicine. He completed a residency in Emergency Medicine at St. Luke's–Roosevelt Hospital. Scott is the former director of the Emergency Department at East Orange General Hospital in Teaneck, New Jersey.

Monica McAlpine, PhD, age 76, turned to painting and writing poetry in her retirement after a career of teaching and publication in medieval studies. Her paintings have been exhibited by several Boston area art associations and her poems have appeared in *The Aurorean, Wilderness House Literary Review,* and *Poetry Quarterly.* An additional poem was chosen for a public reading at Boston City Hall. Monica is Professor Emerita of English at the University of Massachusetts (Boston).

Sherri L. Meade lives in Hatfield, Massachusetts, with her husband, Ian Smith. Her blended family—six adult children and nine grandchildren—is scattered across the United States. Sherri grew up on Long Island, New York, graduated from Stony Brook University with a BS in Mathematics, and dove into a career in the then-new field of computer software. After deeply technical product development experience, Sherri turned to executive management. She successfully completed more than 35 years in management, launching hundreds of new products ranging from large data servers to PCs to handheld devices. After retiring from her technical career, Sherri obtained her real estate license and remains active as a real estate agent.

Catherine Cobb Morocco, EdD, has published two books for educators on using writing to teach for deep understanding with adolescents. Her first poetry book, *Moon Without Craters or Shadows,* was published in 2014 (Aldrich). "Son's Story," from that volume, was the winner of the Dana Foundation (Neuroscience) Foundation prize for poetry about the brain. Her poems have been published in *The Massachusetts Review, The Spoon River Poetry Review, Prairie Schooner, Salamander, The Sow's Ear Poetry Review, The Hamilton Stone Review, Comstock Review,* and in a recent chapbook, *Prairie Canto* (Dancing Girls Press, 2016). Cathy lives in Newton, Massachusetts, and has five grandchildren. She is 76.

Talya Oded, MS, grew up in New Jersey in a lively household with a Yemenite father, a Hungarian mother, three siblings, several cats, and assorted adopted family friends. She lived in Israel for seven years after finishing high school, returning to New Jersey after marrying Effie. In 1997, she moved her family to Memphis, Tennessee, where she teaches at the only Orthodox boarding school in the Mid-South. She holds a BA in English Education and a Master's in Early Childhood Education, and proudly teaches the next generation to embrace diversity, appreciate and strengthen their individual identities, and explore human behavior through an intellectual study of the Holocaust and the civil rights movement. The mother of three, at age 50, she is patiently waiting for grandchildren.

Barbara F. Okun, PhD, is Professor Emerita of Counseling Psychology at Northeastern University and an Emerita Clinical Instructor at Harvard Medical School, where she trained psychiatry fellows in family therapy. She has maintained a Clinical Psychotherapy/Family therapy practice for over 40 years and is coauthor of *Saying Good-bye: How Families Can Find Renewal Through Loss* and of *Conceptualization and Intervention Skills for Effective Helping.* Additionally, she is the author of *Effective Helping: Interviewing and Counseling Techniques* (in its eighth edition), *Understanding Diversity, Seeking Connections in Psychotherapy,* and *Understanding Diverse Families.* She has trained family court judges in family systems perspectives at the National Institute for Family Judges and their state associations and has trained mental health workers in Israel, Kuwait, and Central and South America. Currently, Dr. Okun consults for hospice, Jewish Vocational Service, and other elder care services. She is 80 years old.

Helene G. Oppenheimer is 82 years old and lives happily at NewBridge on the Charles with her husband, Martin. They have been married for 57 years. Also in residence is her 12-year-old cat, Plato. She earned her BS from Simmons College, class of 1956, and, until her retirement, she worked as the Director of the Tax Library at BDO Seidman in New York City.

Aladdin Ossorio, PsyD, is the founder and coordinator of the SageMind Program at William James College. His work integrates geropsychology (the study of aging and behavioral health), neuropsychology (assessing brain-behavior interactions), and health psychology (the relationship of mind, brain, body, and health). Dr. Ossorio presented on issues of neurobiology, memory, and reasoning at the 2014 and 2015 National Society of Descriptive Psychology conferences and recently presented on developmental neurobiology and substance use at the Massachusetts Psychological Association annual conference. He is a member of the National Society of Descriptive Psychology, the American Society of Aging, and the Massachusetts Assessment Society.

Laura R. Reiter, MA, is a writer, researcher, and educator. She calls herself a "late bloomer of life." After 20 years of marriage, she continued her education while working full time. She has academic degrees from Harvard University Extension School, the University of Notre Dame, and the University of Southern California (USC). She was a visiting scholar at Notre Dame while working on a research grant, "Well-Being Among Single Adults," funded by the Retirement Research Foundation in Chicago, Illinois. After receiving her MA degree at USC, she worked as a visiting scholar, researching infectious diseases among Native Americans. She is 78 and currently lives on Cape Cod in Massachusetts.

Adrienne Richard, age 95, is the author of four novels; short stories for young adult readers; numerous newspaper, magazine, and travel articles; and a medical book. Her first book of poetry, *Looking for Flannel Pajamas,* was published in 2013. Adrienne has led workshops in autobiography and spiritual autobiography in New York City and throughout New England, as well as at the Ghost Ranch Retreat Center in Abiquiu,

New Mexico. Since 2003, she has also lectured on Architecture & Design in her eight-course series, Origins of the Arts and Crafts Movement in Architecture & Design (1850–Present).

Stanley P. Rosenzweig, PhD, has been a practicing Clinical Psychologist for well over 60 years. In addition to his private practice, he most recently was Special Assistant to the President of the Massachusetts School of Professional Psychology (now William James College), a school that he founded in the early 1970s and then served as its first Chief Executive Officer. He was affiliated with the Veterans Administration in Boston for over 35 years, where he directed the Psychiatric Day Treatment Program. Dr. Rosenzweig received his BS and Master's degrees in Psychology from the City University of New York, and his PhD from Michigan State University. He has held academic appointments at Harvard, Boston University, Northeastern University, and Suffolk University, and served as President of the Massachusetts Psychological Association.

Erlene Rosowsky, PsyD, divides her time between clinical consultation and supervision, education, and research. She is a Teaching Associate in the Department of Psychiatry at Harvard Medical School and a Core Faculty member at William James College (WJC), where she serves as the Director of the Concentration in Gerontology and also as the Director of the WJC Center for Mental Health and Aging. She is the past Chair of the editorial board of *Generations*, a Fulbright Specialist grant recipient, and the author of three books and numerous professional chapters, articles, and columns. She was honored in 2012 with the American Society on Aging Award for outstanding contributions to the field of aging.

Gregory Ruffa was born in New Jersey in 1925 to parents who had emigrated from Calabria, Italy. He enlisted in the U.S. Air Corps in 1943, serving until 1946, and then entered art school in New York. After working in other advertising agencies, he started his own agency, Gregory Ruffa Associates, in 1950, and grew the company to a staff of 32, with major blue-chip companies as clients. He is 91.

Gerald Sands was born in Boston and educated at the University of Rhode Island, where he earned his BS in Business Administration in 1956. He served in the U.S. Navy from 1957 to 1960, and then founded his own business, CCS Companies in Norwood, Massachusetts; he is now Chairman Emeritus. Gerald also served as International President of the American Collectors Association. He lives at NewBridge on the

Charles with his wife, Lucille, and has three children, seven grandchildren, and one great-grandchild.

Laurie Schreiber has written for publications in Maine and beyond for more than 25 years. Her new book, *Boatbuilding on Mount Desert Island*, is a collection of historical profiles with a touch of contemporary activity.

Harriet Segal is a native of Wilkes-Barre, Pennsylvania. After graduating from Wellesley College, she became a journalist and freelance editor. Her first novel, *Susquehanna*, was set in the anthracite coal regions of northeastern Pennsylvania. It was soon followed by *Catch the Wind*, the story of two doctors working on the campaign to eradicate smallpox. Next came *Shadow Mountain*, which was a Book-of-the-Month-Club selection; and *The Skylark's Song*, a *Good Housekeeping* novel of the month. Her latest work, *The Expatriate*, is set in World War II Europe. A grandmother of seven, Harriet lives in Dedham, Massachusetts, and summers on Cape Cod. At age 85, she is at work on a new novel about the world of medical research.

R. Peter Shapiro, Esq., a graduate of the University of Pennsylvania (Wharton, BS) and Boston University Law School (LL.B. and LL.M), practiced law in New Hampshire from 1962 until his retirement, with a specialization in civil litigation. He served in the New Hampshire National Guard and was activated from 1961 to 1962 during the Berlin Crisis. He has also served as President of Temple Beth Jacob in Concord, New Hampshire, a member of the Union for Reform Judaism's National Board, a Trustee of New England College, and a City Councilor in Concord, New Hampshire. At age 79, he is married, with three children and six grandchildren.

Lynne Sherman, MA, LMFT, was born into a large extended family in Chicago and grew up listening to multiple generations' stories and cautionary tales of their daily lives. She developed an appreciation for the importance of the story that we tell about our lives and about how this story can change us over time. Lynne earned her BA from University of Vermont and her MA in Clinical Psychology from Antioch University. She is a retired marriage and family therapist. As a therapist, she has helped her patients realize and shape their own life stories. She has also taught classes in elder-care issues. Lynne is 71 and lives with her husband in Santa Barbara, California.

Ben Slomoff was affected during his teens by the Great Depression, which limited his education beyond high school. A half-semester at the University of Pittsburgh opened the door to training with Brown Shoe Company. Following six years of service in the Air Force during World War II, Ben returned to Brown Shoe Company, and then went into business for himself, buying Milford Shoe Company. After selling his company, Ben finally completed his education at the University of Massachusetts, majoring in Public and Community Service and earning a BA in 1993 at age 80. He received a Master's in Conflict Resolution at age 84. Ben then moved to California, where he served as a mediator in small-claims court and an arbitrator for Financial Regulatory Administration (FINRA). Ben was married in 1938 and has two children, six grandchildren, and four great-grandchildren. He published his first book of poetry in 2012 at age 99, and his second in 2015 at age 102. He is 103 years old.

Irene F. Smith, RN, was born in 1924 and grew up in a working-class row house neighborhood in West Baltimore, Maryland, just a few blocks from her future husband, Ray, whom she married in 1946. After attaining her Diplomate in Nursing from Sinai Hospital, Baltimore, in 1945, she worked full time as a nurse until the birth of her first child in 1950. She raised three children, returning to work part time in 1960 and full time in 1973. Irene retired from nursing in 1987. Her main focus has always been her family and home: her husband, her children, and her extended family. Yet Irene has found time for participating in community events, her synagogue, and doing volunteer work. She has six grandchildren and two great-grandchildren and is 92 years old.

Nancy Lelewer Sonnabend earned her BA from Sarah Lawrence College in 1957. Herself dyslexic, she received the Alice H. Garside Award for her outstanding contribution to the field of learning disabilities. She currently serves on the Executive Advisor board of the Asperger/Autism Network and the national board of Hearing Loss Association of America. She has written two books and a number of national and international scientific articles, and has guest-lectured at many conferences and schools. A contributor to dyslexia research at the Massachusetts Institute of Technology and Harvard Medical School, she is also the creator of a children's temporal learning program and holds patents on nine children's board games. She was a founding director of Permobil of America, Inc. (now Permobil USA), the world's leading manufacturer of power wheelchairs. Nancy lives at the Prudential Center, Boston,

Massachusetts. She is the mother of four grown children and grand-mother of eight and is 82 years old.

Murray Staub, JD, moved to NewBridge on the Charles in Dedham, Massachusetts, with his wife, Rhoda, in 2013, after spending most of their lives in New Jersey. A graduate of Rutgers University, at age 42, he changed directions and went back to school, graduating from New York University's School of Law. He used his law degree in a practice primarily devoted to municipal law; however, most of his business career was in the menswear industry. Murray and his late wife, Rhoda, have three children, seven grandchildren, and three great-grandchildren. He is 91.

James Van Lanen, Sr., the owner of the Lighthouse Inn on Lake Michigan, is a former real estate broker. He has served as President of the Two Rivers Historical Society and was influential in developing five museums in the city of Two Rivers, Wisconsin, including the Washington House 1880s hotel, bar, and dance hall and the Hamilton Wood Type and Printing Museum. In his retirement, he enjoys violin making, playing first violin with the Manitowoc Symphony Orchestra and volunteering with the Two Rivers Historical Society. He is 84.

Glorianne Wittes, LICSW, is a retired social worker and still-active artist, the lone survivor of a wonderful marriage, and a grateful mother, grandmother, and great-grandmother. Though increasingly limited by Parkinson's disease and other age-related ailments, she is still searching for and expressing joy in her life despite her losses, and despite the troubling world in which we are living. Where there is joy, there is also passion and the urge to connect with others. So here she is, in one of life's greatest transitions, one step closer to the end, making art, mourning her losses, and still seeking moments of joy each day.

Natalie M. Wolf is a graduate of the University of Pennsylvania and is a National Master Flower Show Judge. Natalie took on the enormous volunteer task of selecting, arranging, and curating all the art and decorative objects at NewBridge on the Charles and the other Hebrew Senior Life communities. She is 96 years old.

Arthur Wood, MS, was born in Providence, Rhode Island, in 1941 and is the youngest of three children, spoiled and influenced by his older sisters, who convinced him to play the trombone just like their hero, Glen Miller. So, the trombone it was. His parents placed a high value on education, and the end result was an absorption in lifelong learning, which still encourages him to read books and avoid television. Arthur is a biochemist by training. He has three wonderful children and one grandchild and lives in a large Victorian house with seven unrelated housemates, a style of living that he credits with avoiding depression. He is 75 years old.

Louis J. Woolf, MBA, is President and Chief Executive Officer of Hebrew SeniorLife (HSL), a Harvard Medical School affiliate and New England's largest nonprofit provider of senior housing and healthcare. Mr. Woolf received his BA in Economics from Brandeis University and MBA from Columbia University Graduate School of Business. Prior to joining HSL, he served in leadership positions within the CareGroup Healthcare System, including Chief Operating Officer (COO) of New England Baptist Hospital and Senior Vice President of System Development and Communications for CareGroup corporate. He also served as Executive Vice President and COO of North Shore Medical Center. In 2009, Mr. Woolf came to HSL as President, and was elevated to President and Chief Executive Officer in 2013.

Genevieve Geller Wyner, EdM, grew up in New Rochelle, New York. She is a Wellesley graduate, class of 1952, and earned her EdM from Harvard in 1982. She married her husband, Justin, in 1955. Although bringing up her three sons was her "very best job," along the way, she became a licensed mental health counselor and a Vice President of Human Resources in the family business. She published a memoir entitled *GellerGirl* in 2011. Genevieve has always enjoyed sailing and was a tournament tennis player. Her interests now, at age 86, include writing and current events, especially politics.

Justin L. Wyner, MBA, graduated from Roxbury Latin School, Tufts University, and Harvard Business School. For many years the Chief Executive Officer of Shawmut Corporation, a family-owned manufacturing business now in its 100th year, he is currently Chairman Emeritus. Justin has served in leadership positions locally and nationally, including as Moderator of the Brookline Town Meeting, President of Temple Israel of Boston, President of the Jewish Community Council of Boston, President of the Wharf District Council of Downtown Boston, and President of the American Jewish Historical Society. His hobbies include sailing, golf, and genealogy. He is 91 and is currently writing a memoir.

Jenny Yen, PsyD, graduated from William James College in 2017 with a doctoral degree in Psychology and a concentration in geropsychology. She obtained her BA in Psychology at the University of California, Davis, and her Master's degree from William James College. Her doctoral research is entitled "Let's Talk About Sex: How Older Adults Communicate About Sexuality Issues with Their Friends". Jenny is completing a Clinical Psychology postdoctoral fellowship with a geropsychology focus at the Department of Veterans Affairs Palo Alto Health Care System and plans to pursue a career serving the aging population.

Geraldine Zetzel, MEd, has been in love with poetry since fifth grade, when she produced her first sonnet. In addition to her full-length collections, *Mapping the Sands* (Mayapple Press, 2010) and *Traveling Light* (Antrim House, 2016), she is the author of two chapbooks, *Near Enough to Hear the Words* (Pudding House Publications) and *With Both Hands* (Finishing Line Press). Currently, she teaches courses in the Tufts Osher Lifelong Learning Institute, the most recent being "African-American Poets." A longtime practitioner of Theravada Buddhism, she leads several ongoing meditation groups. She lives in Brookhaven, a retirement community in Lexington, Massachusetts, and is 89.